## ALSO BY ELLEN BROWN

With the Grain: Eat More, Weigh Less, Live Longer (1990).

The Informed Consumer's Pharmacy (with Dr. Lynne Walker, 1990).

Menopause and Estrogen: Natural Alternatives to Hormone Replacement Therapy (formerly Breezing Through the Change: Managing Menopause Naturally, with Dr. Lynne Walker, 1994, 1996).

The Key to Ultimate Health (with Richard Hansen, D.M.D., 1998).

The Alternative Pharmacy (with Dr. Lynne Walker, 1998).

# FORBIDDEN MEDICINE

*Is Effective Non-toxic Cancer Treatment Being Suppressed?*

by

Ellen Hodgson Brown, J.D.

## Forbidden Medicine

*Is Effective Non-toxic Cancer Treatment Being Suppressed?*

Published by:
**Third Millennium Press**
40960 California Oaks Road
Suite #122
Murrieta, CA 92562

ISBN: 1-879854-28-7

Additional copies of this book may be ordered directly from the
publisher for $19.95 each, by calling:
**1-800-891-0390**

PRINTED IN THE UNITED STATES OF AMERICA

# DEDICATION

*To the 44,000 American women*
*who died from breast cancer in 1991,*
*including Selma Meyers and Olga Quijano,*
*who pleaded in court unsuccessfully for*
*the natural serums they believed*
*were keeping them alive.*

# ACKNOWLEDGMENTS

This book would not have existed in its present form without the patience and support of my husband, Cliff, and children, Jeff and Jamie; the insightful comments of Georgia Wooldridge, Nancy O'Hara, Linda Forbes, Winnie Edgerton, Mimi Hatch, Carley Dillon, Trish Rhodes, Karen Novy, Sherry Pasquale, Shelley Parker, Elisa Irwin, Red Hebert, and Paul Ciotti; the eye-catching artwork of Gaye Lub, who donated the cover design; and the kind hospitality of the Keller family. Thanks.

# Table Of Contents

# PREFACE

Imagine you had spent thirty years working with cancer patients and developing a unique treatment protocol. You had repeatedly seen it work and were convinced of its effectiveness. Friends and relatives who had been given a medical death sentence desperately sought this treatment. But a federal judge had told you that if you dared treat them, you would be in jail essentially for the rest of your life.

That is the dilemma Jimmy Keller has faced for the past five years. And as the judge acknowledged when the court was deluged with hundreds of letters in 1991, Jimmy has a lot of friends. Some of the letters were from professionals, like the Beverly Hills M.D. who wrote:

> *James Gordon Keller is no killer, but a healer of men. I have seen his miracles. In less than 24 months, he has dissolved cancerous tumors in 2 patients miraculously, without Western medicine. He is indeed a pioneer of a new practice, however unorthodox by current standards, a new medicine and a new hope for men once diagnosed incurable of cancer.*

More letters were from patients and their relatives, like Don McBride, a bank chairman and real estate developer from Brea, California, who wrote:

> *The majority of the people at the clinic when I was there, and there were over twenty people, all had all of the chemotherapy and radiation and recommended treatment that comes under the AMA auspices in the United States. Yet after all of this, some of them were so weak they were wheeled in and had to be helped by someone. Many of them responded almost miraculously to the treatment that they received.*

Many patients wrote that they were treated for free.

This book was already in press when, on January 15, 1998, Jimmy was arrested for a second time, for treating cancer patients in violation of a court order. Besides being forbidden to treat patients, he was under a five-year gag order concerning his treatments. He had asked to hold publication of this book until that order expired, an event scheduled to occur only a week after his second arrest. The government alleges violations before that, but it waited until the last week to act.

This is the story of a man who cared too much and dared too much. In the struggle to keep his clinic open, Jimmy has survived raids and robberies, a near-fatal beating, a kidnapping, and a jail sentence many called justice gone wrong. Before that, he was saved from a near-fatal cancer by unconventional remedies after conventional medicine had failed. The therapies that saved him and that made up his treatment protocol were an eclectic assortment that covered the gamut and drew from the best of the available natural cancer remedies. The details of his therapies, and the history and vicissitudes of the non-traditional health care movement that his life personifies, are woven through his story.

The facts in the following pages are true. Liberties have been taken with the dialogue and with the sequence in which I learned the facts in order to make them easier to follow. Names have also been changed where indicated. Otherwise, the facts are as I saw, heard and read them. I am using the real name of Jimmy's principal M.D./attorney, William Ginsburg, since his representation of Monica Lewinsky has suddenly made him a public figure.

Appendix A includes further information based on my own need to know -- about the cancer statistics and their manipulation, the anti-quackery campaign, the war on cancer, and their political agendas. Appendix B presents verbatim excerpts from hundreds of letters to the U.S. District Court in Brownsville.

*Ellen Brown*
February 4, 1998
Guatemala City, Guatemala

# PART ONE

## PRELUDE TO A FELONY

*Unless we put medical freedom into the Constitution, the time will come when medicine will organize into an undercover dictatorship. . . . To restrict the art of healing to one class of men and deny equal privileges to others will constitute the Bastille of medical science. . . . The Constitution of this Republic should make special provision for medical freedom as well as religious freedom.*

—*Dr. Benjamin Rush,*
Surgeon-General of George Washington's armies
and signer of the Declaration of Independence (1787)

# Chapter 1

## St. Jude

Tijuana, despite its seedy border town reputation, had a certain charm. The weather that November was invigorating, with an ocean breeze to clear the air of traffic fumes. The streets were cluttered with old cars, makeshift shops and busy tourists. Compared to Kenya, where I lived at the time, the place was affluent. The weather was good but the tour had been a disappointment. The bus had left Los Angeles early in the morning and shuttled us from one Tijuana clinic to another, where we listened to cancer theories and statistics and got a "clinical" view. I wasn't totally disillusioned, but I was tired and ready to go home.

The last clinic on the itinerary was the only one we never got to see. Instead, we got the presentation in a restaurant. I wondered skeptically if this was because it was dinnertime, or because the clinic was unsuitable for entertaining guests. At least, we were being treated to a meal; and if anything was lacking in the cuisine, it was made up for by the program. Suddenly, something was happening.

A man in his late fifties took the podium. He was short and burly, with graying collar-length hair, a beard, and the build of someone who had once played football. There was something wrong with his face, and I couldn't always understand him. Was it his thick Louisiana drawl? Or was it some kind of speech impediment?

He introduced himself as Jimmy Keller, the administrator of the St. Jude International Clinic. He said we would be hearing the stories of some patients, and the first story would be his. In

1968, he said, he had developed a malignant melanoma the size of a golf ball. It was in his left ear and had spread to the lymph gland. He was told radiation wouldn't work on this type of cancer, and neither would chemotherapy. Surgery was his only hope, and that was a slim one.

He turned sideways and lifted his hair. Gasps came from the audience, as he revealed the gaping, twisted hole where his ear should have been. His ear and the surrounding lymph glands had all been removed. The muscles had also been cut on the left side of his face, making his eye droop and his left cheek and the left side of his mouth sag.

I shuddered. That explained the speech impediment. But he didn't seem depressed. He was cheerful and enthusiastic, and there was something appealing about him. At least, the pretty Mexican woman clinging to his arm seemed to think so. She was petite and well groomed, and looked to be fifteen or twenty years his junior. He introduced her as Alma, his wife.

After he had agreed to the amputation of his ear, Jimmy went on, painful tumor nodules had grown back on his neck. Radiation was then recommended, but his relatives were told that even with it, he would be lucky to last six more months. His parents were making novenas to St. Jude, patron saint of the impossible, when they got an unsigned letter from San Antonio. It was a city where they knew no one. The letter told of a clinic in Dallas that administered an unconventional treatment for cancer. I made a note to find out which treatment it was.

More to please his parents than because he thought it would help, he said, he had agreed to go. For three weeks, he forced down the bitter herbal tonic. To his surprise, the nodules on his neck softened up and his excruciating headaches went away. It was his initiation into the world of non-toxic cancer therapies. He branched out into other natural treatments. Soon, his "hopeless" cancer had gone into remission.

Feeling he had been saved so he could help other people with the disease, he set out to explore and test every natural therapy he came across. The ones that worked he combined into a protocol. Its success, he said, could be judged from the testimonies that followed . . .

First up was a woman named Lois. She stated that she had been diagnosed with colon cancer that had metastasized (or spread) to the lungs. She was given only three to six months to live. That was a year ago. She had gone to Jimmy's clinic and now felt wonderful.

Next was a woman who said she had been diagnosed with breast cancer. She too was given only three to six months to live. That was two years ago.

Amelia was another breast cancer case. "They put me through hell," Amelia said. "I couldn't function for three days after I got chemo. I told my husband I'm not going through that anymore. That was six years ago. Jimmy's treatments make me feel energized. I feel great."

Karen testified that she'd been diagnosed with breast cancer and had undergone a modified radical mastectomy. Then she had gotten the bad news: she had a fast-growing malignancy for which chemotherapy wouldn't work. It was her own doctor who recommended Jimmy's clinic. She stayed a month and went home cancer-free.

I was wondering if Jimmy treated anything besides women's cancers, when John stepped up to the podium. He said he had gout. Using conventional medicine, he knew from experience, he would have suffered for at least a week; but Jimmy had gotten rid of his symptoms in a day with an injection.

Howard then testified that he had heart problems. His blocked arteries had been opened up with chelation, and with a remedy called Sulconar. "Jimmy gets remedies from all over the world," Howard maintained. "You can't get them in the United States because they would impair drug profits. The drug industry is controlled by I.G. Farben. It's the largest cartel in the world."

I wasn't familiar with the name, but I wrote it down.

A third man testified that he was diagnosed with non-Hodgkin's lymphoma that had metastasized to the bone marrow. Before he began treatment at the St. Jude Clinic in 1987, his doctors pronounced his cancer untreatable. After three weeks of Jimmy's treatment, his American doctors told him he'd had a "miraculous spontaneous remission."

Jimmy's wife Alma also spoke. She said she'd had breast cancer that had metastasized to the liver, bones, colon, and lymphatic system. She was now going on seven years' recovery.

There were thirteen passionate testimonials in all. The speakers cried, they laughed, they hugged, they talked of love and caring and miracles. They all had stories that would be considered incredible by conventional standards. It reminded me of a religious revival. But I wasn't ready to admit the miraculous.

Was the man really reversing cancer? Or was he merely trading on charisma and snake-oil claims?

"It's always like that," said one of the tour guides on the bus ride home. "We do this tour every two or three months, and Jimmy always puts on a string of exciting testimonials."

"From different patients?"

"From different patients."

I inquired about the clinic. The guides said it wasn't in the best part of town. The premises were small and thread-bare.

"So which clinic do you think is the best?" I asked.

The guides looked at each other, and said they couldn't say.

I cornered them in private. "Then where would you go if you had cancer yourself?"

The guides looked at each other again, and agreed on the St. Jude Clinic. When long-term cancer survivors were presented at the 19th Annual Cancer Control Convention in Pasadena that year, they said, 26 of 30 speakers had been treated there.

Odd, I thought. Other clinics were bigger and better known. I wondered what this one had that the others lacked.

When I got back to Los Angeles, I posed that question to Vaughn, a dentist friend who knew the Tijuana health care scene.

"Keller is the only practitioner down there who tests his substances individually on each of his patients," Vaughn said. "He uses muscle testing and radionics. He doesn't have any big money backing him, so he doesn't have the facilities of some of the others; and he's not a physician. But he has the necessary practical skills, and he has some very effective treatments. His fees are also more reasonable than the others. His patients love him. I think he's probably the best in Tijuana." Vaughn added with a meaningful look, "I guess you know he has survived several assassination attempts."

"Really!" I said. I didn't know. I asked for the details, but Vaughn didn't know any more.

The week after the Tijuana tour, I met a striking-looking young actress named Cherise who said Jimmy had saved her life. She'd had no money to pay him, so he had treated her for free. "I love that man!" she had gushed in her exuberant Hollywood way.

It was a chance meeting, and I didn't expect to hear from her again. I went back home to Kenya, where my husband was then an attorney for the U.S. Agency for International Development.

Six months later, in May of 1991, my family returned to Los Angeles for summer vacation. We hadn't been at my parents' home for more than a week, when I got a frantic phone call from Cherise.

"Jimmy's in jail!" she exclaimed. "They set bail at five million dollars cash!"

"Five million dollars cash?!" My recollection was that serial killer Jeffrey Dalmer had gotten hit with a mere million, and he had had to come up with a mere $100,000 in cash to post a bond. "I thought excessive bail was unconstitutional," I said. "What did Jimmy do, kill his patients?"

"No!" said Cherise. "They called it fraud. A lady who was helping him supposedly told people over the phone that he had a high rate of cure for cancer."

"But he was working in <u>Mexico</u>. How did the U.S. government get jurisdiction?"

"I don't know. They said it was a conspiracy to commit wire fraud. Jimmy was named as one of the conspirators."

"In fact, how did they even serve the <u>warrant</u> in Mexico?"

"All I know," said Cherise in a tumble of run-on sentences, "is that they burst into his clinic and grabbed him at gunpoint and took him across the border. His patients are frantic! He uses his own serum, and they think it's the only thing keeping them alive. He makes it up for them individually. They don't know what to do!"

She said a weekly newspaper had agreed to publish an article about the case. She knew I was doing research in the field. She wondered if I could write it.

My interest was definitely aroused. I wondered why the government wanted Jimmy so badly that they would go to the trouble of kidnapping him in violation of national and international law. Why were they so afraid of his escape that they set bail at $5 million cash? He hadn't actually "fled" the jurisdiction. He wasn't even in the United States when the indictment was issued. He wasn't charged with murder or any other heinous crime. Five million seemed like overkill. Who was it he was threatening? And did that threat outweigh the harm closing his clinic would do to people like Cherise, who desperately wanted his help?

I told her I'd write the article.

A week after I submitted it to the paper, I got a call from Brownsville, Texas.

"I want to thank you for your help," Jimmy drawled on the phone.

"Sure," I said. "Where are you?"

"In the Cameron County Jail."

He explained that he had already been in jail for nearly three months, and that his high-priced attorneys hadn't gotten him out even on bail. He was trapped behind bars, at the mercy of counsel who weren't communicating and seemed to lack interest in his case. He was convinced he was the victim of a drug industry plot. The federal government, he maintained with cynical humor, was the finest money could buy; and there was a great deal of money in the cancer industry. He said he had heard I was an attorney. He felt I understood his treatments and his plight. He wondered if I could represent him.

The man was obviously desperate. Still, I was interested. I just had two problems. One was that I had never done a criminal case in my life. I wasn't one of those Amazon women trial lawyers with Lauren Bacall nerve. At 46, I was still waiting for my voice to change. The other problem was the commute. I was then living on the other side of the world.

# Chapter 2

## In His Defense

When we bailed out of L.A. law in 1988, it was mainly for the sake of the family unit. Our too-charming children, Jeff and Jamie, were growing up while we were busy at the office. Often, we didn't manage even to have dinner together. The kids ate in front of the TV off their "My Little Pony" and "Transformers" trays. I was noticing how atrocious their table manners were at about the time my husband announced he was using his mind for unworthy ends and wanted to join the foreign service. He was then a partner at a Beverly Hills law firm, where he was smothering in securities transactions and bankruptcies.

My own field was commercial litigation -- not the sexiest of issues, but at least I didn't have to get emotionally involved -- no murders, no divorces. I generally managed to avoid speaking in court through meticulous paperwork. Practicing law was an intellectual exercise, research and writing about hypotheticals. The pay was good, but I had the nagging sense that I was caught up in the world of externals. Commercial law was all about money.

What I really wanted to do was to write. I had been an English major at Berkeley. College hadn't taught the important things, like what happens when you die, or how you should live, or what you were supposed to be doing here. That was what I wanted to write about. But first I had to do some research. And in the meantime, I was having problems with my body. My research had wound up focusing on matters of health.

When I hit 29 and still hadn't reached enlightenment, I succumbed to social pressure and took the Law School Admissions

Test. I was dating a law student at UCLA who thought if we went there together, it would be "fun." I was living with my parents and working part-time in a music library. When I got a good score on the test, I got little nudgings from home. "There's not a lot of future in the music library," my mother had hinted in her tactful way.

That was how I wound up at UCLA Law School. The first thing I had published was a law review article on the legal restrictions on unconventional medicine. I graduated and married Cliff, another law student, in 1977. We worked as attorneys for the next ten years, until Cliff decided to go into the foreign service, and we escaped to Kenya.

We envisioned tightening our belts, living like Peace Corps volunteers, and trekking off to the wilderness; but not much belt-tightening was actually entailed. Nairobi turned out to be a thriving metropolis with the majority of modern conveniences. I became a lady of leisure and learned to play bridge. The four of us religiously ate dinner together at 6 p.m., and on weekends we took off for the game park. I was the first of my friends to get my Christmas cards in the mail. I had time to read, write and think. The city sported a university with a medical school and an adequate library in English. I got a couple of books published, not on law but on health.

I hadn't thought much about cancer, however, until a shocking video came from a friend in the mail. ("You've got to see this!" she said.) It was about Harry Hoxsey, "the worst cancer quack of the century." That was what the American Medical Association called him, but scores of patients testified in court that he had cured their cancers. Hoxsey, in turn, said the AMA was a monopoly, a doctor's union setting medical policies in its own interests. Surprisingly, the federal court had agreed with him, and he had prevailed. Yet the Food and Drug Administration had still managed to put him out of business in the United States. That happened half a century ago, but the narrator maintained that cheap, effective natural cancer treatments continue to be suppressed today.[1]

Some preliminary research confirmed this claim. I decided to check out the non-traditional cancer treatment scene. While visiting in California in November of 1990, I signed up for the tour sponsored by the Cancer Control Society, a non-profit organization set up to disseminate information on cancer alternatives.

The tour had then prompted more research. I learned some interesting facts. One was that by 1990, the cost of getting FDA approval for a single remedy was up to more than $100 million; and manufacturers normally had to pick this tab up themselves. Natural products, which couldn't be patented, were generally out of the running, since they weren't lucrative enough to support the investment. Natural products weren't written up in medical journals for the same reason: there was no one to underwrite the studies. That meant interested and well-meaning oncologists might never even learn of their existence.

I also read that after twenty years and a 100 billion dollar investment, we were still losing the war on cancer. The National Cancer Institute had made it seem otherwise, but according to the General Accounting Office, this sleight of hand was the result of manipulating critical data. The GAO had told Congress that the NCI had "artificially inflate[d] the amount of 'true' progress," apparently for the purpose of justifying massive government and private funding.[2]

I had a fairly good grasp of the issues but wasn't sure what to do with them, until Cherise called and asked me to write an article on the Keller case. Then Jimmy called and asked if I could represent him. I thought about it, but decided I had to decline.

In the meantime, I was exploring a book collaboration with Vaughn on dentistry. When I met a physician/attorney who specialized in non-traditional medicine at Vaughn's house the next weekend, it was sheer coincidence. The attorney's name was Bill, and he was with his girlfriend/secretary/paralegal wrapping up Vaughn's license review action. Vaughn had been charged with removing mercury amalgam fillings for health reasons, a practice the American Dental Association staunchly maintained was quackery. Bill had represented Vaughn against the licensing board, and Vaughn had prevailed. Bill was a licensed M.D., but he said he had come to favor natural "alternative" medicine.

I eyed the attorney discreetly as he spoke. He didn't exactly fit my stereotype of a health fanatic. At 64, he sported a voluminous pot belly and was a chain smoker. His conversation was peppered with expletives. "So how did you get into natural medicine?" I inquired.

Bill explained that he had gotten his medical training after World War II in the military in Germany, a country that led the non-traditional medical field. He went to medical school because German girls wouldn't date American servicemen but they would date medical students. He wasn't particularly interested in the profession, so after the service, he switched to law.

I pictured him in a uniform in his younger, thinner days. He was probably rather dashing. His arched eyebrows gave him an intelligent look, and he had a substantial head of hair.

More to the point, he was versed in unconventional medicine. He was also an experienced criminal defense attorney, who knew the tricks of the trade. He was suspicious of the government and told a good story. He said he had developed his courtroom style in the South at a time when corruption was rife, in the days before elaborate pretrial discovery procedures had taken the surprise out of courtroom practice. "In those days," Bill dryly remarked, "nobody knew what evidence would come up, so it was common to hire a few 'witnesses' to wait in the hall who would testify to anything."

"Common for whom," I asked, "the government or the defense?"

Bill smiled. "Both."

I mentioned the Jimmy Keller case. Bill agreed it was an interesting one. He said he had considered bidding on it. At the time he had been busy with Vaughn's case, but now he was free. He added that he knew the good reputation of Jimmy's clinic, and that he could produce experts to testify to it.

"The kind who will testify to anything?" I asked.

Bill laughed. "That won't be necessary. His clinic actually has a good reputation -- depending on who you ask, of course."

"Of course."

"I've gotten to know almost everyone in alternative health care over the last fifteen years," Bill explained, "and I've represented a good percentage of them. We're on a crusade. Health care should be a matter between the doctor and the patient. A lot of doctors now have new ideas about natural, drugless therapies. But drugs are big business, and the drug people aren't about to let these mavericks start a stampede away from their products. The mavericks don't just lose their licenses. They've been winding up in jail. Jimmy's case is rife with government misconduct, like the kidnapping and the five million dollar bail. It's characteristic of cases that are politically motivated. The government is spending a lot of money to get him on contrived charges. It's a $30,000 case that should be worth a $100,000 bond. But this is their test case. They want to put all the Tijuana clinics out of business."

Bill made the case sound pivotal. Obviously, we had to volunteer to help. I wasn't so brave or foolhardy as to take on the matter myself, but I was willing to stand behind a competent man. I hardly knew this one, but the meeting was so coincidental, I took it to be fate. I had already heard enough favorable testimony to think the jury would have to be swayed. I confidently assumed the case would be over by the time my family went back to Kenya at the end of the summer. I suggested we could work together on it, and Bill agreed. "I already know our government lies, cheats, and swindles in these cases," he said. "I like to expose them when I can."

We contacted the defendant and offered our services, and he accepted. It was an impulsive venture, but summer vacations were generally too busy to leave much time for reflection. The first thing we had to do was to "come up to speed" on the case. We got the file in a box by Federal Express.

Topping the imposing stack of documents was one called "Superseding Indictment." It had been issued in 1991 and named not only Jimmy but eight other "co-conspirators" (mainly the employees at his clinic). The indictment charged the defendants with eleven counts of wire fraud and one count of conspiracy to commit wire fraud, carrying a maximum potential sentence of 55 years. The principal fraud involved a remedy called "Tumorex." The representation said to be fraudulent was that "the success or cure rate for cancer victims taking their 'Tumorex' treatment was anywhere from 80% to 100% for cancer victims who had not had conventional medical treatment and from 40% to 65% for those who had already received conventional medical treatment." In fact, said the indictment, "Tumorex" consisted of nothing but water and the common amino acid L-arginine.

I was starting to see what we were up against. How could a common amino acid shrink tumors? And even if it could, how were we going to convince a jury of it?

Bill didn't seem worried. He said a nutrient that was natural to the body was more likely to help it than something lethal like chemotherapy.

"I suppose," I said. "But what about this?" Jimmy was also charged with representing that a radionics device called a Digitron "D" Spectrometer could diagnose cancer in a patient, "by either having the person hold a plastic plate attached to the machine by two wires or by placing the same plastic plate over a polaroid photograph of the person." I stressed "polaroid photograph" as I read this allegation aloud.

"That's how it's done," Bill said nonchalantly. He directed me to some books on the subtle energy technique known as radionics.

I wrote these leads down, resolved to be open-minded, and dug further into the box. Under the indictment was the transcript of an earlier trial involving three of Jimmy's co-defendants. Thumbing through it, I learned that the government's chief witness was the manufacturer of the suspect remedy "Tumorex." This man, whom I'll call Rudnov, had been named as a co-defendant; but he had been given immunity from prosecution in exchange for testifying for the government. I flipped through his testimony, curious to know how he had developed the remedy. Under penalty of perjury at the earlier trial, Rudnov had told this story . . .

In 1975 or '76, he said, he had met a doctor named Shang, who had escaped from Czechoslovakia in the World War II era. Rudnov himself was a Slavic immigrant who was raised in China. Both men spoke fluent Russian and German, and their meeting was an opportunity for them to practice languages they were rusty in. Shang was an M.D. at a cancer clinic, but he wanted to switch to geriatrics. He therefore had no further use for the Tumorex formula, which he had acquired earlier from his colleague, Wesley Irons, M.D.

Dr. Irons, in turn, had originated the formula in the 1940s while working under a grant from the American Cancer Society (ACS). When, two years into his grant, he announced he had found a cure for cancer, the unexpected reaction of the ACS was to cut off his funding. Dr. Irons then got sponsored by the Mormon Church, and then by Presbyterian Hospital in Los Angeles. The hospital did a study on 700 cancer patients, in which Tumorex proved to be highly effective. But this study too was mysteriously terminated, and its results were never reported. There was only rumor: the head of radiology complained that his department was losing $1.5 million a year as a result of the newer, cheaper treatment.

Dr. Irons died a heartbroken man. His formula would have died with him, if it hadn't been reactivated twenty years later by Dr. Shang. As originally devised, it was very difficult

to make. But Dr. Irons later discovered a simple substitute
that functioned the same way. It was this simple formula that
Dr. Shang had passed on to Rudnov.

"That's pretty hard to believe," I remarked to Bill, "especially
the part where the ACS cut off Dr. Irons' funding."

"That sort of thing happens," Bill maintained with a telling
look from under his pointed eyebrows. "It happened to Joel
Wallach." Dr. Wallach was one of the doctors Bill hoped to line
up as an expert witness.

"What happened to him?" I asked.

Bill proceeded to relate the incredible story of Dr. Wallach's
career as a medical researcher. At the time, I wasn't sure whether
to believe it. But I read it in detail later in a book the doctor co-
authored with his second wife, Ma Lan, M.D.[3] . . .

> Before he switched from conventional to unconventional
> medicine, Dr. Wallach said, he had been a pathologist
> employed by the Cystic Fibrosis Foundation, an organization
> set up to find a cure for that troubling childhood disease. His
> job was to autopsy a number of caged primates that had died
> mysteriously in what appeared to be an epidemic of it. When
> he made the first universally accepted diagnosis of cystic fibrosis
> in a laboratory animal in 1978, experts from the Foundation
> and from the National Institutes of Health were ecstatic. But
> that was before they learned that he could reproduce the same
> changes in almost any animal species, merely by inducing a
> deficiency of the mineral selenium. The disease appeared to be
> the result of a simple nutritional deficiency. Dr. Wallach cured
> the "epidemic" merely by correcting the animals' diets.
>
> In humans, the treatment was more complicated, but it
> still involved selenium deficiency. For infants, he recommended
> first determining if the child was allergic to wheat, cow's milk
> or soy, since these allergies can cause selenium malabsorption.
> Then the infant's diet was supplemented with selenium and
> flaxseed oil.
>
> The response of the Foundation to these revelations was
> to fire Dr. Wallach with only 24 hours' notice. He was
> blackballed from further research in the field. He realized then
> that the research industry has a vested interest in <u>not</u> achieving
> its goals. The Catch 22 of any foundation set <u>up</u> to find a

*"cure," he said, is that if its mission is accomplished, its personnel will be out of a job.*

*Dr. Wallach was terminated by the Cystic Fibrosis Foundation ten days after his first wife died of cancer. She had been treated conventionally with chemotherapy. The crushing impact of these two experiences drove him to unconventional medicine, making him a rare and valuable find as an expert witness for the defense.*

But Bill was concerned with more immediate matters. "Son of a bitch!" he exploded as he handed me a document. "Look at this!"

It was a memo addressed to Jimmy's lead counsel. This man, whom I'll call Silversmith, was reputed to be one of the finest criminal defense attorneys in Texas. The problem was that he didn't know medicine. The memo was from William Ginsburg, an attorney retained to advise Silversmith on the medical issues. Like Bill, Ginsburg was not only an attorney but was a licensed M.D. The difference was that Ginsburg had gotten his medical training in a conventional medical school. He gave the conventional diagnosis. In his memo, he opined that Jimmy's methods could not work. A crucial corner had already been turned, or so Bill surmised. Based on Ginsburg's advice, Silversmith had concluded his own client was guilty. He was therefore taking the tack normally taken with guilty defendants: he was playing his cards close to the chest. The court thus had no reason to think Jimmy was anything but a crook.

"We'll have to educate the judge," muttered Bill. "Silversmith has never handled a non-traditional health care case. In the natural health movement, we don't believe our clients have broken any laws; or if they have, the laws are unconstitutional. That's how we want to characterize the issues. We can do it in a motion to dismiss for failure to state a claim."

"Good idea," I said. "What will the grounds be?"

Bill shrugged. "We can find that out in Texas." He added, "You can draft the motion."

"Okay." I was still reading. "But we might have another problem. Look at this!"

At the earlier trial, the head of medicine at M. D. Anderson Hospital in Houston had maintained:

*It [arginine] has been studied as part of this drug development process in animals with cancer and has been found*

*in all of the tests that were done by the National Cancer
Institute to be negative, that is, to have no effect in the treatment
of animal cancer.*

This, Bill finally conceded, could be a troubling detail.

He did not like flying, mainly because of the new no-smoking
rule on intercontinental flights. But I was only half listening to
Bill grumble as we waited for takeoff. I was having second thoughts
myself. What was I doing flying off with a man I hardly knew, to
a remote border town 1,000 miles away, to get involved in a
criminal case? I thought of the pro bono divorce I had once done
for my housekeeper. She turned out to be a bigamist, and her
husband was concealing his assets. I had sworn I would never
again take a case that wasn't in my field.

I remembered the M. D. Anderson doctor's testimony:
arginine didn't work. Then I remembered Jimmy's eager, excited
patients insisting that it did. Something was happening at his
clinic. I wanted to know the details.

I was abandoning my family, but my husband didn't seem to
mind my getting involved. He considered it summer employment.
He was in Washington D.C. then working himself; and the kids,
who were twelve and ten, were in Los Angeles being doted on by
Grandma and Grandpa.

I wondered if Jimmy were really being made an example of
for political ends. Bill thought he had been separated out from
the growing throng of unconventional health practitioners by a
medical/pharmaceutical establishment with pervasive, entrenched
political support, which was bent on annihilating the competition.
Non-prescription nutritional supplements, herbs, homeopathy,
chiropractic, and a host of other natural therapies had increasingly
encroached on the established turf of conventional medicine.

The other possibility, of course, was that Jimmy's therapies
were indeed quackery. But his patients certainly hadn't thought
so. Didn't they have a right to the treatment of their choice,
whether or not it was considered quackery by convention-bound
medical interests? I remembered the holding in a precedent-setting
case: "Every human being of adult years and sound mind has a
right to determine what shall be done with his own body." In a
country where clandestine drug tests had been conducted on army
enlistees and unsuspecting private citizens, it seemed irrational

that willing and eager volunteers couldn't test "unproven" natural remedies. If found consistently effective, they could later be disseminated to the general public.

As the plane lifted off the ground, my thoughts rose to the loftier issues. Heretics and maverick thinkers had always suffered abuse for their non-conformity. The medical profession's dogged resistance to anything new went back at least as far as Robert Koch and Louis Pasteur. At the turn of the millennium, we seemed to be undergoing a paradigm shift away from more materialistic ways of thinking. Rationality was giving way to less familiar modes. Perhaps we were on the verge of celebrating the type of maverick we once burned at the stake.

Anyway, the case was an adventure. I fantasized what it would be like to play the hero and save the day. I hardly imagined I would be a witness to a classic miscarriage of justice. Nor could I conceive how crushing it would be to watch the inquisition of a man who, by most accounts, was successfully prolonging the lives of cancer victims . . . a man who, I would become convinced, was dedicated to the service of humanity.

# Chapter 3

## The Cameron County Jail

Brownsville, at the southern tip of Texas, has the dubious distinction of having hosted the last battle of the Civil War -- dubious because it was fought four weeks after General Lee surrendered at Appomattox. News traveled slowly to Brownsville in those days; and even today, this remote border area has been described as only nominally a part of the United States. The situation, I thought ominously, boded ill for finding a progressive, open-minded jury.

A travel brochure glamorously described the area as "the Texas tropics." There weren't many palm trees, but there was plenty of heat. Brownsville was an inferno. The thermometer registered a humid 100 degrees. We were met at the airport by Jimmy's Uncle Harold and Aunt Lou, who drove us to the condominium where members of the Keller clan took turns keeping vigil. We met Jimmy's sisters Gwen and Diane, his sister-in-law Cita and her children, and his 84-year-old father Guy. Their down-home hospitality was more inviting than the Cameron County Jail, but Bill was eager to interview the defendant, and Harold had volunteered to drive.

We thanked him and hurried from the air-conditioned car to the air-conditioned jail. I didn't notice how sinister it was until the sliding bars rolled closed behind us. While we waited for the guard to bring in the prisoner, Bill amused himself by telling tales of ominous ends that had come to women who ventured alone into jails. His eyebrows leered diabolically as he warmed to the subject. My sense of adventure was fast turning to dread.

Jimmy shuffled in wearing sandals and an orange prison jumpsuit. Either the outfit didn't flatter his figure, or he had put on weight. His glasses were askew, but I soon realized why: he lacked an ear to hold them up. The red inner flesh under his left eye was visible through their thick, distorting lenses. It should have been concealed by his lower eyelid, but the muscles had been cut by surgery. Fortunately, he still had a full head of hair, which fell like a lion's mane over his missing ear. He was carrying a brown paper bag full of papers, which he set on the table. He pulled a comb from his pocket and tidied the part in his hair, making it fall to the left, where his ear wasn't.

Disconcerting as his looks were, I soon forgot them. The prisoner spoke with insight, humility and Southern charm. He became inexplicably appealing, and an air of excitement began to pervade the meeting. Heightening it was the fact that Bill was convinced the attorney/conference room was bugged. We talked in low conspiratorial whispers, as if we were plotting an escape, while my new $29.00 tape recorder whirred away in the background.

Jimmy had charisma, but then we knew that. We wanted to know if he had anything else. After some polite, ice-breaking conversation, I decided to take the bull by the horns. "The indictment says this 'Tumorex' you were using is nothing but a common amino acid and water," I said. I tried to look the defendant in the eye, but his bloodshot eye was magnified by his glasses, and I had to look away.

"That's what it was -- arginine," Jimmy congenially agreed. "I was glad to find that out, too. At least that's something I can thank the FBI for. My serum got a lot cheaper after I could make it from scratch. Arginine wasn't all there was in it, of course. I just used it as a base. I added all kinds of things to my serum. I had 300 possibilities to choose from. I customized it to the patient and potentized it like a homeopathic remedy. It had an amazing ability to shrink tumors." He added, "But arginine alone will actually shrink tumors."

"That's not what the government's expert said," I dubiously observed. I dug into my briefcase and pulled out the 1985 trial testimony of the head of medicine at M. D. Anderson Hospital. It was apparently based on this testimony that the "Superseding Indictment" had made the categorical assertion that "Scientific studies show that L-arginine, when tested, has shown a lack of any significant antitumor activity."

Jimmy had anticipated the issue. He ceremoniously emptied his brown paper bag on the table. "Then what do you make of these?" he asked.

Bill's eyes lit up as he started to read. Soon, he was like a pirate digging into a treasure chest. The bag contained studies -- over forty of them -- all demonstrating the tumor-shrinking and immunity-building effects of L-arginine.

One article summarized the literature. Of 25 studies reviewed, fully 20 -- or 80 percent -- had found a significant favorable tumor response to arginine treatment. "Favorable response" was defined as tumor regression, slower growth, or decreased incidence. The review concluded, "The role of arginine in . . . cancer requires further clinical studies, based on the available strong experimental data."[4] But we didn't find much in the way of clinical studies on humans. I wondered why they hadn't been pursued.

"Researchers can recommend all they want," Bill said, "but if nobody puts up the money, the studies won't get done. Arginine is a natural product, and it's already on the market. It's not going to be profitable to drug companies to test it on cancer."

He handed me a study. "Notice anything special about this one?"

The date on it was 1980. The gist of it was that daily injections of L-arginine into tumor-bearing rats consistently inhibited the growth of tumors. The researchers wrote, "Within 2 weeks, tumor size was reduced to 80% of the initial size."[5]

"Pretty remarkable results," I said tentatively.

"Notice who sponsored it," Bill coached me along.

"Amazing!" I agreed. In small print was written "the National Cancer Institute." The NCI was the same agency the government's expert had claimed had gotten only negative results. It was also a branch of the same government that was now prosecuting Jimmy for making claims its own studies evidently supported. "Legally," Bill observed, "the knowledge of different agencies is imputed to other agencies of the same government."

We came across another NCI study, dated as far back as 1969. It found that feeding acetamide to rats caused liver cancer in 50 percent of the animals after 12 to 15 months. Feeding arginine with the acetamide, however, "led to virtually complete inhibition of the carcinogenic process."[6] Arginine evidently worked not only as a treatment but as a cancer preventive.

I looked for some mention of Wesley Irons, M.D., the doctor who supposedly developed Tumorex in the forties, but I didn't find it. I did find a study, though, from the forties. It demonstrated that an animal extract of arginine and some other amino acids could make rat tumors completely disappear. Injections of the amino acid mixture were said to be 60 to 83 percent effective in eliminating tumors. Merely putting the amino acid solution in the rats' drinking water caused 69 percent of the tumors to disappear.[7]

We were excited. Our prospective client had more going for him than mere charisma! We also had good grounds for bringing a motion to dismiss: the government's claim was belied by its own studies. Smugly, I was starting to think this case was going to be a lead pipe cinch.

While we were reviewing the studies, Jimmy was studying the trial transcript. "M. D. Anderson is the largest private tumor center in the world," he said. "How could its head of medicine have missed these studies?"

"He couldn't have," Bill flatly maintained. "That indictment was returned on perjured testimony. The doctor was lying."

"How did you find the studies?" I asked.

Jimmy looked out of the corner of his better eye in a gesture of amused skepticism. "My daughter-in-law Suzanne found them in the medical library, when I asked her to have a look."

"Sharp woman," Bill said. "Do you mind if we copy this stuff and return it?"

"No."

"Good," said Bill. "I've got more questions. Besides arginine, what remedies did you use?"

Jimmy started naming his popular favorites. He could think of them faster than I could write them down: live cell therapy, Alivizatos' treatment, DMSO, vitamin and mineral therapy, hydrazine sulfate, Pau d'Arco tea, proteolytic enzymes, sublingual free amino acids, Lugol's solution, Carnivora I.V., injectable Essiac tea, levamisole, mistletoe, cesium chloride, GH3 . . . For a 57-year-old man under the stress of prison, I thought, his memory was good.

"You didn't use all those things on every patient, did you?" I asked.

"I just used what tested out."

"How did you test them?"

"By muscle testing. Before that I used a radionics machine called a Digitron. And before that, I used a pendulum."

A pendulum?! I decided my assessment of "lead pipe cinch" could be over-optimistic.

"But I quit using it," Jimmy added, "because it was too weird for some people."

I was thinking that was an understatement, as Bill reached into his briefcase. He pulled out a shiny object on a string. Looking around furtively, as if he were about to make a treasonous statement, he said, "Pendulums work. I use pendulums all the time."

I was floored. I had some understanding of the technique -- the subtle movement of the pendulum acts as a bridge between the conscious and subconscious minds -- but I hardly expected this gruff and street-wise attorney to be sensitive to subtle energy fields.

Bill dropped his voice, apparently in deference to the bugged walls. "If someone wants me to take a vitamin or a mineral, I say just a minute, and I put it in my hand, and I put my pendulum over it, and I watch it. If I start getting a clockwise rotation, I put it in my mouth; and if it starts moving back and forth, I throw it away. Of course, you've got to take your conscious mind out of it, or it won't work."

"Of course," Jimmy agreed, obviously pleased to find someone on his own wavelength. "Anyone could cheat. I used to teach patients to use it themselves. But then I realized it wasn't good, because they'd say, 'My pendulum says I can have ice cream' or something. So I got out of that and went into muscle testing, and that's what I've done in the last few years. I wish I'd been doing it earlier. I wouldn't be in so much trouble now. It's best when you get the patient involved. He can feel his own arm getting weaker or stronger, depending on the answer."

I would have probed for more details, but Bill had already moved on to his next query: "Were you actually promising the rates of 'success or cure' alleged in the indictment?"

Jimmy sighed. "I did gives those figures once, in a speech. But I was just repeating what Rudnov said -- and I never said 'cure.' I didn't expect patients to live forever. I was only trying to relieve their pains and extend their lives beyond the death sentences their doctors had already given them. I told them the disease could always return. They had to watch their diets, take supplements, quit smoking. I think the word 'cure' just came in because the government needed it to build a case."

"That's how they usually do it," Bill said ominously.

My assessment of "lead pipe cinch" was fading fast. Proving arginine could shrink tumors was one thing; proving Jimmy had never promised anyone a cure was quite another. The charge could as easily be made against oncologists who said they "got it all," whose patients later died. But oncologists had convention on their side. As G. Edward Griffin, author of <u>World Without Cancer</u>, would later frame the issue in a letter to the court:

> *There is not one AMA/orthodox physician in the entire United States treating seriously ill people who has not lost many patients. Are they now to be tried for quackery, for making money out of the illness and death of others? I think not, because the AMA lobby has skewed the laws to favor their type of medicine. . . . [I]t is selective persecution and a travesty of justice to punish men like [Jimmy] whose only 'crime' is that he is not a member of the orthodox medical fraternity.*

Bill suspected it was some anti-competitive element of the orthodox fraternity that had set this case in motion. He asked Jimmy if he had ever heard of the National Council Against Health Fraud.

The prisoner rolled his eyes in a disconcerting way. "I've been on their hit list for years," he said. "Whenever I wound up in court, one of their experts would be there to testify against me. One of them called me 'the most notorious quack in the country' on national TV." Jimmy grinned. "I was kind of proud of that."

Bill looked interested. "When was that?"

"1982, I think."

Bill nodded. "That was when federal anti-quackery bills were pending in Congress."

"Interesting!" I agreed.

Since then, Jimmy said, his name had come up regularly at NCAHF meetings. He had heard that shortly before his arrest, an entire meeting had been devoted to the threat represented by his clinic.

"The National Council Against Health Fraud sounds like a government agency," I remarked.

"It isn't," Bill assured me. "It's private. It represents medical industry interests. You can read about it when we get back to California."

"So how did you get on their hit list?" Bill asked Jimmy.

"It's a long story. I embarrassed one of their big guns in front of the Georgia Legislature."

Bill looked at his watch. "We've got time."

# Chapter 4

## Embroiled in Politics

"In 1975," Jimmy started in with his tale, "I was state chairman of the Committee for Freedom of Choice in Cancer Therapy. It was an organization that was trying to get laetrile legalized. Laetrile was the big natural cancer remedy in the seventies."

Bill nodded, evidently familiar with the organization. I was at least familiar with the legal issues surrounding laetrile, from my law school research in the seventies.

Jimmy chuckled. "I wasn't elected. I just read I was the state chairman in <u>Choice</u> magazine, so I figured I was. Mike Culbert wrote it. He helped found the Committee, and he was my good friend."

Bill nodded again.

"I didn't have time for the job," Jimmy said, "but I felt there was a need for people to be informed. I wasn't actually treating anyone then, but I was very vocal. I went around speaking, and I made laetrile available to people. When someone needed treatment, I sent them to a nurse I'd gotten connected up with -- a Ms. Ivy, the sister of Billy Williams. Billy had had colon cancer that had metastasized to the liver. Ms. Ivy had given him laetrile injections and he'd gotten on the whole program, the diet and so on. The cancer had gone into remission and had been in remission for a couple of years, and they had the blood work to prove it. I was referring patients to her, but then somebody scared her. They were putting some kind of pressure on her and her husband."

"What kind of pressure?" Bill asked.

"I don't know, but all of a sudden she quit."

Bill nodded again. "They have their ways."

"Around that time," Jimmy went on, "there was a big ground swell for a freedom of choice bill. Woody Jenkins was my representative in the Louisiana House of Representatives, and I was active in supporting him. Woody was a Democrat by party but conservative by philosophy. He's for freedom in everything. I went to him and said it's time for freedom of choice in health treatment. He says sure, and he drafts a strong bill. It gave everyone the right to use any treatment for any disease he wanted, but laetrile specifically -- provided that if it was an oral remedy, it had to be over-the-counter, and if it was an injectable, it had to be prescribed by a doctor. Of course, the bill ran directly counter to FDA regulations. Woody planned to present it to the House Health and Welfare Committee. He said they'd pass it maybe next session. I said, 'No, Woody, we're going to pass it this session.'"

Jimmy shook his head. "I don't know why I said that. It wasn't going to be an easy thing to pass. At that time, people didn't know anything about this issue, so we were going to have to do some pretty heavy lobbying. There was no viable Republican Party in Louisiana then, just Conservative Democrats -- which I was -- and Liberal Democrats. I felt the opposition would come from the liberals, who were controlled by the medical people. The third camp was the Black Caucus. They could go either way, but I felt I could get them. There were only 12 black representatives, out of 92; but the population was 25 percent black. There weren't that many white liberals, so for a liberal to win, he'd have to have most of the black vote. The sickle cell thing was my ace in the hole. I had helped get a free clinic going in the health department, where we were using laetrile to treat cancer and sickle cell anemia. It was under the auspices of the state."

"Laetrile works on sickle cell anemia?" I asked.

"It does," Jimmy said, and cited some research on it.[8] He said he had persuaded Dr. Pichnich, an M.D. who headed the West Baton Rouge Health Unit and directed three parish health units, to open a free clinic that would administer laetrile to black children with the disease. Jimmy volunteered his time and free laetrile. The Health Unit furnished materials and medical help. The results were remarkable: sickle cell symptoms were immediately relieved by a treatment that was simple and inexpensive. Dr. Pichnich was so impressed that he got on the alternative-care bandwagon.

"That was what first got the conventional people riled up," Jimmy said. "It was pretty threatening to them, getting an unconventional clinic in the health department. We had infiltrated their stronghold. Dr. Pichnich was one of their best doctors. He was well known by the governor's people. They said, 'Dr. Pichnich's been with the health department 35 years. We know who he is, we know what he does, we know how sane a guy he is. If he's doing it, it can't be crazy.'

"So I went around to all the black churches showing the film World Without Cancer, which talks about laetrile. Then I'd bring in a sickle cell testimonial -- a woman whose daughter had it so bad she couldn't go to school; whenever she had a period she had to go to the hospital; she couldn't hold a job. Now she's got a boyfriend and a job, etc., etc. They'd just be cryin,' and they'd be ready to do whatever I asked. Then I told them to send letters to their legislators. The legislators got hundreds. They couldn't figure out what was happening. Before that, the black representatives wouldn't have anything to do with this bill; but I had a reputation with the blacks. I did business with them and they liked me. My granddaddy was a sort of champion of black people. His mother had died in childbirth, and he'd been raised by a black nanny. He had a big plantation in St. Charles Parish. When he died, there were 5,000 black people at his funeral.

"Anyway, the black legislators realized they better take care of their own people. Then fate brings me this lady, the head of the NAACP in New Orleans. She says, 'Don't worry, we'll get your bill passed,' and she contacts all the black people she knows in politics. So we had created popular support, or at least the semblance of it -- the bandwagon effect. But we still had the problem of getting patients to testify. A lot of people had taken laetrile by then and had done very well on the treatment, but it was illegal, so it was hard getting people to speak. They said, 'If we get up there and testify, the government is going to come after us, because we're making public that we're disobeying the law.' I had a dozen witnesses listed who had agreed to appear before the Health and Welfare Committee. I was to meet them on the steps of the state capitol, and guess what. I was standing on the capitol steps waiting for them, and the only one who showed up was Billy Williams. Someone had been making anonymous phone calls saying they weren't going to be able to get their medicine anymore if they testified. I only had Dr. Pichnich and two other doctors, and myself and Billy and another patient. I needed more patients. So guess what I did."

Jimmy grinned, or tried to. Only half his mouth went up, giving him a wry, rakish look. "I called the guy from Lafayette who was the head of the John Birch Society there. He's a Cajun and one of my own people."

"The John Birch Society?" I repeated warily.

"Yep." Jimmy laughed. "They're opposed to regulation in any form. They didn't even need to know what it was all about. I just said, 'Those liberal son-of-a-bitches don't want us to have our medicine,' and they were ready to do anything I asked. I made big yellow posters that said 'Legalize laetrile now!' and I had as many buttons as I could get. I filled the whole hearing room up with people and they all had their buttons on. They weren't patients, but nobody knew that. We had patients, but they'd been scared off, so I had to create the semblance of it.

"The three doctors testified and then the three patients, which included me. Then I said, 'This has gone on long enough. We have all these people here who have used laetrile, but we don't want to take any more of the Committee's time up, so we're going to rescind our right to speak; but I'm going to give you a raise of hands of everyone who's used laetrile and thinks it's of benefit.' And all these people raised their hands. They all really had taken it, or at least had eaten apricot pits; and if they hadn't, by the day they got there I made sure they had."

"How many people?" I asked.

"I'd say about sixty. The legislators thought they were all cancer patients, and they were scared. You can just project that out to the families and the friends, people you would have alienated just like that. The bill went through the House 91 to 1. Then it had to go before the Senate. I was doing tremendous lobbying, and everything was going my way. People got over being afraid to testify. I could present 25 witnesses now. I only had one problem -- there was still one committee member opposed to the bill. He was bought and paid for by the AMA. He happened to be from my mama's parish. So I said, 'Mama, I'm gonna need you to do some politickin.' I need you to go around your old home areas. All you gotta do is tell 'em your son's on laetrile, and they need this legalized for him to live. You know all these people and you tell 'em could they please get to their senator, because he is votin' against the bill.'

"My daddy's from St. Charles and my mama's from St. John, and those were the two parishes that this senator represented. My parents knew everybody everywhere, and everybody knew them. It's just an old thing. My granddaddy on my mama's side had the biggest country store on the river down there. In the Depression, he sold to everybody on credit when they were going bankrupt, until he went bankrupt himself. He could have foreclosed on their property, but he wouldn't do it.

"Anyway, my mama went to all the people she knew and asked them to go to people they knew, and it just erupted from there. The poor senator didn't know what hit him. He changed his mind just like that. He came and apologized and wanted to have all the information we had. If you get pressure coming from the voters, the politicians don't care what the AMA's giving them, because they know at election time what counts is all those people pulling those levers. During this whole time we had a tremendous pressure coming in from all over the state, people calling in and writing in through different groups that were allied with our effort.

"So I came to the Senate Committee meeting and was ready to go, when the Committee people said the government hadn't brought in any witnesses. 'You're unopposed,' they said. 'There's no use for you to present any witnesses, we're going to put your bill through.' So I told everyone, 'We won! The bill's going out of committee.' And guess what happened. After I told everybody not to come, at the last minute, here comes the FDA from Washington. They slipped in unannounced so they could speak last. The chairman apologized to me but said if representatives from the U.S. government come, he can't stop them from speaking. I said okay, but I get to talk last. The chairman agrees. I already knew what they were going to say, and I had already distributed apricot pits to all the members of the Committee.

"I was standing behind the FDA man eating apricot kernels while he was saying they were toxic. He didn't know why everyone was laughing. Senator Campbell gets up -- he's 6'5", in boots and a cowboy hat -- he gets up in front of the FDA man who is speaking and turns his back on him. Then he says to the chairman, 'Mr. Chairman, would you call me when it's time to vote?' and clomps out in his big boots. The FDA man turns around and sees me. I hold up my bag of apricot pits, and he's speechless. He couldn't finish his speech. So the chairman calls a vote. It's a voice vote, and there's no dispute. It's 7 to 0. The FDA men left. My people went after them to debate, but the FDA men took off running."

When we had recovered from that bit of comic relief, Jimmy went on, "The medical people were furious about it. After that I was told by a number of people that I was being investigated by the district attorney, but he wouldn't do anything. It turned out he was on something from Mexico himself, an arthritis medicine."

"So the FDA man was the person you embarrassed from the National Council Against Health Fraud?" Bill asked.

"No, that was in Georgia. I'm getting to that . . . Do you have time?"

Bill looked at his watch. "Go on," he said. "It's interesting."

"Okay," Jimmy went on, "after the Louisiana legislature passed their laetrile bill, the Georgia legislature decided to hold hearings on one. The proponents of the bill called and asked if I could find a doctor to testify for them. I called Dr. Pichnich, but he said he just couldn't anymore. Evidently they'd already started on him. Later he got in big trouble with the medical people. I don't know what, but he's in hiding now. He won't talk to me. I had to get Doc Dotson again, one of the doctors who testified in Louisiana. Dotson's a guy who will take a chance for the cause and do what's right. Then the Georgia people asked me to come and testify too. At first I said, 'No, I couldn't. I'm too busy.' But then I said, 'I have to go. It should be done. It's one of those things you should do.' So I went.

"The Georgia hearings weren't just in front of a committee. It was the whole House of Representatives. In Georgia you speak according to who gets there first, and everyone is heard. It could go for two or three days, non-stop. So Doc says, 'We better get up there so we can get out of here. It's going to be a long thing.' But just then I got an emergency telephone call. It was like the Lord intervened, because all of a sudden I was down at the bottom of the list. What the government had done was to wait to testify last so they'd have the last word.

"So Dotson testified, and a number of proponents. All our big guns were shot and nobody could rebut. In the meantime, I had gone out meeting the members of the Committee and telling them what had happened in Louisiana. I had a bag of apricot kernels, and I was having them eat them. Then the doctor for the medical people gets up and says if you eat six apricot kernels and six five-milligram laetrile tablets, and you eat them all in one day, you'll die of cyanide poisoning. That was ridiculous. I knew without even tasting them that I could eat six or seven, and as many pills, and not hurt myself. So when he said that, I told

Dotson, 'Doc, I got 'em.' He said, 'I know you got 'em.' He already knew what I was going to do.

"When it was my turn, I got up and made a big show of it. I said, 'I'm going to commit suicide in front of the House of Representatives. I'll need some identification here. I want you to identify what I have.' I had a bag all sealed up with apricot kernels in it, and I had a bottle of laetrile tablets that was sealed and had never been opened, and they took it and opened it in front of the Committee. I said, 'Okay, now what I'm going to do is take seven apricot kernels and six tablets.' I put them all in my hand. I said, 'The reason I'm taking seven apricot kernels instead of six is I don't want the FDA to say I had an underweight apricot kernel.' I put it all in my mouth, and you could have heard a pin drop. The galleries were full, with TV cameras rolling; and before that, there was a lot of noise. I was chewing and chewing and everybody was waiting for me to die. It took me awhile to chew all that up. Finally I got through and one of the members of the committee said, 'You want some water, Mr. Keller?' I said, 'No, thanks. I'm going to give my testimony now, and if I die while I'm giving it I want you to make sure that Dr. Dotson, my friend, signs my death certificate.' Then a few people kind of snickered. I hadn't even got started and a little old lady went, 'They been a-lyin' to us!' And a guy hollered out, 'The FDA's the enemy! That's the real enemy!' And pretty soon everyone was shoutin' and goin'.' And the Speaker of the House, instead of gaveling them down, he turned his back on them. I never saw that before. Up till then, he'd been gaveling them down and keeping order; but he was irritated.

"The Committee had already had a straw vote. It was 10 for, 10 against, 1 abstention -- 21 members. It wasn't going to get out of committee. But after I spoke it was 20 for and 1 abstention. (One guy was going to abstain no matter what.) Every member of the Committee came over and thanked me for giving the correct information. Then the Speaker of the House got up and demanded an apology from the federal government to the State of Georgia for insulting the intelligence of the people of Georgia, by sending people down here to give them information that something was poisonous when it wasn't. That was dramatic. The government was really embarrassed. Then I looked up and the TV cameras were all on me. I said, 'Hey, what're y'all doin'? You want me to eat some more apricot kernels?' They said, 'Yeah! Eat some more!'

So I pulled the bag out and started eating some more. I was like a big hero all of a sudden. The next week, there were laetrile hearings in West Virginia, but the government didn't send any witnesses. A lady wrote me and said she guessed they thought I was coming."

We all laughed. "So the doctor you testified against in Georgia was the one who turned out to be the member of the National Council Against Health Fraud?" Bill asked.

"That was the one." Jimmy gave the doctor's name. I'll refrain from repeating it, but Bill said he knew the man. The doctor was still active in the quackbusting business, and he was a popular expert at trials. Bill fully expected to see him in action in this one.

"So what happened to Dr. Dotson?" I asked.

"He lost his license to practice medicine in Texas. He's practicing in another state now, and toeing the line. I've got an article about him somewhere."

Jimmy dug through his papers and produced a 1981 article from the <u>Baton Rouge Morning Advocate</u>. In it, Jimmy's laetrile treatments had been favorably reviewed. Dr. Dotson was quoted as saying:

> *I was deliberately entrapped by my board which sent in examiners to ask for diet pills and tranquilizers, then accused me of non-therapeutic prescribing because I was not able to figure out these people were lying and not sick. . . . Texas has a Laetrile law which would prevent the board from doing that to me for using Laetrile, but would not prevent them from setting me up some other way, with Laetrile being the reason. This is the fear factor in using anything.*[9]

I asked what had become of Woody Jenkins. Jimmy said he was still a member of the Louisiana House of Representatives. (Representative Jenkins' supporting letter to the Brownsville District Court is excerpted in Appendix B.)

Bill looked at his watch again and reached absent-mindedly for the cigarettes in his shirt. No smoking was allowed in the conference room.

"I guess you know," Jimmy got to the business at hand, "that I'm not happy with my lead counsel. He never comes around, and he doesn't understand my medicine. His office is in San Antonio. I've got a local attorney who comes once a week, but I don't trust him. He keeps making promises he doesn't keep. And

Ginsburg doesn't believe in my remedies. I'm thinking of firing the lot of them and putting you two in their place. You understand my medicine and listen to my ideas."

I wasn't sure Bill wanted to be lead counsel, but he didn't actually have to decline. There was another problem with the plan. Jimmy had already paid his bevy of attorneys more than $200,000 up front for taking the case all the way through sentencing. It seemed in his best interests to get value for what he had paid. In the end, it was decided that Bill would just replace Ginsburg in handling the medical issues. Silversmith would remain lead counsel, in charge of determining the strategy and developing the witnesses. My job would be to draft a tentative motion to dismiss, to be presented to Silversmith for filing with the court.

That was the plan, but as it worked out, Ginsburg had more to do with the medical issues than Bill did. When it was all over, we wished we had agreed to take the whole case.

The business arrangements being settled, Bill carried on with his queries. Eventually, he was satisfied that he had enough information to do what he needed to do -- line up medical experts for the defense. He said he was ready to go back to California. He had other clients.

"Do you have to go too?" Jimmy asked me. His voice sounded small and pathetic. "There's more you might need to know."

Bill repeated his warning about women venturing alone into jails, but his patronizing tone only succeeded in convincing me to stay. I didn't have any more pressing cases to worry about, and Jimmy told a good story. The judge hadn't yet heard the defendant's side of the case. I planned to open our motion with a statement of facts that told it in a favorable light; and for that, I could use more facts. Besides, if Jimmy had a collection of little-known remedies that really worked, I wanted to probe for the details. Someday, somebody else might want to know. I was a competent professional . . .

Okay, I was a coward who preferred to stand behind a man. But there was nothing more aggravating than the chauvinistic assertion that I needed this buffer in a man's world. Hoping I looked more confident than I actually felt, I smiled and waved good-bye to my new partner, and carried on alone.

# Chapter 5

## Death Sentence

Going back two centuries was probably delving more deeply than I needed to for legal purposes, but it helped me understand the defendant's character and motivation. I learned that his family was old and established. They had been in the South since before the American Revolution, and they had been active in the Civil War. During Reconstruction (which lasted until 1878), Jimmy's grandmother, who was then a young girl, had been kidnapped by the Yankees. She was held hostage for a week while they tried to get information about her uncle, who headed guerilla activities in their region.

Jimmy had what he called a "conspiratorial view of history." The strings, he was convinced, were always pulled by the moneyed interests. "It was a banking conspiracy that bumped Lincoln off," he confided in the hushed tones of a spy revealing a State secret. "Lincoln signed his own death warrant when he went outside the banking system and printed U.S. notes backed by the faith and credit of the United States. He was trying to keep the government from having to pay interest."

Jimmy had a similar theory about Jack Kennedy: "Kennedy was going to call off the Vietnam War, so they bumped him off. He was the only president who didn't need the oil-drug-bank-labor-agribusiness-munitions-CIA coalition to get elected. His daddy bought him in. If the special interests control both parties, it doesn't matter which candidate gets in; but Kennedy really thought he was president. They showed him he wasn't. The first thing Johnson did when he got in was to escalate the war. He knew why he was in the White House."

I thought of a book I had read by an M.D. who treated AIDS unconventionally, who called himself a "conspiratorialist." I had to laugh. It was a good word, and it definitely fit Jimmy. Needless to say, he considered himself the victim of a drug industry plot. What I wanted to find out was whether it was true, and whether and how his remedies worked. But he had a tendency to wander off into politics and history. I decided to start from the beginning and get the whole story, deposition-style.

"Where and when were you born?"

"1933, near Baton Rouge."

"Brothers and sisters?"

"Five."

Jimmy spoke wistfully of his star-studded youth, when his looks were still intact. He said he had played football in high school, and that he had married his high school sweetheart. He was only 5/8", but his coach said he was the toughest player the coach had ever coached. Jimmy spent 22 months in the naval reserve, then went to Louisiana State University. He majored in economics, in which he made straight A's. He finished in three years while working full time at night.

"What was your first job after college?" I asked.

"Door-to-door salesman."

"Really! Why didn't you do something with your economics degree?"

"Because I didn't believe in Keynesian economics, which is what they were teaching then. I didn't believe you could spend your way out of a depression. I'd have had to go on and get a master's degree in economics, and the only jobs available were for the government. I needed to get out and make some money. By then, I already had a family of six to support."

"You had four kids?"

"In five years."

He described them as good years. His wife was gorgeous and fun-loving, and sales was an occupation at which he excelled. Blacks bought from him because he had been raised to treat them as equals. Cajuns bought from him because they were his own people. He explained that "Cajun" comes from "Acadian," which comes from "Arcadian." The Acadian French had emigrated to the South from Nova Scotia. Jimmy's people weren't technically Cajuns, but his mother's family had come from France.

"What did you sell?" I asked.

"Insurance. Then I got into water conditioning. I built water softening units in my garage and sold them unlabeled. It was a good business. It kept me going when I was doing volunteer work with cancer victims."

"And you never had any medical training?"

Jimmy shook his head. "But I had a sort of instinct for it."

"How do you mean?"

"Like one time, I was visiting the university campus in Baton Rouge selling insurance, when this woman smashed her car into a tree. She was on the ground waving her arms and legs and bleeding all over the place. People were panicking and screaming and running away. I just instinctively jumped on her and held her down so she'd quit moving. Then I stopped the bleeding with a handkerchief that I wrapped around her arm. I talked to her very gently. I told her she'd have to be still if she wanted to survive. I ordered people to get blankets and call the local ambulances. When the paramedics came, they said she could have bled to death if I hadn't come along."

"So how did you know what to do?"

"It just came naturally. People called my mama a natural healer. She helped a lot of people, but she did it with herbs and things, and with the force of her personality. I didn't want to go into medicine. I didn't believe in it either."

"Why not?"

Jimmy looked away. "For one thing, our youngest son Dale died right after he'd gotten polio vaccine. The doctor said there was no connection, but I didn't believe him. It was the vaccine on the little sugar cubes. He got spinal meningitis and was dead the same week. He was only five."

"How tragic!"

Jimmy nodded. "It affected my wife a lot. She got moody and depressed."

Apparently, they were both moody and depressed. In the late sixties, he said, their marriage broke up. Later, his wife would attribute his stormy moods to his cancer. In 1968, he discovered that a black mole in his left ear was growing. It pressed on his earlobe, and sometimes it would bleed.

"They're now calling the area where I grew up Cancer Alley," Jimmy remarked. "They've traced an epidemic of cancer and leukemia there to all the chemical pollutants around."

I nodded. "From the oil companies, I suppose."

"That's what they say, but agribusiness is actually the worst polluter in the area. Baton Rouge is in the rice and sugar cane and cotton belts. One herbicide was so toxic, workers weren't supposed to go into the fields for five days after it was sprayed. Whenever the crop dusters flew over, my mama had to stay in the house to keep from choking. She suffered from chemical sensitivity. My papa suffered from lead poisoning. He was a chemist for Ethyl Corporation, which made a lead additive for gasoline."

"What are your parents' names?" I asked for the record.

"Guy and Beatrice. Mama's no longer living."

"I'm sorry. I guess you probably learned some chemistry from your dad."

"Some, and there are medical people in my family. My brother Mike is a doctor, and my brother Ron is a medical physicist. He worked at M. D. Anderson Hospital in Houston. He figured the doses and angles of the beams for their radiation treatments. That's where I first went for advice about my cancer. Then they referred me to the Veterans' Hospital, which is affiliated with M. D. Anderson. My oncologist was Howard Tobin. He diagnosed malignant melanoma in May of '68."

"How terrible!" I said, doing a quick calculation. "That would have made you about 34."

Jimmy nodded. "Tobin said radiation and chemotherapy wouldn't help. Even with surgery, he said, 'I won't say you'll have a 50/50 chance, but you'll have a chance.' I got the surgery in August of '68. They took my left ear and the muscles in my neck. My eye was all drooping and bloodshot, and my mouth didn't work right. I felt like a monster. I couldn't face my customers."

The excised tumor was sent out for an experimental procedure, he said, in which a vaccine was to be made from it to prevent further recurrences; but the specimen died and the procedure failed. On top of everything else, within two months cancer nodules started growing back in his neck, arms and groin. The surrounding tissue was biopsied when he went for reconstructive surgery. His new doctor then recommended radiation, but Jimmy had already been told it wouldn't work. He walked out of the hospital in despair.

(Later, I got an explanation for this apparent anomaly from an M.D./friend over lunch. Surgery, she said, is always the first treatment for melanoma. If the cancer then spreads, radiation is done to shrink the tumors, not as a "cure" but for palliative purposes -- to reduce the pain that can result if a tumor is pressing on a nerve, or the possibility of a stroke if it is pressing on an artery. But Jimmy was evidently looking for more than palliative treatment.)

"The worst thing was when I looked at myself," he said, turning away. "Before that, I thought of myself as a good looking guy. My worst year was 1969. I was drinking and going to night clubs. I let my business go to hell. I was living alone in a tiny house. I never cleaned it. It was a big mess."

When he survived two serious auto accidents that year, his mother took it for a favorable omen. "Someone must be saving you for something," she said.

"The first accident," he recalled, "I was with my son David in a '68 Ford van. A fifteen-year-old girl ran a red light and stopped in the intersection. I had to swerve around her. I missed her but rolled down the road. The truck spun over three times. We weren't wearing seat belts, so we were lucky we survived. The hood opened and caught me in the nose and broke it, and the bandage around my head had fallen off. My nose was hanging crooked, and I had no ear. The girl looked at me and said 'It's all my fault!' and she fainted. The policeman was telling me, 'You got to lie down. You're in bad shape.' I said, 'I'm all right. Look at the girl.' The girl kept crying, 'Look at the poor man!' She thought she was responsible for my ear and all. But she was all right. David didn't get hurt either. The policeman said if I'd hit the girl, I would have killed her. Her father paid for the hospital, and for some expensive plastic surgery on my face. The doctor at the hospital told Pops I'd last maybe six months, but he had a notion I'd survive."

"How traumatic!" I said. "What about the second accident?"

"That time, I was in the car alone. It was 2 or 3 a.m., and I'd been in a bar drinking. I was very depressed. I probably was trying to kill myself. I ran off the road into the ditch and smashed into a concrete culvert. I was down where no one could see me. I stayed there unconscious till the middle of the next morning. When I woke up, I got out of the ditch and waved someone down. My forehead was cut open, and I was dirty and bloody. My ribs were all bruised up, and I hurt pretty bad in the chest. I was treated at the clinic in Baton Rouge. An old doctor I knew saw me there. He said, 'What are you trying to do to yourself?' That was when Mama got an unsigned letter recommending the Capital Clinic in Dallas. She thought it was an answer to prayer."

"What treatment did they do there?"

"The Hoxsey treatment."

"Really!" I said. "It was a video about Harry Hoxsey that first got me interested in unconventional therapies. But I thought they shut down all his clinics in the fifties."

"He was technically retired," Jimmy explained, "but he was still around. His clinic operated under an osteopathic doctor named John Durkee, but we met Hoxsey when we got there. He was a down-to-earth, likeable guy, in his sixties or seventies. When he saw my face, he said, 'Look what those SOBs did to you! And all you needed was some of my tonic.' He was driving into town and invited us to come along. He talked the whole time. Mama ate it up. He said Dr. Durkee was the best in the business. Durkee wasn't afraid to speak his mind. At medical meetings, he'd call the other doctors murderers for giving their patients chemotherapy."

"Wow! That took some nerve."

It struck me that Jimmy and Hoxsey had a lot in common. Both men were branded the most notorious quacks of their time. Both treated patients who couldn't pay for free. Neither man was an M.D. Each seemed to have been singled out for his uncanny success with cancer. Both were charged, not with bodily harm, but with fraudulent representations about cure. I wondered what the legal issues were in Hoxsey's suit, and how the government had prevailed. I made a note to have another look at the Hoxsey film when I got a chance . . .

# Chapter 6

## Hoxsey

By the 1950s, Harry Hoxsey's Texas clinic was the largest privately owned cancer clinic in the world. Its treatment was practiced in seventeen states. Its unparalleled success made Hoxsey the principal target of the anti-quackery campaign of AMA head Morris Fishbein. Fishbein branded Hoxsey the worst cancer quack of the century, and had him arrested more times than any other man in medical history.

The outspoken Texan proved to be a formidable opponent. The son of an ex-coal miner who never made it past the eighth grade, Hoxsey was the first man to win a judgment against the AMA in court. His conflict with the AMA began after he demonstrated his methods on a police sergeant who was a terminal cancer patient. The method was strikingly successful in shrinking the man's tumor. The following day, Fishbein and his colleagues attempted to buy Hoxsey's secret formula. But while Hoxsey wasn't averse to selling, he insisted that the treatment be given to the indigent free of charge. He said the herbal formula had been developed by his grandfather, a veterinarian, while treating a prize stallion for cancer. His grandfather had passed down the formula with the proviso that no one should be denied treatment merely because he couldn't afford it. When Fishbein refused this condition, Hoxsey refused to deal. Fishbein then began a hostile series of defamatory articles in which Hoxsey was branded a quack.

That was Hoxsey's version of the incident, but the AMA denied it. Only the demonstration on the police sergeant and the ensuing Fishbein vendetta were matters of record.

Hoxsey fought Fishbein's attack by extensive publicity. His radio broadcasts soon drew 300 patients a day. In his most dramatic public demonstration, he removed a tumor that comprised the top of a man's skull. The man lived another thirty years and credited Hoxsey with the cure. This did not, however, win Hoxsey medical support or an investigation. Instead, the next night during his broadcast, the radio station was sprayed with gunfire. Hoxsey repeatedly sought an investigation from the National Cancer Institute or any other wing of organized medicine. After striking oil in Texas, he even offered to pay for it himself. His request was repeatedly refused or ignored. The NCI said Hoxsey's medical records were incomplete. Hoxsey said that doctors, influenced by Fishbein, refused to supply the necessary records.

When Fishbein published an article calling Hoxsey "a ghoul feasting on the bodies of the dead and dying," he went too far. Hoxsey sued for libel and slander. Against a formidable array of reputable medical experts, he pitted the testimony of his patients. Day after day, witnesses testified that their doctors had given them only a short time to live, that they had been treated at Hoxsey's clinic, and that they were alive years later to tell about it. Hoxsey won. In 1949, Fishbein was finally forced to resign from his position as AMA head, after he not only was defeated in court but was caught cheating on his expense accounts.

The attack on Hoxsey, however, continued. The FDA filed suit in Texas district court to enjoin his shipment of mislabeled drugs in interstate commerce. In a single day, Hoxsey clinics were padlocked in seventeen states. FDA agents peppered post offices with posters declaring that the treatment had been found by the Fifth Circuit to be worthless. In 1963, Hoxsey's nurse took the treatment to Mexico, while Hoxsey himself went into retirement.[10]

The legal issues I read about later at the law library . . .

The mislabeling alleged against Hoxsey consisted of a booklet included with his herbal formula. The booklet did not make any claims of cure. It merely listed the names and addresses of satisfied patients. But the FDA contended that the inclusion of this list implied that the formula cured at least some cancers, a fact that had not been proved.

The Texas district court disagreed. It found on the basis of personal testimony that the treatment cured at least as many patients as surgery and radium, without their "physical suffering and dire consequences."[11]

Undaunted, the FDA filed an appeal with the Fifth Circuit Court of Appeals. The FDA contended there was no admissible evidence the herbs worked, despite testimony by numerous patients of alleged cures. Its argument was based on a technicality: laypersons were legally incompetent to determine whether or not they had cancer or had been cured of it, and testimony that their doctors had told them so was inadmissible hearsay. Expert testimony was also introduced to the effect that no substances taken internally were known to be effective against cancer. (Ironically, this was only shortly before chemotherapeutic drugs became standard cancer therapy.) In 1952, the case was reversed and remanded with directions that an injunction be issued. The FDA had prevailed.[12]

I asked Jimmy if the Hoxsey treatment had cured him.

"Not exactly," he replied, "but it helped a lot. The thing was, I wasn't expecting anything. It opened my eyes to the possibilities. After that, I tried every natural remedy I could get my hands on."

Too bad, I thought, that he hadn't heard there were viable alternatives to surgery before he lost an ear to it. But I knew why from my law school research. The remedies were underground commodities. Doctors experimenting with them ran the risk of malpractice actions or loss of their licenses. They could go to jail simply for using remedies other doctors weren't using. The statutory test wasn't whether a remedy worked, but whether its use was standard practice in the medical community.[13]

The other statutory barrier to free speech was the Food, Drug and Cosmetic Act. It gave the FDA the power to regulate "articles (other than food) intended to affect the structure or any function of the body of man or other animals," a broad category that included not only synthetic pharmaceuticals but herbs and other natural remedies.[14] If health claims were made for food supplements, the supplements could be reclassified as drugs.

Manufacturers could be fined or jailed for making health claims without FDA approval; and since substances found naturally in plants or animals weren't patentable, they weren't lucrative enough to fund the multi-million-dollar clinical tests required to get FDA approval.

Jail wasn't just a hypothetical possibility in these cases. It had happened. Wilhelm Reich, M.D., had died in prison after making unapproved claims about a medical device that worked along the lines of radionics. Dr. Ruth Drown died at the age of 72 after being jailed for the same crime.[15] John Crane served three years for helping develop the "Rife generator," a bio-electronic instrument said to painlessly destroy viruses.[16] John Richardson, M.D., and James Privitera, M.D., both spent time in jail for using laetrile, while Bob Bradford was tried for smuggling it into the United States. Bruce Halstead, M.D., had gotten a four-year sentence for recommending an herbal tea to cancer patients, in violation of a California law that forbids treating cancer with anything but surgery, radiation or chemotherapy.[17]

"Halstead's stuff worked," Jimmy maintained. "I know because after he was arrested, the guy who put up the money and ended up with a big supply of it brought it to Mexico and traded it with me for treating him and his wife. The guy just wanted to get rid of it. Halstead was head of the American Association of Preventive Medicine and a topnotch doctor. But they wanted to get rid of him, and they did." Jimmy dug into his stack of documents. "Here's an article about his trial. You can take it with you and read it."

"Thanks," I said. "So how did Harry Hoxsey manage to keep a clinic going in Texas, when he wasn't even a doctor?"

"Hoxsey owned the clinic," Jimmy explained, "but it was run by Dr. Durkee, who was a licensed osteopath."

"It was Dr. Durkee who called the other doctors murderers for using chemotherapy, right?"

"Right."

"And that didn't get him in trouble?"

"I didn't say that," Jimmy hedged.

"Why? What happened?"

He looked around furtively. "I don't often tell that story," he said.

"Why not?"

"A lot of people won't believe it. But I confirmed it through reliable sources. Pops confirmed it too."

I had met Jimmy's father. He was a sincere, white-haired elderly gentleman with the pink cheeks of a child and the countenance of a saint. "I'm pretty open-minded," I said.

"Okay, it was my brother Ron who heard that the Capital Clinic was closed. He phoned Dr. Durkee to find out why, but the voice on the line was so thick and muffled, Ron couldn't understand him. He had to find out what happened from a woman who worked at the clinic. She said armed men had broken into Dr. Durkee's house, and that they had tried to cut his tongue out with a knife. They didn't succeed, but they cut it up pretty bad. They poked his wife's chest with an ice pick, and she lost a lung. She was still alive, but later we heard that her wounds had gotten infected, and she had died."

"That is hard to believe," I agreed.

Jimmy nodded, adding ominously, "I've seen a lot of things you wouldn't believe."

Making a mental note to pursue that provocative statement later, I asked, "Was it a burglary?"

Jimmy shook his head. "They didn't steal anything."

I recalled what Hoxsey had said: Dr. Durkee was quite outspoken. Was the attack simply a gruesome warning?

"Did Dr. Durkee actually call the other doctors murderers to their faces?" I asked.

"Probably not in so many words. He probably said something like, 'You gentlemen think you're going to be able to poison the body into good health, but it's not going to happen. You may reduce the tumor initially, but you're going to leave the body in such a weakened state that it will succumb to the next bacteria or virus that comes along. The immune system won't be able do its job any more. You're going to wind up killing your patients."

I thought it sounded pretty innocuous. I had seen the same charge expressed in more inflammatory terms. Dick Richards, M.D., had written in The Topic of Cancer in 1982:

> It is no longer a rarity to find patients at autopsy who have died not of their cancers, but of the means used for treating them. This is not a theory. It is already a matter of widespread medical record. Opinion could quite reasonably see this state of affairs as legalized manslaughter.

"So after what happened to Dr. Durkee," I asked, "weren't you afraid to start treating people yourself?"

"I wasn't treating anyone at first. I just made a lot of noise. I went around telling everyone I'd been helped. But after Dr. Durkee's clinic was closed, there wasn't any place to tell people to go, so we started treating each other. What we had was more of a club than a clinic. We met in each others' living rooms and exchanged treatments."

"Did you use the Hoxsey tonic?"

"Not then. We didn't have the formula. We got it later, but then we were mainly using laetrile."

I nodded. "I wrote a law review article on laetrile in the seventies."[18]

The official consensus was that it was a quack treatment that didn't work, but what I had read made me wonder . . .

# Chapter 7

## Laetrile

Like the Hoxsey treatment, laetrile wasn't a cure-all; but it had helped enough people to make its availability a political issue. Other innovative treatments had been suppressed by the FDA and the medical establishment, but so quietly that the public was hardly aware of them. Laetrile stirred so much controversy that lawsuits were brought testing whether cancer patients had a constitutional right to its use. In 1979, the U.S. Supreme Court ruled they did not.[19] But the issue lived on as newer therapies took the stage, and as AIDS patients joined cancer victims in demanding to have control over the medical treatments used on their own bodies.

Laetrile wasn't actually new. It was a form of an ancient remedy called amygdalin, which was used as a cancer treatment by Native American Indians, the ancient Chinese, Asian Indians, and Europeans. Amygdalin is a chemical found naturally in over 1,200 plants, particularly in the seeds of certain fruits and nuts (apricots, peaches, plums, cherries, and bitter almonds). What was new was the form developed by Ernst T. Krebs in the fifties. "Laetrile," which stands for "laevo-rotary nitriloside," is amygdalin prepared in such a way that when light is refracted through it, it turns only in a leftward ("laevo-") direction.[20] Dr. Krebs said it worked by releasing cyanide and benzaldehyde. These cytotoxic chemicals kill cancer cells without harming healthy cells, which are protected by the enzyme rhodanese. Only left-hand-rotating amygdalin, however, was said to work for that purpose.

The FDA's authority for keeping laetrile off the market was again the Food, Drug, and Cosmetic Act. Under the original Act, products intended to affect health could be marketed if they were merely shown to be "safe." Effectiveness was left to the marketplace: ineffective products wouldn't sell. But in 1963, the Kefauver-Harris Amendments added the requirement that before the products could be sold, they also had to be proven effective. The Amendments were ostensibly passed in response to the thalidomide scandal, but critics said this was just an excuse. Thalidomide _was_ effective: it prevented nausea in pregnant women. What it wasn't was safe; and for that reason, it had already been banned from the American market. The real target of the Amendments, suspicious critics suggested, was a popular cancer treatment called Krebiozen.[21] Showing that natural remedies like Krebiozen were safe was fairly easy; but to prove their effectiveness took many millions of dollars, an insurmountable hurdle for struggling entrepreneurs developing inexpensive products. Critics maintained that conventional treatments were so much more toxic, so much more expensive, and so much less effective than the natural alternatives that if left to the forces of the market, they wouldn't stand a chance. Conventional cancer therapies had to maintain their market positions through legislation that made them the only legal options.

The upshot of this legislation was that Krebiozen was prohibited in interstate commerce, and so was laetrile. Doctors using laetrile on cancer patients risked losing their hospital privileges and their licenses. Drugstore owners who displayed pro-laetrile books were notified that they would receive no more prescriptions from doctors who were members of the AMA. A major television network that arranged for pro-laetrile advocates to appear on one of its shows was told that if the show went on, no member of the AMA or the FDA would appear on the program in the future. The show was subsequently canceled.

In the late sixties and early seventies, laetrile's promoter was the McNaughton Foundation. It tried to get FDA approval for the substance but immediately ran into political problems. In 1970, the FDA granted it permission to investigate the drug in the treatment of cancer; but a week later, this permission was mysteriously rescinded. The McNaughton Foundation responded with a modified application, which the FDA also rejected. The FDA contended the drug had never been proven completely safe, and that the application failed to explain exactly how it worked. Laetrile proponents responded that aspirin, penicillin, and tranquilizers had also been approved for clinical investigation before anyone knew exactly how they worked; and they weren't completely safe. The debate looked less scientific than political.

Laetrile's growing popularity finally forced the National Cancer Institute to conduct clinical trials on cancer patients. The results of studies conducted at Sloan-Kettering Memorial Hospital were reported in 1981. The patient/subjects received laetrile intravenously for 21 days. Many reported feeling better at some time in the study; but eight months later, only 20 percent were left alive. The treatment was pronounced a resounding failure. By 1990, however, some thirty clinical studies had been published supporting laetrile's effectiveness.[22] What had gone wrong in the NCI study? Critics said the researchers had not used the pure laevo-rotating laetrile of Dr. Krebs. They had used a degraded product that would not release cyanide into cancer cells. Another problem was that the patients chosen were those given up as incurable by orthodox medicine. NCI statistician Dr. Irwin Bross noted in a letter published in the New England Journal of Medicine:

> All that has been learned from the Laetrile study is that there is a class of patients whom no treatment -- orthodox therapy or Laetrile -- can help . . . It would have been ethical . . . to give the public a fair answer to its questions about orthodox versus unorthodox cancer therapy. It is unethical to claim that this highly publicized study gave any such answers.[23]

Coincidentally, Dr. Bross was one of the expert witnesses Jimmy hoped to have testify at his trial. But the testimony he wanted the doctor to give wasn't on laetrile. Like Dr. Wallach, Dr. Bross had lost his government funding for research after publishing an outspoken series of scientific articles critical of the NCI, his own agency. He had publicly charged the NCI with a fraudulent coverup of its dismal results.

"He's a statistician who can show their whole conventional treatment is a fraud," Jimmy said. "That's why people were flocking to my treatments. They worked when conventional treatment didn't."

Jimmy talked about how he'd gotten into cancer treatment. "I got into working with cancer because I saw a problem I felt needed to be corrected," he said. "People should be able to choose treatments they think will help them -- especially if the conventional treatments haven't worked, and the patients have been declared terminal, and the treatments they want are non-toxic. Doctors agree. Almost every doctor I've talked to thinks patients should have the right to have any kind of treatment they want. I used to tell my patients, 'I know you're mad at your doctor, but he's as much a victim as you are. I've got a brother who's a doctor. He wants his patients to get well. But doctors can't do things they haven't been taught or aren't allowed to do. They're victims of the information they get from medical school, and it's controlled by the drug industry.'"

"In fact," I said, "people in the drug industry are probably well-intentioned too."

"Sure," Jimmy agreed, "they're all just doing their job. It's just the way the system works. Drug companies have to push their products, and they can't push products that are too cheap to be worth developing."

"Still," I said, "plenty of cheap products are on the market. They must be profitable to <u>someone</u>."

"True, but they aren't subject to FDA approval. Drugs are a special case because of regulation, which defeats the forces of the marketplace."

"Good point."

"Working with cancer patients wasn't something I chose to do for a living," Jimmy went on. "I felt I'd been led to it. Believe me, the water softening business was a much safer and less stressful occupation. I had the market cornered, and my business was set up so it pretty much ran itself."

I did believe him. I knew alternative practitioners who actually <u>had</u> licenses, who refused to take terminal patients because it was too risky. When the patients died, the relatives were liable to sue the "quack" who saw them last. But Jimmy was evidently marching to a different drummer. The terminal patients were the ones he couldn't turn away. Their very desperation had driven him to abandon the security of his business, taking a substantial cut in pay and risking arrest. He had been in their shoes . . .

As I was pondering the defendant's character and motivation, a large, dark, threatening-looking guard appeared. "Dinner," he said gruffly, and escorted Jimmy out.

Dining alone at the Fort Brown Hotel, I was glad to have something to read. I flipped through the article on Dr. Halstead . . .

*The professional credentials and accomplishments of Bruce Halstead, M.D., went on for thirty pages. They included publishing approximately 200 scientific works, serving as a consultant to the Encyclopedia Britannica, and consulting for the World Health Organization and the United Nations. Despite his impressive credentials, after more than five years of harassment and attempts at entrapment, approximately 25 armed officers had broken into the doctor's home in 1983. His clinic was raided and the doors were barricaded, preventing patients, some of whom had driven hundreds of miles, from receiving treatment. The charts of 98 patients were seized, leaving no medical records for their treatment. A formal complaint against the officers alleged that "the technical files, letter files, telephone records, and financial records were ravaged in a manner reminiscent of Gestapo storm trooper tactics in Nazi Germany."*

*The indictment against Dr. Halstead alleged that he had fraudulently recommended a Japanese herbal tea called "Agua del Sol" to enhance the immune systems of cancer patients. The prosecutor called it "worthless swamp water." Yet substantial evidence was presented at trial for its effectiveness, including research showing it to have an active anti-leukemic effect in laboratory animals. Dr. Halstead had also taken the legal precaution of having his patients sign waivers stating no therapeutic claims had been made for the tea. And 500 of his patients and supporters had written supporting letters to the court.*

*The jury nevertheless found the doctor guilty on all twenty felony counts, one for each patient who had taken the tea. The letter of the law is that non-government-approved remedies are illegal in the treatment of cancer, no matter how effective or non-toxic they are. The defendant was fined $10,000 and sentenced to four years in prison, was ordered never to practice* medicine or engage in any health-related professional activity again, and was ordered to close his clinic and relinquish his passport.

Dr. Halstead had made political enemies. He had reported toxic waste dumping in the Santa Ana River and the Los Angeles basin, and he had alienated the American Cancer Society. He was notoriously outspoken, calling the people who control the economics of medicine "the most vicious criminal element in the world today," who "make the Mafia look like a group of Sunday school teachers by comparison." He made bold statements like:

> [I]t is well documented that there are methods within the field of nutrition and electromagnetic therapy which, if made widely known, could probably cut the national health budget in half. But that would erode the economic base of a multi-billion dollar industry backed by vested interests. The hospitals, doctors, drug companies and allied health industry only make money when people are sick.

In 1985, documents were uncovered showing that Dr. Halstead was one of several prominent leaders in the non-traditional health care field who had been targeted by an underground medical network including the National Council Against Health Fraud (NCAHF), the FDA, the ACS, and the American Pharmaceutical Association. The network, which met secretly, was said to use tactics reminiscent of the Communist witch hunts of Joe McCarthy.[24] Dr. Halstead wrote in 1987:

> The legally well-documented activities of the NCAHF show beyond any reasonable doubt that they are deeply involved in prosecutorial activities to suppress all forms of alternative health care throughout the United States, all of which is in violation of the Civil Rights, RICO, Sherman, Clayton and Patman Antitrust Acts. . . . The NCAHF is directly affiliated with both the AMA, CMA [California Medical Association] and its allied drug industry. The AMA

*operates the largest drug sales force in the world. They are also the purveyors of medical services that now threaten to bankrupt this nation and completely destroy our social security system -- most of which can be prevented. Health costs could be cut by 70 percent in this country.*[25]

In the Texas heat, I suddenly felt a chill. If Dr. Halstead couldn't prevail, was there any hope for our maverick client?

# Chapter 8

## Eclectic Therapies

Prisoners at the Cameron County Jail could be visited by their families for only fifteen minutes a day, four days a week, talking through a glass over a phone line that was barely audible. But this wasn't true for their attorneys. Criminal suspects, says the Constitution, have an inalienable right to counsel. Attorneys can see their clients face-to-face twelve hours a day, seven days a week. Jimmy's attorneys had rarely capitalized on this opportunity; but I was virtually retired, and this was my only case. I had a "captive" audience with a cutting-edge non-traditional cancer therapist. I decided to plumb the depths.

Counting the number of audio tapes I had already filled and pondering the ominous task of transcribing them, I decided it was time to upgrade my electronic capabilities. Browsing at the local Brownsville mall after dinner, I chanced upon this cute little laptop computer on sale for only $1,299. Naturally, I had to have it. The next morning when I visited the jail, the machine was in my briefcase.

The jail was getting to be less forbidding with familiarity. The personnel were mainly of Mexican derivation, and so were most of the prisoners they were guarding. Some of the men smiled and joked, in Latin live-for-the-moment fashion. There was even a tiny, shy Mexican woman sitting behind the bars, clutching her purse and waiting patiently.

That was my perspective, but for Jimmy his new quarters were not improving with age. "They say this is the worst jail in the U.S.," he whispered. "There's constant tension in here. There's one tiny cell near the front with no bed in it, only a bench, and it always has three or four men in it. They get left there for months, I guess to punish them; but it's cruel and unusual punishment. A lot of guys crack up under the strain. They just put them in a padded cell and throw their food in and leave them there for days." He added what would become a familiar refrain: "I've got to get out of here!"

"Maybe you could escape through your mind," I tried to be helpful. He had mentioned he engaged in meditation.

Metal clanged in the background. "Gimme the goddam keys!" someone yelled.

"Maybe not," I conceded. I wanted to say not to worry, we would bust him out, but I wasn't sure it was true. So I said what any woman would say in those circumstances. "Do you want to see what I bought?"

I pulled out my new battery-powered toy and fired it up, as Jimmy obligingly expressed his admiration. Fingers poised on the keys, I got to work. "So after laetrile you got into arginine, right?"

"Well, not exactly. I was doing a lot of different therapies, but it got to where I was doing more chelation than anything else."

"Wait. I've got something on that." I pulled out some notes.

They were from a discussion over lunch with Bill, who had explained, as he doused his cigarette and dove into his Texas-sized steak, that chelation is an unconventional treatment for blocked arteries. He was enthusiastic about the therapy, having had more than fifty treatments himself.

"Maybe that's why you're still alive," I remembered thinking. For a man who lived in a perpetual cloud of smoke and had a fondness for red meat and drink, I had to admit that Bill seemed to be in relatively good health.

He had proceeded to expound on the treatment. He could swear a blue streak when he wanted to, but he could also spout fluent prose; and he happened to be in a professorial mood.

"Chelation," Bill began his discourse, "was first developed as a treatment for cardiovascular disease in the fifties. A conventional M.D. named Dr. Clarke was treating tenants in a World War II tenement house in Detroit who had gotten lead poisoning from the paint used on the building. They were treated in a charity hospital with EDTA, the conventional treatment then and now for lead poisoning."

EDTA, I learned when I looked it up later, stands for disodium ethylene diamine tetra-acetic acid, a substance that binds with heavy metals and allows them to be excreted from the body.[26]

"The patients were all elderly," Bill went on, "and many of them had cardiovascular problems. To Dr. Clarke's surprise, their cardiovascular troubles went away. This accidental finding generated a lot of interest, and enthusiastic papers were written. But for mysterious reasons, the papers were abruptly retracted by their authors. The studies weren't rediscovered until the late sixties, after many years of obscurity. Chelation for cardiovascular disease eventually became a medical specialty, with well-researched protocols. I represented Ray Evers, an early pioneer in the field. He was an M.D., but he wound up losing his medical license."

I smiled. "I guess that means you lost the case."

"It was Evers' own fault," Bill defended his professional honor. "We got the case kicked out of court. It wasn't chelation he got in trouble for. He was left alone until he branched out into cancer. He rediscovered the black and yellow salves. They're herbal folk remedies that have the remarkable property of attracting cancerous but not non-cancerous tissues. We nearly had the Board convinced to let him go, because the salves were covered by the covenants and standards of eclectic physicians -- which Evers was. But then he got on the stand and said he'd never seen all those eclectic books till his lawyers showed them to him. He didn't have to testify at all, but the truth was going to set him free. He undid two years' hard work by his attorneys. He was an unregenerate rebel to the last -- but a great intuitive clinician."

Bill added, "At least we got one favorable ruling that has helped other doctors since."

"What was that?"

"A ruling that once a drug has been FDA-approved for some purpose, it can be used for any purpose that a doctor, in his best professional judgment, deems appropriate. Evers was using EDTA, an FDA-approved drug, to clear the arterial system, something the FDA hadn't approved it for. Of course in practice, that just meant the prosecutor wasn't as likely to be the FDA. It was more likely to be the state medical board, suing under medical practice acts that say doctors can only do what's 'standard practice' in the community. And that was how they got Evers. Case closed."

When I repeated Bill's story to Jimmy, he just laughed. "You could count on Evers to say the wrong thing. Whenever he got up to speak, he got himself in trouble."

"You knew him?"

Jimmy nodded. "I was hoping he'd teach me something about chelation -- and that he would take some patients off my hands. I already had more than I could handle alone. But you know what happened instead. I wound up teaching him and taking some of his patients, after he lost his license and left Louisiana. I showed him some cancer remedies -- laetrile, DMSO, and some others."

DMSO, or dimethylsulfoxide, Jimmy called "the world's best solvent." He explained that it doesn't actually shrink tumors, but it carries other remedies into the cells and makes them more effective.

"Then how did you learn chelation?" I asked.

"From Doc Dotson. I got interested in it when Pops developed three huge melanomas on his neck in the seventies. Mike, my brother who is a doctor, had scheduled him for surgery. But I didn't want Pops going through what I did. I put my business on hold, jumped in my truck and went. I took him to Doc Dotson, who was doing chelation in Texas. Doc did a blood test and hair analysis that showed high lead and cadmium levels. He did the chelation and then prescribed the ingredients so I could do it at home."

"I thought chelation was for heart problems."

"It's for lead poisoning, and that's what I figured Pops had. He worked for a company that made the leaded part of leaded gasoline. I'd read that one cause of lymphatic cancer can be lead poisoning. Lead completely compromises the immune system. I checked it with a pendulum. It tested out. I gave him other things besides chelation -- laetrile and some other stuff. In two or three weeks, the tumors completely disappeared; and they never came back. Pops never had to have surgery. Mike couldn't believe it. I was impressed myself. That's when I got into doing chelation for other people."

(Later, I found a study suggesting that chelation could, indeed, reverse certain types of cancer.[27])

"So how did you get into using a pendulum?" I inquired.

"I read a book on it."

"A self-taught man."

Jimmy ran his fingers under the collar of his faded orange jumpsuit. "You see where it got me. My chelation treatments did win me some political protection though. I treated the governor's executive secretary with it, and some friends of the district attorney's; and they were happy with my treatments."

"I was wondering how the medical board managed to entrap Dr. Dotson, who was an M.D., and they couldn't get you. Who was the governor?"

"Edwin Edwards. The D.A. wouldn't touch the case. I was accused of bribing him, but I didn't. It turned out he'd been to Mexico himself for unconventional treatments. I was living on the edge though. One time I came home and found the house surrounded by police cars. Someone had broken a window and the police had come to investigate. I came in and found all my things on the floor and a number of shotguns and pistols pointed at me. The police had found something they thought was marijuana."

"What was it?"

"Pau d'Arco. It's a Brazilian herb that builds up the immune system. I kept it in five-pound bags for making into a tea. One policeman also found some bottles of injectable vitamin C. He read the label and said, 'Acid! Ascorbic acid. We've got him!' I said, 'That's vitamin C.' He said, 'Don't get smart with me.' They finally decided they didn't have anything and left. I said, 'Come back here and put my clothes back,' but of course it was wishful thinking."

I laughed. "So after chelation you got into arginine?"

"Not exactly. I was into a lot of different things before that. One was hematoxylon."

More remedies. I was tempted to move him ahead to the kidnapping and $5 million bail, but I decided it was best to be methodical. I didn't have any urgent appointments to keep, and he wasn't going anywhere either. "So what's hematoxylon?" I asked.

"It's a natural dye or stain that comes from a tree. It's used conventionally to pinpoint cancer in the body. A Texas M.D. named Tucker experimented with it and found that it worked not only as a test but as a treatment. He started with animals, then progressed to humans. He found there was a non-toxic amount of it that would actually regress tumors. He was treating patients free of charge, but the other doctors started calling him a quack, so he escaped the heat by going to Panama. Later, though, he came back to Houston and went on quietly treating cancer patients. I heard about him, and we developed a mutual admiration for each other's work. But then Dr. Tucker got cancer himself. He called me from the Baptist Hospital in Houston and said the hospital wouldn't let him have his own remedy. He wanted me to give it to him in his hospital room. I went, but our phone conversation must have been overheard, because when I got there, a sheriff was guarding the door and said no one could enter. Within a week, Dr. Tucker was dead. He was in his late sixties or early seventies."

"Tragic. So what did you think of his remedy?"

"It worked. I used it with a ruby red laser. I injected the hematoxylon first, then shone the laser on the area about a half hour later. It got great results. One woman had a carcinoma of the skin that had eaten a deep hole in her forehead. I used the ruby red laser and it went away."

Later, I read research confirming the effectiveness of both hematoxylon and the ruby laser in shrinking tumors.[28] One writer wryly commented that Eli J. Tucker, M.D., was at one time known as the grand old man of Texas medicine. He was even presented the "Award of Merit" by the AMA. But that was before he discovered a viable, non-toxic treatment for cancer.[29]

"I had two of those ruby red lasers," Jimmy went on, "but they both eventually broke. My brother Ron called a professor who had started his own electronics business, and asked him to make us another one. But when the professor tried to get the components, federal agents descended on him. He called Ronnie and asked what was going on -- the professor didn't see the problem with getting a 10 amp ruby laser -- but he didn't pursue it."

Jimmy then recalled another doctor who had fled to South America, William F. Koch, M.D. Dr. Koch headed the Michigan State University Medical School in the 1920s. Jimmy had never met the doctor, but he had used Koch's "glyoxylides."

"The establishment destroyed him," Jimmy said. "They ridiculed him and exposed him in the media. He was establishment himself, and they were afraid of him. The government dragged him through some very expensive lawsuits. There was even a threat on his life. He wound up fleeing to Brazil."

I would have questioned this unlikely story, but I had come across it before in what appeared to be well-researched sources.[30] I wondered where Jimmy had gotten Koch's products, which were off the market.

"I had a supplier in Michigan," he explained. "There are brokers of these things. The remedies were disguised as copper and zinc. They were injections. You'd begin with the one called copper on the first and third day. Then you'd give the zinc. When it worked, it was very powerful. It was a rapid oxidizer. If it didn't work, it was like getting a shot of water. Of course, the FDA claimed it was water. They were right in a way -- all homeopathics are basically water -- but studies show that they work."

I nodded, having read some of the studies.[31] The underground brokers of unconventional medicines reminded me of Prohibition in the 1920s.

# Chapter 9

## Arginine

Jimmy was a walking encyclopedia of natural remedies, but the government seemed to be interested in only one. For legal purposes, I decided it was best to hit on it before indulging my curiosity in the rest. "So when did you get into arginine?" I inquired.

"It must have been late 1981," Jimmy said. "I was looking for something new. I was worried about a particular patient, Carolyn Creighton. It was in her home that I was treating people in Baton Rouge."

He described her as a beautiful, fair-haired, fair-skinned mother of three in her mid-thirties. Her skin was her problem. In 1978, she developed malignant melanoma from a mole. Eventually, it migrated into her lymph nodes and her lungs. Her doctors in New Orleans removed a large tumor on her leg and cut off her moles, but they still gave her only six months to live. She got chemotherapy after the surgery.

"They put a tourniquet around her leg and injected the vein with chemo, and said it would stay in her leg," Jimmy said. "It was crazy. The vein goes right to the heart. The poor woman vomited 24 hours straight and split all her stitches. Then the melanomas grew back where the surgical scars were. When I met her, her leg had swollen up like she had elephantiasis. She had to lift it with her hands to move. I treated it with a paste of laetrile and DMSO applied right on the tumors, along with laetrile intravenously and a lot of other things -- vitamins, proteolytic enzymes IV, Wobe-mugos enzyme, natural progesterone cream. After awhile, I had her out dancing."

"You were dating her?"

"No, she was married. It was a hoe-down to kick off Woody Jenkins' campaign for the Senate. She danced nearly every dance -- and could she dance! She kind of went wild after she came through all that."

"If she was doing so well, why were you looking for something new?"

"Her leg had gotten better, but a big black melanoma tumor had come up on her back. Nothing I used would make it go away. That was when Rudnov was lecturing on Tumorex. He said five American doctors were using it on cancer patients and getting great results."

Jimmy said he was impressed by a collection of photographs taken by one of these M.D.'s, a doctor named Doug Brodie. One series of photos involved a 90-pound boy with a 120-pound abdominal tumor. (A 120-pound tumor? I had my doubts, until my daughter later showed me a picture in the Guiness Book of World Records of a tumor weighing in at 300 pounds.)

"Water just poured out of the boy," Jimmy said, "as the Tumorex shrank the tumor. It was incredible."

"What happened to him?"

"His body couldn't support such rapid detoxification, and he died."

"Too bad."

"But it was still an unprecedented case. Nothing else could shrink tumors so fast or so well. Dr. Brodie has agreed to testify at my trial. He saw a number of dramatic Tumorex cases, and he's a clinician. I've got half a dozen other M.D.'s lined up who sent me patients as well. They've got before-and-after records, and they can testify to how well the patients did."

"Sounds good. So you were impressed with Dr. Brodie's photos," I led the witness, "and invested in some Tumorex."

"Two vials at $450 each," Jimmy said. "I got them from Frank Cousineau, who got them from Rudnov."

"Frank was one of the guides on the Cancer Control Society tour," I remarked. "So then you tried the Tumorex on Carolyn," I led the witness again.

"Well, first I tried it on myself. I tried everything first on myself. I had some tumors that had come up, and I had a tumor here that had gotten hard." He pointed to the back of his neck. "I could feel the Tumorex pulling and grabbing at the tumors after the first couple of shots, and I actually had some that went down and went away. Then I tried it on Carolyn. She could feel it grabbing and popping and punching, and within a week the tumor was completely gone, just down to nothing. It was amazing."

"So what happened to her?"

"She lived 3-1/2 years longer than expected . . ." Jimmy looked away.

"I guess she died," I said after a respectful silence. "Then the Tumorex didn't work?"

"It did. It shrank her tumors. But what I didn't know then was that it doesn't necessarily work forever. Rudnov said a three-week course of it would reverse the disease. I discovered later that a lot of patients need more than that, so I had them come back for boosters. But Carolyn was my first arginine case."

That was how it was, I thought, when you broke away from the conventional and proven. You had to work by trial and error. You didn't have established protocols to fall back on.

"My serum got more effective after I improved on it," Jimmy went on. "I began with a base of all the amino acids. Then I added arginine to protect the patient from the toxicity of the others. Then I added two or three or four other amino acids, depending on the patient; plus a lot of other things."

"Which other amino acids?"

"It depended, but L-cysteine and L-glutathione came up a lot."

He looked pensive. "There were other problems in Carolyn's case. She smoked too much. I couldn't get her to quit. And she'd gotten chemotherapy. Rudnov said Tumorex was only 40 to 60 percent effective for patients who'd had prior conventional treatment."

"That seems a bit anomalous," I remarked. "Most people would say you'd have better luck if you'd already had surgery to cut out the malignancy, or chemotherapy and radiation to stop it in its tracks."

"But you know that isn't true," Jimmy said, looking out of the corner of his eye. "The fastest way to cause cancer in laboratory animals is with radiation. My brother Ronnie was a medical physicist at M. D. Anderson. He said the average tumor dose when he worked there was 6,000 rads. The mean lethal dose of whole body radiation is 500 rads. That's what they teach you in physics class. Ronnie got totally disillusioned with radiation when he worked there. He had to quit going through the front lobby because he couldn't stand to see what the treatment was doing to the patients. I remember him describing a man who had cancer of the sinus cavity, who basically had no face left. The man was smoking a cigarette through a hole they'd made in his trachea so he could breathe. Ronnie spent four years at M. D. Anderson working on his certification as a medical physicist, but he gave it all up because he didn't believe in it."

"You Keller boys think alike," I said. "But if radiation is so toxic, why do they use it?"

"It shrinks tumors. That's why it's considered effective. The problem is the long-term effects. It destroys the immune system and causes secondary cancers later. But oncologists don't have anything else to use. If they try anything besides radiation and chemotherapy, they can lose their licenses."

I nodded. "Like Dr. Halstead."

"Yep." Jimmy added, "The fact that radiation shrinks tumors is deceptive. Radiation makes the tumor go down at first because ninety percent of the tumor is somatic cells. They're the normal cells that live by oxidation and divide one at a time, and they're non-malignant. Malignant cells live by fermentation and divide geometrically. They're the ones that wind up invading the body. But Krebs postulated that a tumor is at most only ten percent malignant cells."

I knew the name. Ernest T. Krebs Jr. was the biochemist who developed laetrile. But I didn't know what Jimmy was getting at. I said, "So?"

"So malignant cells are much more resistant to radiation than non-malignant cells. The radiation destroys the non-malignant capsule, so the tumor appears to shrink. But that just allows the malignant cells to escape and spread. That's why secondary tumors tend to form after you get the radiation."

For a snake oil salesman, I thought, the man knew a lot about his subject. But his view of cancer certainly differed from the conventional one. Ninety percent of the tumor he thought was something good, a protective shell. If he were right, it meant you couldn't just measure tumor shrinkage to determine the benefit of a cancer remedy. You had to look at how it made the patients feel, and whether they outlived their prognoses. Tumor shrinkage was irrelevant if the patients died. I made a note to myself to do some research on whether tumor shrinkage actually increases survival.

"So how do you feel about surgery?" I asked. I thought I might as well cover all bases.

"It's better than chemo and radiation. At least it doesn't directly attack the immune system. In fact," Jimmy said cryptically, "it's probably safer than a biopsy."

"Why do you say that? In surgery, they cut out the whole organ. In a biopsy, they just take a sample."

"That's the problem. In surgery, they try to 'get it all.' They know that if they accidentally cut into the tumor, the cancer is liable to spread and they'll have a dead patient on their hands. But that's just what they do in a biopsy. They cut right through the capsule and expose the malignancy. The cancer can escape and spread -- and that's when it kills you."

I added this controversial theory to my research list.

"I think I could have saved the patients 100 percent of the time," Jimmy went on, "if I could have gotten them before they'd even had a biopsy. Back in 1983, they didn't come to Mexico until they'd been through all the conventional treatments their insurance would pay for, and their immune systems and their bank accounts had been wiped out and they'd been given up for dead. But later, when people got more enlightened about cancer treatments, some people did come who hadn't had even a biopsy. And those patients are all alive and well."

"If they didn't even get a biopsy," I asked, "how could you be sure they had cancer?"

Jimmy sighed. "That's the reason those cases aren't going to do me much good in court. But in my work, I didn't need to know if they had cancer or not. They came in with lumps and feeling bad and losing weight. They went home well. That was all I needed to know."

It was what they meant, I thought, by "wholistic" therapy. You looked at the patient as a whole and fixed whatever was out of balance. You didn't even need to be able to name the disease.

"Doctors need biopsies for legal purposes," Jimmy observed. "It's only after they've proven that the patients have cancer that they can cut, burn and poison them without getting sued for it. The difference is, their treatments are toxic and mine aren't. The problem is in the courts. There are other reliable tests for cancer, but the courts have ruled that a biopsy is the only legally acceptable test."

"What other tests are there?" I asked. We were drifting far afield, but the prisoner seemd glad for the diversion. He was evidently more comfortable thinking about cancer than about his ominous predicament.

"One test is hematoxylon," he said. "When it's injected, the dye will only clump up where there's a malignancy. X-rays can then show the location of the cancer. Another test is HCGH hormone in the urine. It's the old rabbit test for pregnancy. It showed either pregnancy or cancer growth."

"What does pregnancy have to do with cancer?" I asked.

"The trophoblast produces HCGH in pregnancy. It's the first cancer we have. Trophoblast cells are the ones that grow geometrically and give the fetus its huge growth during its first few months. After that, the cells convert into normal cells that grow arimethetically. Our first cancer is at conception, and our first cure is the transformation of these cells into normal cells. Cancer consists of trophoblasts in the wrong place at the wrong time. The pancreas should inhibit the trophoblast's growth in the 56th to 60th day of pregnancy. If the pancreas doesn't activate, you get chorionepithelioma, the most virulent cancer there is. John Beard showed that it and the trophoblast cells of pregnancy are identical."

"You should have been a professor," I said. "Who's John Beard?"

"He was a researcher in Scotland in the first part of the century."

"How do you spell 'chorionepithelioma'?"

"I don't know."

"I'll look it up." I also made a note to look up the statistics on radiation and chemotherapy.

# Chapter 10

## Carport Clinic

No sunshine found its way into the windowless fluorescent-lit conference room, but I could tell by the state of my stomach that it was about noon. I wanted to wrap up the Louisiana phase of Jimmy's cancer career before lunch. "So Carolyn Creighton died," I said. "Then what happened?"

"After Carolyn died . . ." Jimmy gazed through the walls into the past. "It was like a big piece of me died with her. It was very, very hard watching her die."

I felt a story coming on. We probably weren't going to get through the Louisiana phase before lunch.

"After that," he said, "I lost my enthusiasm. I really was hurt, like I'd failed. I was just going to do my water business. I could hardly do anything."

Practitioners who dealt regularly with death, I reflected, learned to distance themselves from their patients. But it wasn't Jimmy's style. He hugged them all and said he loved them and seemed to mean it. It was a rewarding approach until he lost one. Then it was devastating.

"So how did you get your enthusiasm back?" I asked.

"Junie showed up. She was a nurse from Costa Rica."

"The Junie in the indictment?"

Jimmy nodded and waxed lyrical. "She was like four nurses in one person, a perfect organizer -- just what a disorganized guy like me needed. Good with books and good with patients. Nobody could find veins with a needle like she could. One time I clocked her. We had 35 chelation patients that day. She found their veins and had them all hooked up to IVs in an hour -- Junie and the tape girl who followed behind her. We had fourteen cancer patients the same day. That was probably a record, but we had a lot of patients. We didn't need to advertise. They just found us by word of mouth." Jimmy sighed. "Junie was pretty too -- good body, nice skin, very strong. She protected me."

Love had struck. Together, he said, they found a large house in Baton Rouge with a four-car carport and parking areas nearby. They enclosed and carpeted the carport and converted it into a clinic. Soon they were living happily together in it, catering to a carport packed with patients.

It wasn't long before they were seeing some dramatic recoveries. As evidence, he produced a battered envelope full of letters and affidavits from former patients and their relatives.

"Lunch," signaled the large, dark guard.

"I'll read them," I said, grabbing the envelope as I was escorted out. The letters livened up the institutional egg salad sandwich on white bread I purchased at the government cafeteria.

One poignant letter was from a woman named Shirley Hubert, of Kenner, Louisiana. In 1981, she said, she was diagnosed with lymph gland and bone tumors. A tumor on her arm had grown to the size of a lemon. Her doctor had scheduled surgery for the following day, intending to amputate her arm. But Shirley was understandably reluctant to agree to this radical procedure. When she refused, her doctor said he would no longer treat her. He gave her only six months to live. In her letter, dated a year after she was treated by Jimmy, Shirley wrote:

> . . . *February, 1982 was the sixth month, pain was so intense I was taking a bottle or more of pain pills each week . . . . We finally found Jimmy Keller, in Baton Rouge, La. treating cancer patients with Tumor-X and getting outstanding results even though some of the patients had been given up by their Doctors . . . . On February 6, 1982, I received my first injection. Before I had received all of the first injection (about 1/2 of it) my pain was gone, and my complexion was coming back (it had been ashen color). By the time six days passed, I had received 6 injections, I was cured of my cancer; by the end of 12 days my tumors were all gone. I have had no pain or recurrence since, nor have I had any side effects from this treatment.*

Another remarkable letter was from a woman named Brenda Laughlin. It read in part:

> Doctors said I had a rare lung cancer [and] had to undergo a year of Chemotherapy . . . . I had lost all of my hair and was so sick I wished I could die. I assured myself I would never take Chemotherapy again. . . . The doctors had told me when I quit taking Chemotherapy that I had about two weeks to live. I have outlived their prediction by nearly two years now. February 22, 1983 I gave birth to a beautiful baby boy . . . . I told [my doctor] what I had done and after the baby was born he did blood tests and x-rays and was amazed to find no sign of cancer. . . . I still do everything Jimmy Keller told me to do and had it not been for [his] program, neither my baby or I would be here.

Two of Carolyn Creighton's siblings had also written letters to the court. Her brother, Norman Cavin, wrote:

> [Jimmy] has been treating my cancer since 1978 . . . and I still lead a normal, happy and healthy life. . . . My father is an example of the effects of radiation treatment. I saw him die a very painful, violent death. I know now that with Jimmy's alternative treatment, my father would not have had to experience that type of torture. . . . Each day that Jimmy is not allowed to continue treating people, they are forced to do nothing or to try radiation or chemotherapy. These treatments take away any type of normal life for these patients. . . . Without Jimmy, we lose our rights to choose a treatment that works.

Faye Franklin, Carolyn's sister, had also contracted malignant melanoma. She wrote:

> In my opinion, [chemotherapy and radiation] take dying cancer patients and torture them for the remaining months. I want to remain healthy and active in spite of my illness and with Jimmy Keller's treatment, this is possible. . . . I have never met a more self-sacrificing person [than] Jimmy.

Back in the conference room after lunch, I pulled out this handful of letters. "These are some remarkable cases," I said. "Can you get these patients as witnesses?"

Jimmy scanned the letters. "Not Shirley," he said. "I don't know where she is. In fact, I don't know where most of my 1983 patients are. The government confiscated all my records when they raided my clinic in 1984."

"Like with Dr. Halstead," I observed. I had read about this constitutionally questionable practice in raids of other practitioners too. Confiscation of patient records compromised not only the practitioner's defense but the patients' ongoing treatments.

Concerning Shirley, all we would know of her subsequent progress was what was later revealed by the FBI: "She indicated that she had been cured by Mr. Keller."

"How about Brenda Laughlin?" I asked.

"She died."

"Too bad."

"But her husband wants to testify. She lived 2-1/2 years longer than her doctors gave her, and she didn't die from cancer. It was from pneumonia. She couldn't fight it. Chemotherapy had destroyed her immune system."

I nodded, having read about that problem too. Serious infection was a recognized risk of chemotherapy. Patients treated with it had been known to die from a cold.[32]

"How about Norman Cavin and Faye Franklin?"

"They've already volunteered. Seven people in Carolyn's family got cancer. Only the ones who got conventional treatment died -- Carolyn and her father. The ones who just got my treatments are alive and well."

It occurred to me that Carolyn's family constituted a small-scale study bearing out Rudnov's claims about the hazards of conventional treatment.

"Norman had the same kind of cancer Carolyn had," Jimmy said, "and he got it at about the same time. But by luck, he didn't have health insurance. One of the most dangerous things you can have today is what we call 'real good health insurance.' They'll hit you with everything they've got."

Jimmy was serious, but I had to laugh. His way of looking at the health care crisis turned everything upside down. People who didn't have insurance or get radiation and chemotherapy were the lucky ones.

"So Junie came along," I got back to the facts, "and you got a carport clinic going in Baton Rouge. Then who was it who committed the alleged wire fraud over the telephone? Was that Junie?"

"No, that was Maxine. It cost her two years in the slammer, too."

"Two years? Even drug dealers get out in a year!" The excessive sentence reminded me of the prosecutorial misconduct Bill had talked about -- the kind typical of cases that were politically motivated.

"Wait till you meet Maxine," Jimmy remarked. "See if you can picture her in prison."

# Chapter 11

## Maxine

She definitely didn't fit the ex-con stereotype. Maxine turned out to be a sincere and personable, white-haired 59-year-old Mormon grandmother of twelve. I didn't meet her until later, but I'll tell her story here as she told it then. She said she was a former pediatric nurse from Sandy, Utah, who had been a victim of cancer herself. Like Jimmy's, it had been put in remission by alternative treatments -- laetrile, colonic irrigations, and a metabolic diet. She had then gotten involved in helping other people with the disease.

When a friend reported seeing a tumor go down in a week from Tumorex treatment, Maxine got Rudnov's tape. Impressed, she volunteered to work with him. Her job was to refer patients to Rudnov's Tijuana clinic and follow up with their treatments after they got home. What would look bad in court was that she took payment for it -- $1,000 per referral. But Maxine said she hadn't asked for the money, and at first she had declined to take it. Rudnov's reply was, "Fine. I'll keep it myself." Maxine decided she could use it to help defray the patients' costs, cover her phone bills, and supply amino acids to the patients after they got home. But she remained uncomfortable with the arrangement. Rudnov "didn't give a hoot for the patients," she said. Worse, few of them had actually recovered. He had testified in 1985 that he had an 80 to 90 percent success rate, but he later admitted that the figure applied only in the short-term. Few of his patients had survived for long.

"He was feeding them steak and hot fudge sundaes," she said cynically. "When I sent down amino acids, he didn't give them to the patients. When I asked him questions, he told me to call Jimmy. He said Jimmy had more knowledge about Tumorex than anyone else."

She decided to make a trip to Baton Rouge. She set out from Utah with her husband Eldon in their motor home, uncertain what they would find on the other side of the Mississippi.

"I had no idea Jimmy was so grotesque," Maxine remarked. His home she described as "very old -- but very clean, and always jam-packed." His truck was old, and so was his car. But she forgot these superficialities when she heard the patients' recovery stories. Jimmy's modest circumstances were explained when several patients revealed that they hadn't had the money to pay him. Their money had gone for conventional treatment. Jimmy didn't ask about money. He just treated. Eldon later wrote to the court:

> Jimmy had an 'open door policy' allowing any and all who needed treatment to come to be treated, no one was barred and I estimate that 30% of the people who came to Jimmy for treatment did not pay for their treatment. . . . [E]very time [Rudnov] came with a shipment of Tumorex he required no less than $30,000 and . . . demanded to be paid up front every time.

"There was no evidence of money in any way," Maxine wrote to the court, "which encouraged my feeling of the care Jimmy had in helping his fellow man."

These observations would be confirmed in other letters to the court. Marjorie Raucher, a registered nurse from Santa Monica, California, wrote:

> The practice at the clinic was not to ask anything about money . . . . On Saturday afternoon the accountant would give each person their bill for the preceding week, that was all . . . . Since I left the clinic on a Wednesday, I did not get my final bill. When I arrived home I waited a week, then called to say I hadn't received it. It didn't come, so I called again. After one month, when the bill still hadn't arrived, I called Jimmy to ask for it -- he said 'Don't worry about it.'

Apparently, he had found other compensation. The work was its own reward. It had become an obsession. "The two or three days we were there," wrote Maxine, "I could only talk with him after 10:30 or 11:00 at night, as we ate dinner. He started early in the morning. Food was brought to him as he worked."

She decided she wanted to work with Jimmy, even if it meant cutting her compensation in half. When she said Rudnov was paying her $1,000 per patient, Jimmy said he would go broke at that rate. He offered her $500. She accepted.

"I thought you already had more people than you could handle," I remarked to the defendant after I heard this story.

"I did," he conceded, "but I reasoned that everyone deserved the chance to get well. And after the move to Mexico, I couldn't keep the communication lines open that I had in Louisiana because of poor phone service. That part of the job fell to Maxine. She was very conscientious and worked very hard. She had costs, and she needed some payment."

They would both regret the deal later. The telephone referral arrangement gave the government grounds for claiming U.S. jurisdiction. But at the time, they felt like kindred souls. Maxine wrote to the court, "I was to encourage [the patients] to stay on their diets, learn to cope with their stress, positive thinking, etc. . . . . I was on the phone from 6 to 7 in the morning until 10 or 11 each night." Her phone bill sometimes ran around $2,000.

"She was pulling them up by their bootstraps," Eldon observed. "It's a terrible thing about cancer. When the family is told one of their members has terminal cancer, sometimes they just want to get it over with. They want the person to die."

I pondered what it would be like to spend a fourteen-hour day tending cancer patients headed for death. Most people would shy away from the task -- unless they were in it for the money -- but Jimmy and Maxine didn't seem to be netting much. For Jimmy, I surmised, it was a way to re-capture what he had lost with his good looks. People now loved him for his work. He had found his identity in being needed.

For Maxine, too, the work seemed to be its own reward. "I really loved the people," she said. "I would tell them to call collect. I knew that's what I was supposed to be doing." It must have been a blow to her convictions, I thought, when the work she felt called to do earned her jail time.

Then another disturbing thought struck me. Her sentence set an ominous precedent for Jimmy's case. If merely talking up his treatments was worth two years in jail, what was in store for the kingpin who had master-minded the whole operation?

# Chapter 12

## Fringe or Cutting Edge?

"That's an evil one," Jimmy whispered as he motioned toward a particularly large and threatening-looking warden. "Think about it. What kind of person applies for prison work? The ones who really enjoy it are into whips and chains. One guard here is nice, but he hates his job. He's been smuggling in serrano peppers for me."

"Why do you want serrano peppers?"

"For the vitamin C. None of the food here has vitamin C in it. They don't let us have fresh fruits and vegetables. The guard says they do it on purpose to keep all the prisoners sick, so we won't cause trouble. I'm pretty sure we're getting salt peter too. You can get all the candy you want though." Jimmy grinned. "So guess where I've been getting my vitamin C?"

"Where?"

"In Skittles. I read on the label that they contain a lot of it."

I laughed. The man was enterprising, even in jail.

It seemed like as good a time as any to delve into his treatment protocol. "I guess vitamins and minerals were part of your therapy," I broached the subject.

"Of course."

"Which vitamins and minerals?"

He listed vitamin A emulsion, vitamin C, vitamin D3, vitamin E, niacin, water soluble beta carotene, choline, selenium, calcium orotate, magnesium orotate, potassium orotate, zinc orotate, chelated trace minerals.

"And you put your patients on a special diet?"

"Right. I customized it to the patients after testing them, but basically it was whole grains and beans; lots of fresh, steamed and raw vegetables, organically grown; sometimes a little fruit; only cold-pressed oils; distilled or bottled water; animal products sparingly -- sometimes they were eliminated for awhile. The animal products we allowed were organically grown eggs, poultry breasts, white scaled fish and lamb. We used a lot of cayenne pepper. But diet wasn't the most important thing in my treatment. It was my serum -- and live cell therapy. That was something I was even more excited about than arginine. My serum got rid of the cancer, but live cell therapy allowed the damaged organs to rebuild themselves. In the U.S., Customs turns it back at the border; but you can get live cells over-the-counter in Germany."

"Okay," I asked, "what's live cell therapy?"

The way Jimmy folded his hands and got settled, I suspected I was in for one of his long professorial explanations. "Live cells," he began, "are genetic material taken from a specific organ of the fetus of a cow or sheep -- except for live cell placenta, which is human. As cells get older, they mutate. Live cells re-code the organ. They're the imprints that create new cells, allowing the cells to rejuvenate themselves. Researchers have followed them with a radioactive tracer and have seen the body take them to the right organ. Then the organ sheds the mutated DNA and RNA and picks up the new. Movie stars have been going to Europe for decades for rejuvenation treatments, and a lot of it is this therapy. But you have to have money to go there. I was making it available just south of the border, and mine were the best prices in town."[33]

"Interesting," I said. "What else did you use?"

"Another great remedy is Alivizatos' Greek treatment. It doesn't work on every cancer, but it's particularly good for liver cancer, which my regular serum wouldn't work on. I had admired Dr. Alivizatos' results with liver cancer for years, but I didn't know what was in his serum."

"So how did you find out?"

"By pure luck. Alivizatos' nurse had married a man whose mother was getting the treatment in Greece, but it had gotten to where it wasn't working on her. She'd heard of my treatment but they were out of money, so they offered to trade the formula for the treatment. I got a good deal there. Some people who checked out for Alivizatos' treatment survived on it and nothing else.

Nobody is using it in Mexico now though, and Dr. Alivizatos is dead. Another doctor still does it in Greece, but you have to go there to get it."

"Another remedy headed for extinction," I remarked. "So what other remedies did you use?"

"Carnivora is another powerful German remedy. It's an extract of a plant -- Venus fly trap. It works on cancer and AIDS. About the only cancer it doesn't work on is brain cancer. It doesn't cross the blood/brain barrier. In fact the only thing I ever found that did was my serum."

"I see."

"I also worked a lot with the subconscious. People won't get well no matter what you give them, unless you clear the subconscious. I programmed everyone to believe they could get well -- and they did, and they stayed well. I had them listen to self-hypnosis tapes. One side had spoken suggestions for reversing cancer. The other side had subliminal messages hidden in ocean sounds. When I couldn't get the tapes anymore, I taught the patients to do affirmations, like 'Thank you for my perfect health.' I'd have them relax every part of their bodies when they went to sleep, then say 'I am perfectly well' over and over. I taught them to do it themselves."

"Why couldn't you get the tapes anymore?"

"Because the FDA raided the company that made them. They seized all the manufacturer's stuff in '83 or '84 and made him take his cancer tapes off the market, after pretty much putting him out of business."

"What was wrong with the tapes?"

"I suppose the fact that they claimed to be treating cancer. It was too bad, too. It was a cheap therapy with no side effects that the patients could do themselves."

"Too bad!" I agreed.

"Another thing I did on all my patients was to unblock the acupuncture meridians."

"Really," I said. I knew that in Chinese medicine, the acupuncture meridians are the set patterns through which energy is considered to flow in the body; but I didn't know Jimmy did acupuncture.

"I did a modified version of it," he explained. "I ran the scars and shins with a needle. I'd find the injured spots by muscle testing and inject them with a local anesthetic. It followed the nerve and unblocked the meridian. I did every patient that way. Sometimes it took me two hours. After awhile I got so I could sense where the weak spots were without muscle testing, but I muscle tested anyway, just to prove to the patient I was hitting them. I'd run the meridian down the shins because it goes to the thyroid and the parathyroids, which tend to get blocked in everybody."

"Really. Where did you learn that?"

"Different places. I learned about the shins from a German doctor. I learned to stick the acupuncture points with xylocaine from a Chinese doctor. I learned about the scars from another doctor."

The man was like a bee, collecting from all the flowers in his path. He kept rattling off therapies. "We did hyperthermia," he said. "We used Ginkgo biloba and germanium and chaparral. We used KCl, arginase, natural progesterone cream, Panama gas . . ."

"Panama gas?"

"It's an inert gas that seems to have an affinity for malignant cells. It interferes with the metabolism of cancer cells but not normal cells."

"I see."

"Another thing that's good is isoprinosine. It's a Mexican anti-viral, though American doctors will tell you there's no such thing. They're raving about it now in Europe, but hardly anybody had heard of it back when we were using it in the early eighties. I learned about it when the AIDS people came to Tijuana looking for it. I read up on it and found it was also good for cancer."[34]

"A man ahead of your time," I remarked.

"I suppose. Co-enzyme Q10 is another thing they're raving about now that was practically unknown back when we started using it." Jimmy rubbed his knuckles. "But I'll tell you what I could use right now."

"What's that?"

"Some DeWitt's Kidney and Bladder Pills. They're good for arthritis and gout. They're made in England. They only cost about $3.00 over-the-counter in Mexico, but you can't get them for any amount of money in the U.S. There's an American product with the same name, but the ingredients are different, and it doesn't do much."

"Why can't you get the British product?"

"I suppose because it competes with the American product."

"I see. So what else did you use?"

"Well, I also used homeopathic medicines. They're a form of vibrational medicine. Vibrational medicine involves transferring certain energetic qualities to the patient, rather than the physical substance itself. You can transfer the radiant qualities of medicine into things, and sometimes that works well. Sometimes the radiant qualities work as well as the substance. But there are some things vibrational medicine doesn't work well on. Sometimes you need physical medicine, IVs and so on. Someday we may not need machines or substances for medicine at all. We'll be able to do it with our minds. But for now, the ticket is to find out what the person needs at that particular time. I got the answers from radionics and muscle testing."

I asked about a remedy I knew other Tijuana clinics were giving intravenously, hydrogen peroxide.

"It's good," Jimmy said, "but it isn't very efficient in an IV drip, because you can't infuse it with anything else. I used electrolytes of oxygen, which can be mixed with other things."

"Did you give arginine in an IV drip?"

"You don't want to drip it in. You have to push it in fast."

"Okay. What else?"

Jimmy thought a moment. "I also prayed a lot." He explained that he rose every morning at 4 a.m. and meditated on his patients and their remedies. Then he called on whatever beneficent entities might be in the vicinity and willing to help, and asked for guidance. Answers would follow. "Sometimes they were totally off the wall," he said. "But when I tried them, they worked." He lapsed into silent thought, perhaps wondering where his beneficent entities were now.

"I was thinking more in terms of particular substances and conditions," I brought him back to the exigencies of the moment. "What would you do, say, for colon cancer?"

"Okay, for colon cancer I used different serums. I had hundreds of remedies to choose from. I tested them all, plus their compatibility with each other. That's why it took me so long. I also used acidophilus -- orally, vaginally, and rectally."

"Rectally?" I wrinkled my nose.

"There are absorption pores in the rectum," Jimmy explained matter-of-factly. "In Europe, many medications are given there. The drug is absorbed instantly, almost as fast as by a shot, and there's no needle."

"Okay."

"Another really good thing for colon cancer is levamisole. It's a regular drug, an anti-parasitic. A lot more people have parasites than you would think. They're a major factor in running down the immune system. Everyone is aware of parasites in Mexico, and they take medicines for them. But Americans don't recognize the problem. Mexicans make a soup out of an herb that helps eliminate parasites. They also have cheap drugs for worms, and levamisole is one of them. It takes care of eight different parasites. I gave it routinely to all my patients."

"Like you do for pets," I said. "I know people in the foreign service who take de-worming medicine whenever they give it to their dogs, just for prevention."

"Same principle. Levamisole is actually used in the U.S. for colon cancer. In fact, it has revolutionized colon cancer therapy -- which is good evidence that the disease can be caused by parasites. But they give too much of it in the conventional treatment. You only need enough to knock the worms out. I gave 150 milligrams for five days every three months. Another problem with the conventional treatment is that it's $1,200 a year. That's for humans. For animals, it's $15 a year. In Mexico, it's $10 a year for both. When a doctor at the Mayo Clinic questioned the price being so high in the U.S., the drug company people said the difference was justified because they had to finance research. But the studies were actually financed by the National Cancer Institute, and the product had already been on the market in other countries for 20 or 25 years."[35]

Jimmy smiled. "I asked a front man for the drug companies once why the same drug costs four or five times as much in the U.S. as in Mexico. He said, 'Because Mexicans don't have much money.'"

I laughed. "So what would you do for prostate cancer?"

"For prostate cancer I gave various live cells. The likely ones were total pituitary, anterior pituitary, adrenal, prostate. I always gave the one called RN 13. It's 13 different live cells, which go to all the organs and rejuvenate them. I also used saw palmetto extract. It comes from a plant. It decreases the swelling of the prostate and blocks the type of testosterone that encourages prostate cancer."

"Okay, what about for breast cancer?"

"It depended on the case," Jimmy said, "but I'd often use live-cell anterior pituitary. One kind of breast cancer, the kind that is estrogen-receptive, can be the result of the body producing too much estrogen. The anterior pituitary is the control mechanism for the hormones. If it's over-active, you have to tune it down. In Germany, they do it with live-cell substances that come from the anterior pituitary of an animal fetus. Sometimes, though, the ovary is under-producing progesterone, which balances estrogen. Then you use corpus luteum and whole ovary. The corpus luteum is the part of the ovary that produces progesterone."

"So how can you tell which problem it is?"

Jimmy smiled. "That's the beauty of radionics -- you don't have to know. You just have to know what live cells test out. If you give live cells for all the things that can go wrong, you cover the whole gamut. I had 240 different cells for different organs or parts of the body. They could take care of just about any problem that existed. They took off the pressure for the tumor to return. I used radionics or muscle testing to figure out which particular remedies the patient needed."

"I see." I could also see that we probably weren't going to avoid the issue of radionics at trial. This most far-out and "fringe" of Jimmy's methods was critical to the success of his therapies . . .

# Chapter 13

## Radionics

Maxine admitted introducing Jimmy to radionics, but she hastened to add that she wasn't pushing it. When he saw her "Digitron 'D' Spectrometer" and asked what it was, she hesitated to tell him. "You won't believe it," she hedged.

"Try me," Jimmy said. Soon he owned one himself.

I considered myself open-minded, but the subject was new to me. Before I had gone to Texas, I had hit the books to find out more. I learned that radionics is based on the following premises: (1) all substances, including the human body, emit subtle patterns of radiations; (2) distortions or disharmonies in these patterns indicate disease; and (3) a skilled operator can, with the help of certain instruments, detect these distortions and treat them. The practitioner is said to use a form of extrasensory perception to "read" the subconscious body/mind of the patient. The radionics machine, like the pendulum, merely magnifies the response, making this subtle body language more graphic and easier to decipher. The body doesn't even need to be present for a skilled practitioner to read its messages. The field through which mind and body operate electromagnetically is shared with the earth itself. The operator can tune into the patient's field and read it through this greater field, even at a distance. To get a "lock" on the patient, a drop of blood, photograph or other "witness" is used. I read . . .

*In this century, the first instrument used to measure distortions in the body's subtle energy patterns was the* pendulum. But long before that, traditional African healers were rubbing two sticks together and getting readings from when they "stuck." Modern-day radionics started with a French priest named Abbe Mermet. He got the idea from dowsing, the mysterious technique used to locate water hidden underground. Mermet reasoned that if he could detect the condition of an underground stream with a pendulum, he might also be able to detect the condition of the human body with it. He proved the technique on hospital patients to whom he had access as a priest. He called it "medical dowsing." Later, it was called "radiesthesia" ("sensing rays").

Mermet lacked credibility because he wasn't a doctor, but this couldn't be said of the next luminary in the field. Albert Abrams, M.D., was a celebrated American neurologist who did his research at Stanford University. Abrams discovered that if he percussed, or tapped the abdomen, of a healthy patient who was holding diseased tissue, the tapping would produce the characteristic sound of a body with the disease rather than that of the patient's own healthy body. Then he discovered that a drop of blood worked as well as diseased tissue. From these discoveries he derived a system of diagnosis using a drop of blood as a "witness" of the patient. It proved to be effective even when the patient wasn't present. Later radionics practitioners found they could successfully diagnose and treat not only from blood but from urine samples, clips of hair, or photographs of their patients.[36]

In 1924, the British medical establishment set up a blue-ribbon committee to investigate the Abrams technique. The committee, headed by Sir Thomas Horder (later Lord Horder, the Queen's physician), intended to discredit the practice in England before it caught on. The committee examined a variant of Abrams' box called an emanometer, operated by a Scottish homeopath named W. E. Boyd. Under scrupulously controlled conditions that eliminated the possibility of fraud, Boyd had to distinguish between apparently identical substances in identical bottles, secretly marked. To the shock and dismay of the committee, he was nearly 100 percent accurate in these tests. Sir Thomas told the Royal Society of Medicine that the odds of this happening by chance were millions to one. Needless to say, this was not the result sought by the Royal Society. While Sir Thomas reported it, he diffused its significance by using the opportunity to castigate radionics practitioners for the "inconsistencies" in their results.[37]

Radionics continued to flourish in England, although practitioners risked civil and criminal prosecution. George de la Warr, its leading exponent, eventually wound up in a very expensive lawsuit for fraud. The complainant was a customer who had bought one of de la Warr's radionics machines and couldn't get it to work. Fortunately for the defendant, the jury focused not on whether the instrument worked but on whether de la Warr genuinely believed that it did, and he was found not guilty.[38]

The American leader in the field after Albert Abrams, M.D., was not so fortunate. Ruth Drown was a chiropractor who devised her own equipment and was highly proficient at operating it. She also developed an amazing collection of photographs of blood spots on which could be seen shadow images of diseased organs. She had had no formal medical training. Her discoveries were apparently based on intuition. By the fifties, Dr. Drown had become the kingpin of radionics. The FDA set out to destroy both her and the technique. When they found a complainant in 1951, they prosecuted her to the full extent of the law. Edward Russell, a British writer, gave this account of her trial by an eye-witness:

> [M]any in the court had formed the impression that the charge against her was trumped up. Efforts to have her patients testify that her treatment was ineffective were a complete failure. All the patients testified to her correct diagnosis and treatment. . . . One after another -- very real and healthy people -- testified that they had been cured of all kinds of diseases and ailments. . . . When the jury went out, the court stenographer was certain she would be acquitted. To everyone's surprise she was not. The best guess as to why was that the jury were more impressed by the radio experts who testified that the instruments could not work as a radio.[39]

Dr. Drown was convicted of medical fraud and quackery. All her equipment was destroyed. Her spirit was destroyed with it. Her appeals dragged on but were unsuccessful. In the

*1960s, when she was in her seventies, she spent a term in a
California prison. A few months after her release, she suffered
a stroke and died.*

That was the early history of radionics, but more recent
researchers made it sound "high tech." In a book called <u>Vibrational
Medicine</u>, Richard Gerber, M.D., related it to the theories of
Stanford University Professor William Tiller. Formerly the
Chairman of the Department of Materials Science, Dr. Tiller had
been a full professor of engineering at Stanford since 1964. He
had published 250 papers on conventional engineering subjects,
and had published another 55 papers involving research in what
he calls "subtle energies" or "energies outside the realm of four-
dimensional space/time." Dr. Gerber said Dr. Tiller had new ideas
about the physical laws of the universe. Using Einstein's equation
relating energy to matter, he had predicted the etheric plane. Dr.
Gerber observed:

> *Up until now most physicists have accepted the seeming
> limitation that one cannot accelerate matter beyond the speed
> of light. This assumption is partly related to the fact that when
> one inserts numbers greater than the speed of light into the
> Einstein-Lorentz Transformation, one arrives at solutions
> containing the square root of -1, which is considered an
> imaginary number. Since most physicists do not believe in
> imaginary numbers, they assume that the speed of light is the
> maximum velocity at which matter can travel.*[40]

Yet, noted Dr. Gerber, these imaginary numbers are used by
physicists with impunity every day. They are necessary to finding
solutions to the equations of electromagnetic and quantum theory.
Physicists have proposed the existence of a particle known as a
"tachyon," which would theoretically exist only at speeds
exceeding the speed of light. Dr. Tiller hypothesized that the realm
of negative square roots, or "negative space/time," predicted by
Einstein's equation is the etheric plane. In negative space/time,
particles move faster than the speed of light and have negative
mass. Where positive space/time matter is associated with the
forces of electricity and electromagnetic radiation, negative space/
time matter is linked to magnetism and what Dr. Tiller calls
magneto-electric radiation. Positive space/time matter is also

characterized by positive entropy: it runs down and becomes less organized over time. Negative space/time matter is characterized by negative entropy: it becomes more organized over time. The most notable exception to the rule of entropy in the physical universe, observed Dr. Gerber, is found in living systems. They take in raw materials and energy that are less organized and build them into systems that are more organized. The life-forces that do this building in human beings emanate from the etheric and astral bodies existing in negative space/time. Under radionics theory, disorganization in the energy matrix of the subtle bodies is the cause of disease. The target of radionics techniques is to balance this disorganization with subtle energies. Noted Dr. Gerber:

> . . . *Albert Einstein proved to scientists that energy and matter are dual expressions of the same universal substance . . . . [A]ttempting to heal the body through the manipulation of this basic vibrational or energetic level of substance can be thought of as vibrational medicine. . . . By rebalancing the energy fields that help to regulate cellular physiology, vibrational healers attempt to restore order from a higher level of human functioning.*[41]

While Dr. Tiller was developing his theories at Stanford, other research in the field was being conducted by Professor Emeritus Dr. Valerie Hunt at the University of California at Los Angeles. For over two decades, Dr. Hunt had been probing the human energy field and its relationship to health and disease, using Kirlian photography, computers, oscilloscopes, "chaos theory," and film from a regular camera enhanced with the aid of a computer that runs amber light through it, making the field visible around the body. Applying cross-plot analysis to graphs recorded by oscilloscope of myograms of muscle contractions, Dr. Hunt had found that all living things have a "chaos pattern," and that "anti-coherency patterns" result in various physical disabilities, including cardiac arrhythmia. She also found something astounding: both disease and healing enter the energetic field before they enter the body. She wrote, "We discovered by recording brain waves, blood pressure changes, galvanic skin responses, heartbeat and muscle contraction simultaneously with auric changes, that changes occurred in the field before any of the other systems changed."[42]

By the time I was done reading about radionics, this technique that had once struck me as "fringe" had taken on the aura of twenty-first century medicine. It was non-invasive and without side effects, satisfying the Hippocratic oath to "First do no harm." Where it could do serious harm, I feared, was to its practitioners. It was this "blatant" quackery, more than anything else, that was liable to keep Jimmy behind bars. We were dealing with a system in which the validity of medical innovation was left to the judgment of the man and woman on the street. Bill had his work cut out for him, I thought, trying to find experts who could make these subtle energy techniques credible to a jury.

It wasn't actually Bill but Maxine, as it turned out, who would line up the defense's most credentialed radionics witness. If we had to go to trial, Dr. William Tiller was a witness I didn't want to miss.

# Chapter 14

## Testing the Tests

Jimmy confided that Junie was jealous. "How can I compete with a machine?" she complained.

Jimmy had become obsessed with radionics. He read everything he could find on it and spent hours practicing. He trained with Peter Kelly, the best radionics man in the country. But mostly, he just practiced. "It's the kind of thing," Jimmy said, "you have to learn yourself."

Lacking the FDA, government standardization, or peer-reviewed medical research, he set out to test everything himself. Every patient was different, and their needs changed from day to day. He tested everything that went into their bodies -- every batch of serum, every bottle of drinking water. Some products were more active than others, and even products from good companies could go bad.

Before he tested the remedies, he tested the tests. His new Digitron he tested with blood samples. He got them from Dr. K., a close personal friend. Dr. K. would consult with Jimmy's patients at night after his regular office hours, and would give them blood transfusions or admit them to the hospital when necessary. When the diagnoses Jimmy got on the Digitron from Dr. K.'s blood samples matched those that came back from the laboratory, he was satisfied his new machine worked.

After he got into trouble for using the Digitron, he got into muscle testing.

I had researched it too. I learned that muscle testing works on similar principles as radionics but has the consummate advantage that it uses no "drugs or devices" that can be regulated by the FDA. The subconscious mind communicates merely through the resistance of the patient's own arm. I read . . .

> *The principles of muscle testing, or "applied kinesiology," were discovered largely by accident. Dr. George Goodheart, a Detroit chiropractor, found that some of the standard chiropractic muscle tests provide clues to the workings of the whole body. His new system combined chiropractic with Eastern ideas about energy flow. Weaknesses were identified and then treated to correct imbalances in the body's energy systems. If the outstretched arm was easily pushed down, something was weakening the body's energy field. If the arm "locked," the field was strong. Where energy was found to be restricted or excessive, Dr. Goodheart discovered that either the muscle might be weak or the patient might be reacting to certain foods or other irritants. The technique was found to be particularly successful in locating and treating allergies.[43]*

Dr. Goodheart's work was refined by John Diamond, M.D. Dr. Diamond wrote:

> *Over the years, Dr. Goodheart had achieved many amazing results -- results that had far-reaching implications. . . . If a particular nutritional supplement was given to a patient and the muscle tested strong, it was the right supplement for that patient; if the muscle remained weak, it was not. Other methods of treatment could be similarly evaluated. With Applied Kinesiology, doctors had a really useful tool, a system of feedback from the body itself. If they gave a patient the proper treatment, the body would respond immediately as if to say, 'Yes, that is what was needed.[44]*

"So how did you check the results of your muscle testing?" I asked.

"With a pendulum," Jimmy replied matter-of-factly.

"I see . . ."

"I wasn't trying to prove it to anyone but myself," he explained. "I did it after I'd seen so many patients that I'd forgotten the results of the muscle tests. When the answers matched, I figured I wasn't just imagining them. If I had been, I probably would have come up with different answers."

He said, for example, that in principle he supported a strict vegetarian diet. But he found when he tested the patients that most of them needed some animal protein, especially eggs or fish. Eggs actually tested favorably for more people than milk did; and many patients tested out on meat. In principle, he also avoided synthetic pharmaceuticals; but some tested out for some patients. He maintained he had never lost a lung cancer patient after he started giving a certain Mexican antibiotic when muscle testing indicated it was needed.

"I could buy that," I hedged, "but I don't know if a jury will -- even if we manage to get one that's honest and uncorrupted and paying attention . . ."

I was sorry I had brought up that potential flaw in the jury system, as Jimmy lapsed into gloomy thought. "I've got some affidavits that are pretty convincing," he finally said. He rustled through his disheveled papers and pulled one out.

It was the 1984 notarized affidavit of a patient from Kaplan, Louisiana, named Laura Hebert. She wrote that Jimmy's Digitron had picked up a medical condition in her body that conventional diagnosis had failed to catch. The machine showed her as having "a heavy involvement of ovarian cancer with metastatic involvement of the pancreas." Laura wrote, "We laughed about the ovarian part, because I didn't have any ovaries." But Jimmy continued to insist that his diagnosis was correct. His treatments did make her feel better, she said, and her blood amylase dropped to a favorable 231.

"What's blood amylase?" I asked.

Jimmy shrugged. "I don't pay much attention to medical tests. I just ask the body, and it responds."

I smiled and read on. Laura said she had then made the mistake of taking estrogen. She had been using the hormone for hot flashes and irritability, but Jimmy strongly recommended against it. She stayed off it for awhile, but finally she went back on it. Each time she got the hormone shot, her amylase rose. Eventually it got up to 2,500, and she had to go back for surgery. When the doctor opened her up, he found cancer. His report, which was attached to her affidavit, said, "the lesion is most consistent with that of an adenocarcinoma probably of ovarian origin." She wrote:

> *If only I had believed the digitron machine, I could have avoided my medical nightmare entirely. [Jimmy's] machine was completely accurate while four CT scans and five ultrasounds were wrong. . . . I am doing much better now, thanks to his treatment and the discontinuation of the hormone shots. . . . It's ironic how we live in the land of the free, yet have to flee our country for successful cancer treatment.*

"Pretty good diagnosis," I agreed.

Jimmy smiled. "Laura's brother thought so. He was so impressed that he did a study comparing my diagnoses with conventional diagnoses. It turned out they matched."

"He'd make a good witness!"

Jimmy sighed. "He would if I could find him. It was seven years ago. His phone number was in the files the FBI took when they raided my apartment in 1984."

Jimmy added after some thought, "But Don McBride can testify about the Digitron. He has volunteered to be a witness, and he's a convincing speaker."

When I read Don's notarized affidavit, I had to agree he was a witness with credibility. He was a real estate broker and developer, president of three companies, and chairman of the board of Founders National Bank in Brea, California. Don wrote that he had been an observer at Jimmy's clinic in Matamoros, just across the Mexican border from Brownsville, when he took his mother Velma there in June of 1983.

The oncologists who diagnosed Velma's breast cancer, Don wrote, had given her three options: surgery, radiation, or chemotherapy. But she had buried three of her closest friends with cancer, and they had all been treated conventionally. When she saw their futile suffering, she made her son promise that if she ever got the disease, he would take her for non-traditional therapy. Of course, that was before she saw Jimmy and his homespun clinic.

"He doesn't look like a doctor," Velma hedged.

"Mom," Don replied, "he isn't a doctor. He's a healer. That's why we're here."

Velma had brought her x-rays and mammograms with her, but Don said Jimmy never looked at them. He just used the Digitron, then pronounced the diagnosis: she had cancer in the left breast under her left arm, entering the chest cavity and the lung, and in the lymph node. "I was amazed," Don wrote. "Jimmy made the same diagnosis as the doctor, and he'd never seen her medical records."

Velma was then sent to Jimmy's brother Ron, who was using a machine called an Accuscope in another room. ("The Accuscope uses footpads," Jimmy explained when I asked. "They make a circuitry between different points on the body and the feet. When the machine beeps, you know there is a weakness or blockage in the circuit.") When the Accuscope got to Velma's left breast, it went "beep, beep, beep." Ron called it a poison area. Don was even more impressed. "They had it on two machines."

Velma was given colonics, huge doses of supplements (vitamins, minerals and Jimmy's serum), and a strict nutritional diet. "After a week of this program," Don wrote, "both my mother and myself felt that the cancer was in total remission and that if she would keep the same nutritional regime she would live much longer than her seventy eight years."

Unfortunately, she didn't; but her death wasn't from cancer. Velma unexpectedly suffered a brain stem stroke from which she never regained consciousness. "They x-rayed her three different times," Don wrote; "all of these x-rays proved according to the doctors she had no active cancer."

He then went on to describe a remarkable case involving the patient who had first sparked his interest in Jimmy's clinic. Clarence Schwartz was the chairman of Founders National Bank and chairman of the board of St. Jude Hospital in Fullerton, one of the largest hospitals in Orange County. He had developed a serious brain tumor in 1982, when he was 69. He had gone to Scripts, then to UCLA Medical Center. Surgery had left him paralyzed down the left side of his body, in his arm, leg and face. Chemotherapy and radiation were tried but were unsuccessful. He was told he would rapidly go downhill.

Clarence wound up in a wheelchair, and the bank meetings moved to his home. His mind was still sharp, but he could not hold up his head or shake hands, and he was on oxygen. After a year, he said he could not carry on anymore. He decided to try Jimmy's clinic. He was so sure death was imminent that he took his funeral clothes with him. He was a retired Navy captain and wanted to be buried in his military uniform in Arlington. Too weak to fly commercially, he had to charter a private plane on which he could get oxygen. He intended for the plane to proceed on to Virginia with his body. He flew to Brownsville and checked

into the Presidente Hotel, across the street from Jimmy's clinic in
Matamoros.

Each day after Jimmy treated him, Clarence's progress was
tested by the strength of his grip. The first day, he could not grip
at all. The second day, he could hold Jimmy's hands. After ten
days, he could make Jimmy drop to his knees. Two weeks later,
he flew home commercially. "It was like a miracle," Don wrote.
"If it hadn't been for the surgery, he'd have been normal. His
brain tumor had totally shrunk. A CAT scan showed no evidence
of it whatsoever. He was fine! One doctor was so upset, he wouldn't
talk to him."

Clarence, like Velma, did die. But his death, like hers, wasn't
from cancer. "His death certificate said he died of a coronary,"
Don wrote. "We thought he just gave up, because he was paralyzed
and unable to get around. He wanted to die."

Don then described another dramatic case involving an
inoperable brain tumor. In this case, the patient was still alive.
His name was Wesley Smith, and in 1983 he was only two years
old. Don wrote:

> His parents, Guy and Didi Smith, together with their baby
> of just a few weeks had for three months been on the road
> taking Wesley to Children's Hospital in Orange, UCLA
> Medical Center, then up to San Francisco and finally to Oral
> Roberts Faith Hospital. At Oral Roberts they tried to operate
> on a tumor in his brain which was inoperable. The surgery left
> the boy paralyzed on the left side of his body. It was a pathetic
> sight to see this little fellow's bald head with the sutures still
> in his head. The doctors had told Wesley's parents that the
> operation was unsuccessful and he would have very limited
> time to live. He was cross eyed, his left foot was turned
> backwards. He could not hold himself upright. Two people on
> each side of him could hold his hands and he could stay erect
> but he was very weak and uncoordinated.
>
> After Wesley's third or fourth day at the clinic, my mother
> noticed that his eyes were no longer crossed and called it to the
> attention of his parents. They hadn't even noticed and were
> thrilled. About the fourth or fifth day he started holding his
> head up and trying to pull himself upright. At the end of the
> first week he could pull himself up and with one person on
> each side he could walk. His foot was straightening out. . . .

*By the end of two weeks when we left, he was chasing the ducks all around our motel. It was absolutely amazing. After his parents returned home with their son . . . they x-rayed the boy and there was no evidence of tumor at all. The treatment he was given in Matamoros had literally shrunk the tumor in his brain.*

I was back to thinking Jimmy's case was a lead pipe cinch. All we had to do was to get these compelling witnesses on the stand. But my job was to try to avoid trial altogether, by crafting a motion to dismiss that would dispose of the issues on paper. And I still hadn't made it through the facts of the case. "What made you leave Baton Rouge?" I pushed on.

"I got enjoined."

"I thought you were protected by the governor."

"He didn't get re-elected."

# Chapter 15

## Exodus

And so the story unfolded. Jimmy said he had always worked closely with Dr. K., Dr. Dotson or another M.D.; but there was no denying he was practicing medicine without a license. The problem for the Louisiana State Board of Medical Examiners was finding a complainant willing to testify to it. They tried for years without success. His efforts on behalf of blacks and cancer patients had won him substantial public support, including a favorable review in the Baton Rouge Morning Advocate. He continued to be politically active and enjoyed the protection of powerful politicians.

Eventually, however, the Board did find witnesses willing to take the stand. They were the relatives of a woman who was terminally ill with cancer. "She was too sick to travel," Jimmy recalled, "so each day, I made the trip to her home. I told the family they could not expect a recovery, only relief of pain and a better quality of life. The family was very poor, so I treated her free of charge. In a few days, she was able to walk and was off pain medication. She lived six months longer than expected; but she did die, and her doctor reported the treatment to the State Board. At the hearing, her relatives admitted she'd been helped by the treatment and hadn't been charged for it. But the judge said it didn't matter. I was practicing medicine without a license. He issued a court order enjoining me from practicing medicine in the state."

"Why do you suppose the family agreed to testify?" I asked.

"I don't know. They weren't hostile, but they were really poor. I got the feeling their testimony might have been bought and paid for."

"I see. But why did the Board have to get an injunction? Practicing medicine without a license is already against the law. Why didn't they just have you arrested?"

"Good question. The problem was, they couldn't prosecute a criminal action without the district attorney; and the district attorney wouldn't act. I was actually told the Board would leave me alone, if I would just keep my mouth shut. I was giving lectures at a health food store that drew a lot of people. But I was young and arrogant and believed in what I was doing, so I kept on doing it."

It was only a matter of time before Governor Edwards finally failed to get re-elected. The Board lost no time moving in. Jimmy was served with a temporary injunction in March of 1983. His impulse was to stand and fight; but then he remembered he had patients in the middle of treatment. He would be putting them in jeopardy. He decided to comply with the injunction by leaving the state. His chelation patients he left with Dr. K.

Like Dr. Dotson, Dr. K. wound up paying dearly for his involvement. The doctor was "disciplined." He was taken off the staff of the local hospitals, leaving him without hospitalization for his patients. He was later institutionalized for a nervous breakdown. Today Dr. K. is an emergency room doctor, without a private practice.

Organizing his fourteen cancer patients into a car caravan, Jimmy blazed a trail to Mexico. The land where the unorthodox Puritans had sought refuge to practice what they believed had become the land of oppression for unconventional medicine. Mexico was the new frontier. Medicine there wasn't allopathically standardized like in the United States, perhaps because the country boasts as many homeopaths as M.D.'s. Its National Homeopathic Medical College is the oldest homeopathic school in the hemisphere, dating back to the 1700s.

"Doesn't Mexico have a regulatory agency like the FDA?" I asked.

"It does," Jimmy replied, "but it isn't as strict or as bent on prosecuting. Every clinic in Tijuana uses medicines that aren't approved. They don't care about little guys like me as long as no one complains -- and no one ever did. The FBI actually went out looking for complainants, and they couldn't find any."

"But don't you have to have a license to practice medicine in Mexico?"

"Of course, but I had doctors and nurses working for me. My clinic was a licensed corporation, and I was the head of it. I could do whatever I needed to to run it. It was a legal entity, and it was squeaky clean. Anyway, they have a looser definition of 'practicing medicine' in Mexico than in the United States. I've seen employees in Mexican drugstores giving people injections and IVs. You can get any drug you want without a prescription, except narcotics; and the drugs only cost about a fourth of what they cost in the U.S. You can get IV solution over-the-counter. In fact you can get it everywhere in the world except the U.S. and Canada. The only thing you can do on your own in the U.S. is swallow pills, which are much less effective than injections. Pills have to go through the stomach, where they get digested. Injections go right into the blood. IV solution is 60 cents a bag in Mexico. It wholesales for $2.40 in the U.S. My daughter got charged $40.00 a bag when she had her surgery. They can mark prescription products up as much as they want. Insurance pays. If we went back to a free market, where you had to pay for your own medicines and services, it wouldn't take long for people to discover the value of natural medicines. The irony of it is that the more unnatural the treatment, the more expensive it is -- and the more disruptive to the body. The cheapest remedies are actually the best."

"You should have run for politics," I said. "So what things can't you do in Mexico without a license?"

"I think you just can't call yourself a doctor, or do invasive things like surgery, that can do serious harm to the body."

"That's how it used to be in the U.S.," I observed, "before the special interests got involved. So you were up to the car caravan to Mexico."

"Right. We drove to Matamoros, just across the river from Brownsville. It was Rudnov who suggested the location. He has a clinic in Tijuana." Jimmy's functional eyebrow arched skeptically. "A mutual friend told me later he heard Rudnov say he could never have a successful clinic in the same town as mine."

Jimmy's clinic was in Matamoros, but the staff and the patients stayed on the other side of the border. The patients needed kitchens to prepare their special diets. He rented apartments for them in Brownsville. For a clinic, he found a stately old three-story antebellum-style house in Matamoros with a tree-lined yard. The price was right: $500 a month. Later, they found out why the price was so low; but by then, they had already moved in.

The house was rumored to be haunted. ("It <u>was</u> haunted," Maxine asserted matter-of-factly.)

Paranoia joined the ghosts in haunting the premises. Dozens of non-traditional cancer clinics had already paved the way in Mexico, but they were in Tijuana. Matamoros was perilously close to Louisiana, where the State Board was still gunning for Jimmy.

"One time," he said, chuckling, "some fanatical woman saw someone and thought the feds were coming. I was in Baton Rouge then attending the injunction hearing, and my brother Ron was in charge in Matamoros. I'd hidden $5,000 in the mantle in the clinic as emergency money in case we needed it. Ron called and I told him to get the money out, and he hid it in the couch in the apartment in Brownsville. But when he went to get it, the couch was gone. The owner was planning to replace it with a new one and had had it hauled away. Ron chased it down and found it in Matamoros, guarded by some large unfriendly-looking Mexicans. Ronnie had to do some fast talking. He said he was a radiation physicist, and that he had dropped a radioactive source in the sofa. It was very dangerous, and he had to get it out before it killed someone."

I laughed. "And they bought that story?"

"They were suspicious, but they let him search the couch. He managed to get the money out with his back toward them. He said 'gracias' and got out of there before they could change their minds." Jimmy laughed too. "It was rough in Matamoros. Some of the patients had cars stolen, and we had a van stolen. One time I had to run a guy off who was trying to steal my car. I said, 'This is my car. You go steal another one.' But that was before we found a guy who wanted six dollars a day to guard the place. He looked like Wyatt Earp and carried a long pistol like you see in the movies. No one fooled with him. He would shoot them and they knew it. He stopped everybody at the front gate, including the FBI and the reporters."

Even paranoids had enemies . . . and Jimmy's, it seemed, loomed larger than mere thieves. In 1983, anti-quackery bills were pending before Congress; and in 1982, the National Council Against Health Fraud had labeled him the most notorious quack in the country. That made him a prize catch . . . .

# Part Two

## The Prosecution Builds a Case

*[T]he people regard it among their vested rights to buy and swallow such physick, as they in their sovereign will and pleasure shall determine; and in this free country, the democracy denounce[s] all restrictions upon quackery as wicked monopolies for the benefit of physicians.*

— 1838 treatise on Jacksonian democracy

# Chapter 16

## The Quackbusters

The anti-quackery bills of the early 1980s were introduced into Congress by Representative Claude Pepper of Florida, who succeeded in becoming the oldest member of the House before he died. His political longevity was attributed to his loyalty to the medical/pharmaceutical complex. No commercial interest had a more powerful lobby. Quackbusting became the order of the day. Promotions were to be had and careers to be made. The bills eventually died in committee, after public resistance was expressed through thousands of letters and petitions. But in the meantime, extensive hearings were held and wide publicity was generated.[45]

Ironically, Claude Pepper had begun his political career on the other side of the fence. When then-Senator Pepper introduced a prototype of the National Cancer Act into Congress in the 1940s, he made the mistake of backing his bill with testimony from patients cured of their cancers by a dietary treatment alone. The therapy was that of Max Gerson, M.D., a German ex-patriot whose daughter now has a clinic in Tijuana. Not only was the bill defeated, but Pepper's support of Gerson and of socialized medicine (a pet peeve of the AMA) actually cost him his seat in the Senate.

When the National Cancer Act was finally signed into law in 1971, the political push came from the drug industry. The industry's answer to cancer was cytotoxic ("cell-killing") chemotherapy, which had burst on the scene at about the time Pepper's cancer bill was being defeated. The drugs originated in World War I with the mustard gases used in the trenches. On victims who survived, these chemical weapons were noted to have the longterm toxic effect of damaging bone marrow and DNA. The drugs were developed in Germany by I.G. Farben, a huge drug cartel that manufactured the nerve poison used to kill six million Jews. With the outbreak of World War II, the use of nitrogen mustard on cancer patients was continued experimentally under the mantle of military secrecy. After World War II, these chemicals were openly tested on cancer. The end-products were the widely-used neoplastic agents in the mustard, or alkylating, group.[46]

By the 1970s, Pepper had learned on which side his bread was buttered. Opposing the pharmaceutical business and the AMA was political suicide. When he finally made a comeback in the House of Representatives, he not only avoided supporting unconventional therapies but actually led their investigation as quackery. The anti-quackery bills he introduced in 1981 and 1982 targeted the competitors of the conventional medical establishment. A 1984 U.S. House Subcommittee report called "quackery" a "$10 billion scandal." Americans, noted the report, spend upwards of $20 billion a year on "unproven" medical treatments.[47] No mention was made of the fact that $100 billion now goes annually for conventional research and treatment for cancer alone.

The most controversial of the anti-quackery bills was what opponents called "the nefarious Post Office 'Thought Police' Bill." It would have given the U.S. Postal Service the power to ban from the mails any book, magazine or other publication that expressed a view about health care or nutrition that was contrary to the prevailing views of the orthodox medical establishment, in evident violation of the First Amendment. It would also have let postal officials seize the records and close the businesses of people distributing or selling such printed materials.[48]

Practitioners of unconventional treatments for cancer were in a particularly precarious position. By the 1980s, the medical/pharmaceutical complex had acquired a legal monopoly over cancer therapies. In many states, a special statute made the use of substances or devices illegal in the treatment of cancer unless their safety and effectiveness had been proven to either the FDA or the State Board of Public Health. Legal cancer

therapies were essentially limited to synthetic chemotherapy
(patentable drugs that could support the cost of FDA approval),
and radiation and surgery (which were grandfathered in before
controlled clinical trials came into vogue).[49]

High on the list of cancer treatments targeted by the
"Quackbusters" was the suspect remedy "Tumorex." In 1983, an
Arizona M.D. named Wickman and a naturopath named Anderson
were arrested for using it. As Jimmy told the story, the bust took
place at Dr. Wickman's office during business hours, when the
door, as usual for a doctor's office, was unlocked. The raiding state
agents nevertheless broke it down with axes, a dramatic entrance
apparently staged for the benefit of TV cameras trained on the
scene. Frank Cousineau, an eye-witness to the transaction, said
Rudnov had delivered the remedy to Dr. Anderson at the airport
in San Diego. Anderson went straight to Phoenix and drove to
Wickman's office. State agents were at the door within minutes.
Rudnov had evidently set the doctors up.

"Wickman jumped bond and left the U.S. and is practicing
medicine in a foreign country," Jimmy said. "Anderson got seven
years and served two, with probation for the other five. He was
the nicest guy -- a real fine man, very honest. He was married and
had children and was a minister of a Christian church. He had a
radio program, and he had a lot of knowledge."

Jimmy thought that may have been why Dr. Anderson was
hit. "He was in a position to tell the public that arginine can
prevent cancer. In the seventies, laetrile was their big competitive
threat. But arginine is twenty times as effective as laetrile, and it's
perfectly safe. It's a common amino acid available in any health
food store. You can't say it's not approved. It's there. It could be
administered by doctors right now if they knew how. They just
don't have the information."

If everyone knew about natural immunity-building therapies
like arginine and used them preventatively, Jimmy thought, cancer
itself might be wiped out. The sinister view was that this result
was not in the best interests of the cancer industry. To Bill (an
avowed conspiratorialist), it explained why Jimmy's crime
outweighed that of the serial killer who got a lesser bail. The
serial killer was a threat to only a few stray youths. Jimmy could
wipe out a megalithic industry. It was an exaggeration, but Bill
liked vivid imagery.

"You don't really think," I said dubiously to Jimmy, "that there are people out there purposely conspiring . . ."

"No," he conceded. "People don't get up and say, 'Okay, we are not going to allow this to be used because it works.' It's just that in a market economy, you've got to make a profit. A pharmaceutical company isn't going to pick some common property of nature that can't be patented and develop it, because they have to make a profit for their stockholders. People are out there busting quacks because they're trying to stop competition, but that's normal. That could happen in any business. It's not that there was a conspiracy *per se* . . . " He added after thinking about it, "But it sure seemed like there was . . ."

"When did you first get that feeling?"

After further thought, he said trouble had first blown into his Matamoros clinic with a Brownsville M.D. I'll call Dr. Marley. Jimmy had met the doctor through a patient named Frankie Kille.

"Frankie had a big tumor on her breast," he said, "a horrible, wide-open thing. Her doctor had given her only six weeks to live. I was treating her by spraying my modified serum right on it. There was a newspaper article written about her recovery. She died later, but she lived a lot longer than expected. She might have lived longer than that, but she couldn't get follow-up treatment after the government cut me off from my patients in 1984. They seized my records and enjoined Maxine from giving out my phone number, then told the patients I'd abandoned them and defrauded them. That was how they built their whole case. As long I was in communication with my patients, they couldn't get a single witness, before or after Matamoros."

I nodded and moved him along. "So what happened with Frankie and Dr. Marley?"

"Okay, Frankie first came after she'd had chemotherapy, and her blood situation wasn't good, so I sent her to the emergency room in Brownsville for blood. She met Dr. Marley there and liked him, and he said he wanted to work with me, so I sent him other patients. He seemed real happy to have the referrals, until Sarah Johnson. She was six years old and had leukemia. She was hemorrhaging and having nosebleeds, which meant she was probably in the last fatal stages of the disease. I'm leary of childhood leukemia, because it progresses so much faster than other cancers. I always ask the parents to go for chemotherapy first and get the child in remission. Chemotherapy can actually do some good in those cases, because it gives you a breather to start working on them. But Becky, Sarah's mother, had already refused chemotherapy; and the girl was in desperate need of blood. Within an hour of when they got to Brownsville, she was hemorrhaging bad. I told Becky to go across and ask Dr. Marley for platelets, but Marley said he wouldn't give the girl blood unless Becky promised not to take her to Mexico."

"That sounds like malpractice."

"It was. But it probably wasn't Marley's idea. I think he was under duress. He never had any problem taking my patients before. With Sarah though, he suddenly started saying he was afraid he might lose his medical license. He might be charged with being part of a conspiracy."

"I wonder where he got that idea."

"You don't suppose" -- Jimmy looked out of his better eye -- "that somebody was talking to him . . ."

"Like who?"

"Well," Jimmy said like a teacher to a slow student, "who investigates conspiracies? I think Marley made a deal with the government. My local attorney told me Marley was involved in some kind of insurance fraud. I think the deal was, they'd drop the fraud claim against him in exchange for one against me."

"I see! Extortion -- although I guess when the government does it, they call it something else."

Jimmy nodded. "If Marley takes the stand, Silvermith plans to impeach him with it."

"That could be some interesting testimony! So what happened with Sarah?"

"Okay, I was up the whole night looking for a Mexican doctor. We had to get whole blood, which is all they had in Mexico. We had to match her up. But before the night was over, the girl was at my clinic getting transfused; and it helped her a lot. Then I started treating her. At first she was afraid of the needle. She was deathly afraid of white coats. She screamed when she saw one -- like the doctor we had working there -- so I didn't let him get near her. I played with her and took my time. I tried to get her confidence. I told her, 'I want you to know that we're doing this to get you well, and I know you will. You're a splendid little lady and we're going to work together to get you well. I'm not going to hurt you.' I'd put the tourniquet on, spot the vein, take it off, pat the arm -- back and forth, till she got used to it. I always used a sock for a tourniquet . . ."

"A sock?" I could imagine this coming up at trial.

"It was a clean sock," Jimmy assured me. "It didn't hurt as much as a regular tourniquet. I slipped the needle in before the little girl realized it. She didn't cry. She wasn't fighting it. Her mind was working to get herself well. She was anxious to do it. The next day it was easier. After the treatment, she was perfect. She was running around and playing. They ran leukemia tests on her three weeks later. They ran a white blood count and checked the immature cells. She was back to normal limits on the white blood, and she had practically no immature cells. She was in remission. It was a perfect test."

Later, I read a letter from Sarah's mother Becky confirming these facts. She wrote:

> [Jimmy] said he didn't want to take my money when he wasn't sure he could help her. I pleaded with him to please treat her because I was so afraid of the orthodox treatment. . . . Sarah became visibly better within the two weeks that she was there. The blood test that she received at the end of her treatment showed no bad blood cells. The treatment had cleared her blood.

Yet Sarah's name now featured in one of the counts of the indictment. If Becky was so happy with the treatment, I wondered, who was testifying for the prosecution?

The answer turned out to be Sarah's father. He hadn't been in Matamoros or seen what went on, but by the time of trial, he and Becky were divorced.

"I guess Sarah died," I said.

Jimmy nodded. "It wasn't from cancer though. It was from chicken pox."

"Chicken pox?"

"Her immune system was shot from chemotherapy."

Maxine later told the story of Sarah's death. Becky had called and asked if she and her daughter could live with Maxine for awhile. Becky was trying to avoid a court order requiring Sarah to get chemotherapy. Maxine agreed, but in the end Sarah got the drugs; and within the year, she was dead. Government experts later conceded that chemotherapy had weakened her immune system so much that she succumbed to an ordinary childhood disease.

Jimmy said Becky had come to Tijuana looking for him, but Maxine had been enjoined from revealing where he was. When

Becky couldn't find him, she wound up going to another Tijuana practitioner; and that doctor had insisted on the chemotherapy. Becky decided she might as well go back home for it.

"She wants to take the stand for the defense," Jimmy observed.

The whole thing struck me as mixed up. Chemotherapy had precipitated the girl's death. Yet it was Jimmy who was on trial for promising to get her better. Her oncologists didn't have to promise anything. They could force their immunity-destroying drugs by court order.

A later newspaper article identified Dr. Marley as the doctor who originally called for the Keller investigation. But Jimmy suspected the government had approached the doctor rather than the reverse. If so, the real complainant was the FBI. The question then was, who had approached the FBI?

# Chapter 17

## The Sting

After Dr. Marley's about-face, Jimmy kept seeing suspicious-looking men driving by his clinic. They appeared to be casing it. He decided it was time to move to Tijuana. He took his last new Matamoros patients in November of 1983, intending to close the clinic in mid-December for Christmas. He would open again in January in Tijuana. Then in the first week in December, Maxine got a call from a couple who said they had a little boy with leukemia. The couple wanted to see the clinic, but they were afraid to go into Mexico. Could they meet Jimmy in Brownsville?

"You know Maxine," Jimmy said wryly, "always eager to help." She told them they could go to his Brownsville apartment early in the morning, before he went over to Matamoros.

When the couple showed up, Jimmy was suspicious. He hastily dialed Maxine. His son David happened to be at the apartment at the time. While Jimmy was on the phone, the couple tried to engage David in conversation.

"If you knew David," Jimmy said, "you'd know they didn't get much out of him. He doesn't talk much."

Maxine confirmed that the woman had called her, but Jimmy remained suspicious. He told the couple they couldn't talk there. They'd have to go into Mexico. The couple followed him to the clinic, but he was busy. He didn't pay much attention to them after they arrived.

He said he finally talked to them briefly. They wanted to know if he could cure their son. He told them he never used the word. The best you could do with cancer was to control it. The problem could always return. Jimmy asked for the child's medical records. The couple said they didn't have them.

"That confirmed my suspicions," he said. "Normally they'd have brought the patient in, but at the very least they'd have brought medical records. Without medical records or the patient, there's nothing to discuss."

Jimmy asked if the child were in remission. The couple said he wasn't. Jimmy said that before he could treat the boy, they would need to get conventional treatment to get him in remission. The couple continued to ask what Jimmy perceived to be leading questions. Finally, he cut them short and showed them out. "They were baiting me," he said, "but they couldn't get me to say what they wanted me to say. They made the mistake of using a leukemia child. Leukemia moves real fast in children. The only way to treat it is to get them in remission first with chemotherapy."

"I thought you were opposed to radiation and chemotherapy."

"I'm opposed to radiation," Jimmy explained. "I don't need it. My serum does a better job of shrinking tumors, and it doesn't burn the patients up or make their hair fall out at the same time. In fact they look forward to the treatment, because it makes them feel good. But chemotherapy can sometimes give a positive short-term gain, because it attacks cells at the point of division, and cancer cells divide faster than normal cells. The problem is the long-term effect on the immune system. It can be so devastating that the patient dies from something else -- pneumonia or some other infection. I sent patients for chemo when I was desperate, but not in more than one case out of a hundred; and I always used my other treatments with it to build the immune system back up. I didn't treat leukemia children, though, until they'd had chemotherapy and were in remission."

"You took Sarah Johnson," I pointed out.

"I did, but I told her mother not to bring her. I had the child against my will."

"So what would you do for leukemia after the child was in remission?" I inquired.

"Then I'd use live cell bone marrow, live cell spleen, live cell multi. I also had a special herbal formula for leukemia that I put together myself. Another thing I found later that's great for lymphatic leukemia is colchicine. In fact it's good for all cancer."

"I thought colchicine was toxic," I said, recalling some research I'd done for a book.

"It's not," Jimmy assured me. "It's a natural herb. I take it regularly myself whenever I can get it."

"Interesting. So what happened with the couple asking suspicious questions?"

"Well,"-- Jimmy arched his better eyebrow -- "we made the news." He pulled out a dog-eared manila folder full of clippings. The one on top was from the Brownsville Herald and was dated December 14, 1983. It began:

> A fraudulent clinic operating in Matamoros for the past 10 months, has been drawing scores of desperate cancer victims here from every corner of the nation to receive injections of suspect drugs.

The reporter maintained:

> The Herald's investigation formed the basis for an undercover sting operation pulled off by an FBI agent and an Texas attorney general's investigator posing as husband and wife. The couple met Keller at Amigoland Villas and followed him to the clinic, where he agreed to treat their 10-year-old son who had leukemia. The son did not exist, but Keller said he could successfully treat the child for $3,000-$3,500, his standard fee for the 'cure,' states an investigative narrative by the investigator who posed as the wife.

Maxine later described the panic of the day. For her, she said, it began with a phone call. "It's all over the newspapers and on TV!" Jimmy exclaimed on the phone. "They say we have a quack clinic and we're robbing people!"

"You've got to get out of there," Maxine urged. She understood there was a warrant out for his arrest.

"What about the patients?" Jimmy hesitated.

"You can't help anyone if you're in jail!"

Maxine said she called a retired CIA agent in Florida. (A CIA agent? She explained that he was a loyal supporter. Jimmy had put his cancer in remission.) The ex-CIA man said, 'Get Jimmy to me, and I'll get him out of the country.'"

Jimmy wasn't keen on running away, but the system had made him a renegade. Huddled in the back seat of a car and covered up so no one could see him, he got as far as Houston. Then he learned from his brother Ron, who had a friend who was a prosecutor in Houston, that at that time at least, no warrant was out for his arrest. Maxine got another phone call in the middle of the night. "I can't do it," Jimmy said. "I can't leave the patients in the middle of treatment."

Jimmy told the rest. "I drove all night. I wanted to finish one more day's treatment, but I couldn't go back to the clinic. Reporters were running around trying to take pictures and so on, so the Mexican health department closed it, though they were actually our friends. They said they'd open it up two weeks later. I had to treat the patients at the apartment in Brownsville. I treated 20 or 25 patients there. The prosecutor made a big deal about this 'crime,' because I wasn't licensed to practice in Texas. But anyone with any compassion would have done the same."

"Compassion and some nerve," I said.

"I suppose. I sued the <u>Brownsville Herald</u> and the reporter later for libel. The reporter wound up losing his job. But it didn't help us much. I don't think he was really behind the investigation anyway."

"Why not?"

"Because the same day the story appeared in the <u>Herald</u>, it also appeared in another paper, and on the radio and on local TV."

Jimmy thought the media blitz had been orchestrated by the FBI, to generate the hostile publicity it needed to build its case.

In January of 1984, Jimmy moved his permanent residence to Tijuana. But the FBI wasn't satisfied with merely chasing him away. They were bent on conviction. According to a California medical fraud advisor quoted in a later article about the case in the <u>San Diego Tribune</u>:

> [A]uthorities on this side of the border have neither the will nor the resources to pursue such cases. . . . The feds could do something with the mails and telephone lines, but somebody has to put a high priority on the matter and have strong feelings about it. Apparently in Texas, somebody had that.[50]

Again the question was, who? Conspiratorially-minded observers saw it as a drug industry plot. Cancer Control Society tour guide John Adderley later wrote to the court, "I believe it to be self evident that these alternative drugs, substances and methods of treatment . . . are competition to a multibillion dollar industry. I believe that this industry, as opportunity presents itself, uses its considerable influence to have one of these drugs, substances, or alternative practitioners, cut from the herd and . . . made an example of."

Charles R. Tessier Jr., who had worked with Jimmy in successfully resisting the fluoridation of Baton Rouge drinking water, wrote to the court, "I believe the establishment (Gov. agencies and medical groups) were trying to entrap him both in Baton Rouge, La. and the area where you are now."

Al Lippman (a retired research scientist who holds 23 U.S. patents and is listed in Who's Who) asked the court, "Who could gain from interruption of Jimmy Keller's unselfish and much needed work? Some opine that those with a strong vested interest in facilities and operations of the older method of treatment might be concerned over the rapid obsolescence that would result from the new technology."

For whatever reason, there seemed to be a vendetta out against Jimmy and his clinic. In 1984, Dr. Marley went to Washington to testify against him in anti-quackery hearings in Congress. A federal investigation was launched against him, handled by the FBI.

The agent in charge was a man I'll call Dixon. He was reported to have two pictures of Jimmy tacked on his office wall, one with a beard and one without. Dixon was heard to say that his sole job for two years was to "get something on Keller." Apparently, he expected to find it in the Matamoros clinic.

"The Mexican authorities had taped up the front of the clinic," Jimmy said, "but they told us they were going to leave the back door open and not come back till the first of the year. The first week in January, they broke the tape and went in. The FBI were there, and so were the TV stations and the press. They were all waiting to get in and go through files and equipment, but there was nothing there. They were furious. They realized they didn't know where I was. They called Maxine, pretending to be looking for treatment. And you know Maxine . . ."

"Not really," I said.

"Well, she's very trusting. She almost fell for it; but luckily, she called me first. It took them months to find me. The trouble was, the patients couldn't find me either."

There was nowhere else to look for evidence but Jimmy's Brownsville apartment. The problem for the FBI was that they couldn't enter without "probable cause." Jimmy had already gone to Tijuana, leaving the apartment occupied only by two Costa

Rican girls. One was Junie's 16-year-old daughter, who had been living with Junie until the sting operation. The other was a 27-year-old woman who had been hired by Junie to be her daughter's companion while she finished school. The ploy used by the FBI was to arrange for a "health inspection" by the health department.

Dixon was present, but he cautiously did not enter. He prepared his inventory outside. This inventory of contraband formed the basis for the criminal search warrant that followed.

"They can't do that," I gratuitously opined.

"They did it," Jimmy replied.

The Brownsville Herald reported on January 25, 1984:

> *The Texas Attorney General's Office has filed suit against the owner of a fraudulent cancer clinic, and a platoon of federal, state and local law enforcement authorities have raided two Brownsville condominiums occupied by his staff, turning up a large cache of illegal drugs.*

On January 26, the series continued:

> *State and federal authorities today were still sifting through boxes of drugs, medical equipment and a pile of documents seized in a search of condominiums occupied by relatives and employees of the owner of the Universal Health Center [Keller's Matamoros clinic] . . . . 'By working closely with the FBI during this very difficult and dangerous investigation,' [Attorney General] Mattox said, 'we hope that enough evidence of federal criminal violations has been gathered so that the FBI can pursue Keller and his bunch wherever they try to hide.'*

The reports, Jimmy observed drily, were exaggerated. The "very dangerous investigation" was opposed only by the two terrified Costa Rican girls, who were neither his employees nor his relatives; and the "large cache of illegal drugs" was nowhere identified in the government's list of contraband that formed the basis for the ensuing criminal search warrant. The warrant listed only "Xylocaine and Magnesium Chloride, which are drugs which are required to bear the legend: CAUTION: FEDERAL LAW PROHIBITS DISPENSING WITHOUT PRESCRIPTION." They were not dangerous narcotics or illegal drugs. They were simply prescription drugs.

Also listed as contraband was the Digitron. "It didn't work," Jimmy said. "It was an old one we left behind. They also got my patient records. Without the names of my Matamoros patients, they couldn't have built a case."

Without his records, Jimmy had another problem. He couldn't call his patients to line them up as witnesses, or prove that his treatments worked. On the bright side, if the search was improper, the indictment could be too. It was the kind of technicality for which liberal courts had been known to dismiss a case. Jimmy said Silversmith was planning to bring a motion on it. Constitutional law was his strong suit. The question was whether the district court in Brownsville was a liberal court.

On February 2, 1984, the <u>Brownsville Herald</u> reported that felony arrest warrants had been issued against James G. Keller and eleven others, who had "lured desperate cancer patients here with claims of an almost total cure rate." But only one "victim" was actually identified, and she wasn't a patient. The patient was her husband. I'll call them Jackie and Tom Turner. The complaint said the suspects "intentionally conspired to commit the offense of theft from Jackie Turner and other persons not known." I had already read Jackie's testimony at the 1985 trial. If we had to go to trial again in 1991, we expected to hear a complete replay of it.

According to her testimony, by the time Tom was treated at Jimmy's clinic in 1983, he had already been through the conventional cancer mill. He was misdiagnosed with Crohn's disease when he was in Saudi Arabia working for Conoco Oil Co. When he was opened up surgically late in 1982 in Oklahoma, his surgeon found cancer of the colon. By February of 1983, the cancer had spread to his liver and his prognosis looked grim. He underwent chemotherapy, but the disease only wound up spreading faster after he took the drugs. His doctor told him there was nothing more he could do. In Texas, another doctor offered Tom a second, more toxic chemotherapy, but Tom refused. He opted for Jimmy's clinic.

"He told me the chemo was just making him worse," Jimmy said. "When he came in early December, he was in bad shape. He was in the back of a pickup truck on a mattress in horrible pain. We gave him the first shots in the truck so he wouldn't have to move. He started getting better and better, and started coming into the clinic. The last time I saw him was the day after the clinic was closed, when I drove back from Houston to do one more day's treatment. We were on the second floor, but by then he was so much improved that he was able to walk up the stairs by himself. He was so happy with my treatments that he wanted to make some video tapes, so the news of what we were doing could get broadcast out. But he always seemed to be strung out on drugs. He was taking narcotics for pain. I told him he should get off them as soon as he could. Narcotics are very destructive. They're the antithesis of getting well. That's what the war on drugs is all about. But Tom said he wasn't in pain. He said he kept telling them that, but they were forcing him to take the drugs."

"Who was forcing him?"

"His wife and the FBI. He said there were FBI agents at their house in McAllen every night. He said I should be careful, because his wife was talking to the FBI."

"You're kidding!"

"No. But she overheard him and denied it. She said he was hallucinating."

I wondered if Jackie had sought out the FBI, or if the FBI had sought her. I also wondered how she felt about her husband.

"If you want my opinion . . ." Jimmy paused and cleaned his glasses.

"I do," I said.

"I don't think she cared very much for him. It seemed like she would be glad when he got out of the way. I don't think she liked taking care of a sick person. No doubt the FBI thing gave her an opportunity to feel like she was doing something for the government. If you're doing something for the government, you can't be doing wrong. And they probably told her there would be some rewards for cooperating. I don't know what, but I do know she got a house in Oklahoma. She was on the government witness protection plan. She said the bank got it for her, but did you ever hear of a bank giving people houses?"

"No."

According to further testimony at trial, in January of 1984, Tom Turner was rushed to the hospital by helicopter. He'd been heavily medicated. He was on narcotics for pain and antiemetics to counteract the nausea caused by the narcotics. Soon, he was dead. The cause of death was listed as cardiopulmonary arrest, with diffuse metastasis from primary liver carcinoma as a secondary cause. But what, Jimmy wondered, had caused Tom's cardiopulmonary arrest? Jimmy suspected narcotics.

# Chapter 18

## Tijuana

When he got to Tijuana in January of 1984, Jimmy first stayed in a hotel on the American side of the border. FBI agents were right behind. They didn't have a warrant or an indictment, but they were making inquiries. The woman who ran the hotel told him they had come around looking for him.

"What did you tell them?" he asked, alarmed.

"I told them," she said coyly, "I didn't know who they were talking about."

He had come to the right place. The woman routinely housed patients and took them to various clinics. Once she had been arrested for it, and had been mistreated in an American jail. But she had beaten the charges and was still engaged in that nefarious pursuit.

"She was hiding me," Jimmy said. "She could keep deep, dark secrets." It reminded me of the Fugitive Slave Law of the 1850s, which made hiding people who were attempting to take charge of their own lives a felony.

Later, I read this imaginative projection of the Prohibition-like scenes to come if the FDA were to get its way in banning therapeutic natural supplements from the over-the-counter market:

> *FDA agents, trained by undercover experts from the FBI, are shutting down holistic medical clinics, raiding warehouses filled with imported herbs, and arresting nutritionists across*

*the country for practicing medicine without a license. Dietary-
supplement prohibition has come to America. 'Speakeasy'-type
underground clubs and brain-nutrient parties are flourishing
-- a sign of deep cultural interest in the banned substances.
Activists scramble to find safe sources for CoQ10, N-
acetylcysteine (NAC), chromium, evening primrose oil, and
smuggled Chinese herbs for people with HIV, cancer, diabetes,
PMS, and a host of other illnesses. Unfortunately, some people
are getting sick and some are dying from contaminated black-
market amino acids and nutrients. Many products are
counterfeit, containing less than the correct potency or
containing none at all. Other people are dying because they
cannot find sources for the nutrients and herbal therapies that
had been benefiting them.[51]*

In the nutritional supplement field, these scenes were still
largely hypothetical. But in the cancer arena, nutrient smuggling
was already big business. Jimmy knew because after he left the
hotel at the border, he stayed with a woman whom he described
as at one time one of the biggest smugglers of laetrile into the
United States. I'll call her Arlene. ("She was just a friend," he
explained. "She was a friend of Rudnov's, who was helping me
because I was still his best customer.")

While Jimmy was staying with Arlene, she asked him to pick
up a shipment of amygdalin from the Mexican federal police. "She
bought it for $5,000," he said. "It was worth maybe $100,000."
The shipment had been sent to Tijuana from Germany by way of
Mexico City, and had been intercepted by Mexican officials at
the border on its way to California. The carrier was a young
unsuspecting American who didn't really know what he'd gotten
himself into. He knew he was carrying laetrile, but he didn't know
how seriously that crime would be taken by the authorities. He
was beaten and tortured by Mexican officials, then arrested again
by the Americans on the other side. Someone had tipped off
officials on both sides of the border.

"The only other person who knew about the shipment," said
Jimmy, "was Rudnov. He diverted it to Arlene. It was enough
raw material to start a business making laetrile, and that's what
she did with it; she started a laetrile factory. Later, I heard about
another case where a man got busted at the border carrying laetrile
that nobody except Rudnov knew about."

"And he was one of your friends?" I said dubiously.

Jimmy looked pensive. "I've been known to make mistakes." He seemed to be thinking of someone else. "Rudnov had a good product -- Tumorex. I wouldn't call him a friend."

I thought of a notorious laetrile case involving an actor. "Didn't Steve McQueen go to Tijuana for laetrile, and then die?"

"He did," Jimmy said, "but he didn't die of cancer. He died of a heart attack after surgery. The way I heard it, the clinic had gotten him better. It was the Santa Maria Clinic in Rosarito. They didn't just use laetrile. They used a lot of different immune-supporting therapies. But he left before they were done with him. He went back to smoking and drinking and his old ways. He had a relapse and had surgery, and died of a heart attack under sedation."

"Like Tom Turner," I remarked.

Jimmy nodded in a meaningful way. "I'm sure there were people who were glad to have McQueen out of the way. He was making a lot of bad press for conventional medicine and a lot of good press for unconventional medicine. After he died, the clinic he went to in Rosarito got so much bad publicity it went out of business."

> *Later, I read a biography of Steve McQueen confirming Jimmy's version of the actor's death.*[52] *Another source stated that McQueen "had been given up by his physicians as a terminal case when he tried laetrile. He was responding well until a physician persuaded him to undergo surgery on a tumor; he then died on the operating table of an embolism. The Establishment proclaimed that this proved the laetrile treatment was worthless."*[53]

"Of course," Jimmy conceded, "he may not have been getting the best laetrile either. The stuff available in Tijuana then wasn't much good. Most of it had been heated and was racemic."

"Racemic?"

"Inactive. The 'levo' form had become partly 'dextro,' or righthand-rotating. The releasing factor that releases cyanide into the cancer cell doesn't work on righthand-rotating amygdalin. The better product came from Germany, but you couldn't get it then; and the injections that you could get didn't do much, so I got suspicious of them. I was using oral laetrile and apricot pits instead. I mixed aloe vera cream with a big laetrile tablet and about half a teaspoon of DMSO to dissolve it. Skin cancers were almost eliminated with this mash. But I still needed a good injectable."

"For someone who majored in economics," I remarked, "you know a lot about chemistry."

Jimmy shook his head. "I don't know so much. All I needed to know was what remedies checked out. What chemistry I did know I picked up here and there -- from Pops, and I listened to people who knew. I got over the barrier of thinking I didn't dare do anything myself. I had all my own formulas. When I found out what was in Tumorex, I improved on it. I added DMSO as a carrier. It was particularly good in brain cancer and scar tissue cases. Scar tissue isn't easy to penetrate, but DMSO will ride through cells without damaging them."

"I see. So did you ever get a good injectable laetrile?"

"I did. I talked to the chemist who was working with Arlene, who supplied all the Tijuana clinics with remedies. I told him the stuff he was making wasn't effective. The most effective kind is a freeze-dried powder that dissolves easily and can be reconstituted right before injection, so it stays biologically active. The chemist said, 'I know.' He was just making what the other clinics had asked for. It was cheaper to make and to ship. I asked if he could make the active form, and he said he thought so. He tried and succeeded, and thus came the first good lefthand-rotating laetrile to Tijuana. I bought from him, and so did some of the other clinics; but some of them just went on using the racemic injections."

It was another downside, I thought, of the black market: government suppression was allowing unscrupulous businessmen to peddle inferior products. Quality was unregulated, since the government declined to recognize the quality of any of it.

Jimmy chuckled as he recalled another incident involving this chemist. It also involved a hot-and-heavy competitor I'll call Dr. Block. "The chemist told me Block told him to snoop around my clinic to see what I was using to get such good results. The chemist told Block I was using the same remedies that were available to all the other clinics."

"So what was your secret of success?"

"Well, we did have some things the others didn't have," Jimmy said, "but it wasn't so much what we had as what we did with it.

Patients all get out of balance in different ways. You can't give them the same remedies in the same amounts at the same times and expect miraculous results. I figured out which and when and how much by radionics or kinesiology. The other clinics wouldn't use anything like radionics, because they were trying to establish credibility with the conventional people. But I was just trying to get people well."

"Interesting. Okay, so the FBI were making inquiries in Tijuana. Did they ever get a warrant for your arrest?"

"They got a Texas warrant," Jimmy said, "but it wasn't enforceable in Mexico."

"That's true." I had actually looked at the treaty between Mexico and the United States. It provided that a fugitive could be arrested on a U.S. indictment only through extradition procedures involving a prior hearing before a Mexican tribunal, and a determination that the crime was one for which extradition was appropriate. Extradition wasn't granted for activities that weren't crimes in both countries. "Did they ever try to extradite you?" I asked.

"I heard they did try a legal procedure once through Mexico City to get me," Jimmy said, "but I never got served with any papers. My Mexican attorney just told me about it. The judge took one look at it and said, 'You can't extradite a person in Mexico for something that isn't a crime in Mexico,' and threw it out. It's not a crime in Mexico to claim a high success rate for natural remedies. Besides that, I had an *amparo*."

"What's an *amparo?*"

It means 'protection.' It's the equivalent of habeas corpus in advance. If you have an *amparo*, they can't arrest you and lock you up without some evidence against you, and they have to give you an appointed hearing to bring the evidence forward. They have to have a complainant, and they can't touch you till the hearing date. Usually, they don't show up at the hearing. But after that, they have to leave you alone."

"So how did they manage to arrest you in 1991?"

"You tell me. There was never any hearing."

"In fact," I asked after thinking about it, "how did they even get a Texas warrant for your arrest? Your clinic wasn't in Texas."

"That's right," Jimmy said. "I think that's why the case got moved to federal court -- and how the prosecutor got promoted to U.S. Attorney. He already had an indictment from the state of Texas, when somebody realized there weren't any grounds for state jurisdiction."

The federal prosecutor in charge of Jimmy's case was a man I'll call Meier. Some private investigation revealed that in 1984, he was a mere assistant state district attorney. He was fresh from law school at the University of Texas, where he graduated in 1980. After that, he clerked in federal court -- for the same judge who was sitting on Jimmy's case now. Needless to say, we did not consider this a good sign. Meier's office was in the same building as the judge's. We had nervous visions of them maintaining friendly relations over lunch.

"I don't know this for a fact," Jimmy explained his cryptic remark, "but I think Meier was bumped up to 'Special U.S. Attorney' just so he could prosecute my case in federal court. Eventually they dropped the 'special' part and he was promoted to U.S. Attorney."

"I see . . . They could base federal jurisdiction on telephone calls that were considered 'wire fraud' in interstate commerce."

"Exactly." Jimmy arched an eyebrow. "Quackbusting is a sure bet, you know, for furthering a government career. The woman undercover agent who did the sting operation got a nice promotion too."

"Ominous. So what happened after they got a Texas warrant for your arrest?"

"Well, they showed up at my brother Ron's house in Houston. His wife was home alone with the children. They said an arrest warrant is a search warrant, which isn't true. And the warrant was for me, and I didn't even live there. Ron lived there, and he wasn't named in the state indictment. But his wife was too intimidated not to let them in. They bullied her, threatened the kids and pulled all their stuff out. Then Dixon used the information he got from the raid to get Ron fired from his job."

"Wow! What was Ron's job? He'd gotten out of radiology, right?"

"Right. He was disillusioned with it, and he could make more money in sales. He'd gotten a job as a sales representative for a company that made radiation measurement devices. He'd been with them for ten years, and they'd just offered him the position of regional sales manager in Denver, when Dixon told his boss it was best if they let Ron go. Dixon said Ron was involved in a big conspiracy, and that the government suspected the company of making the radionics instruments."

"Did they?"

"Of course not. But Dixon said Ron was going to be indicted, and if the company let Ron go, the government would probably forget the investigation against the company."

"How did Dixon know Ron was going to be indicted?"

"Good question. No grand jury had met yet. Ron worked for me in Matamoros, but only for a couple of months, while he was down there getting treatment himself. But Dixon must have made out a convincing case. The vice president of the company met with Ron after that and said he was the best salesman they'd ever had. They hated to see him go, but Dixon had threatened to practically put them out of business and they had no alternative. It was the second job Ron lost to the cancer industry. It cost him his marriage. He couldn't take care of his family anymore. He tried to get another job, but he couldn't. He was blackballed from everything."

"That's awful!"

Jimmy nodded. "But Ronnie was pretty bold in those days, and he was mad. He made up his mind to sue Dixon and some other people for searching his house without a warrant. He went to see Governor Edwards' personal attorney at the governor's mansion. People said, 'You're going to the governor's mansion? You better watch out!' But Ron went. And at first, the attorney seemed interested. He said, 'It looks like we have a good case here.' Then he kept Ron waiting in his office for what seemed like hours, while Ron sat around wondering what was happening. When the attorney finally came back, he said, 'This thing is too big for me. I can't handle it.'"

"Why did he say that?"

"That's what we wondered."

"Your brother sounds like an interesting guy," I remarked. "I'd like to meet him."

"He's in hiding now."

"Maybe after you win this case."

"Do you think I'm going to win?"

"I do," I said.

The successful lawyer assures the client with confident statements like, "It's in the bag!" It was a technique I needed to work on. My assurances didn't sound very convincing even to me.

# Chapter 19

## The Rosarito Raid

Jimmy's pursuers couldn't get him by extradition to the United States, and they couldn't find anyone willing to complain. That left the less savory options -- kidnapping and murder. He was convinced they had tried both. The first time, he said, was during Easter week of 1984. He had a clinic then in Rosarito, a charming resort town on the beach south of Tijuana.

"Nice place," I remarked. "How did you wind up there?"

"I was looking for a place for a new clinic," Jimmy said, "and Betty Lee Morales had volunteered to help. She and Andrew McNaughton wanted to build a hospital in Rosarito and put me in it. McNaughton was the Canadian test pilot who started all the clinics down there. He'd heard Krebs and was impressed with laetrile."

"And Betty Lee Morales was president of the Cancer Control Society," I said. "I heard her speak once, in the seventies."

Jimmy nodded. "She was also one of the founders of the National Health Federation. Thirty years ago, she was the queen of nutrition in the United States." He sighed. "If Betty had lived, I wouldn't be here today."

"Why do you say that?"

"She was my protector in Tijuana. I became known as 'Betty Lee's little boy.'" He laughed. "Do I look like a little boy? To Betty Lee maybe I was. She was an elderly lady, but she was wise! She was the master of the movement. It all fell apart after she died. Once she said, 'Right now I keep them all moving along. Nobody fights. But after I go, they're going to kill each other.'

And she was right. She had the power to arbitrate. She'd say, 'Now you sit down here and you sit down. We're not going to have a fight. We're going to have a united front.' And everybody did what she said. After she died, the NHF split up, and everybody started suing each other. They all thought their therapies were the best and were suspicious of the others."

It was a problem I had read about before. Rivalry had plagued the natural health care movement from its inception. The fierce competition among unorthodox schools contrasted sharply with the cartel-like standardization imposed on conventional doctors by the AMA.[54] The hallmark of the natural health care movement was freedom and individuality, a lack of standardization and rigidity that led to jealousies and rivalries. The closest thing to a united front it had to offer were the National Health Federation and the Cancer Control Society, held together by their "guru" Betty Lee.

"How did she die?" I asked.

"It was in a car accident, in '88 or '89."

"That's too bad. So why had she taken an interest in you?"

"She said she thought I was getting the best results. She came down to Matamoros in '83 to check out my clinic. That was what she did. She'd been all over the world investigating unconventional therapies, and everyone respected her opinion. She started out by asking me what I knew about acid/alkaline balance. It was her thing. I said I'd heard her lecture, and I repeated what she'd said: if your acid/alkaline balance isn't right, you'll never get well. Bad bacteria, fungus, viruses all live in and produce an alkaline base. Good bacteria, like acidophilus bulgaricus, live in and produce an acid base. The good ones and the bad ones compete with each other. Putrifying, undigested foods produce toxicity, making bad bacteria, causing fermentation and putrefaction. You gas up, build up methane gas. Gas is an expression of poor digestion, fermentation, putrefaction. If you have this problem, alkalizers -- especially aluminum-based alkalizers -- are going to hurt, not help. If your first morning urine is alkaline or even neutral, you've got a problem. I was using Betty's urine test papers. The test shows how much hydrochloric acid you need. If you eat wrong, it will always show up in this urine test. I always infused hydrochloric acid the first day the patients came in. It would safely balance the body whether it was acid or alkaline."

I winced. "You put hydrochloric acid right in the vein?"

"It doesn't hurt," Jimmy said. "It's a little-known fact, but there's a type that's specially manufactured for intravenous use.

In fact hydrochloric acid is the <u>only</u> strong acid you can safely use intravenously, because the body produces it. I was using Betty's 'Protagen,' which is hydrochloric acid with enzymes."

"I can see why she liked your answers," I remarked. "They were her answers."

"I suppose," Jimmy said, "but what really convinced her was when she talked to the patients and heard their stories. Then she started sending patients to me, and one of them was her husband. He had a mysterious disease that was finally traced to a spider bite. I helped him recover. After that, Betty told everyone I had the best success rate and was the best place to go. John Adderley and Frank Cousineau said the same thing."

I could confirm that. These two men, along with Cancer Control Society co-founder Lorraine Rosenthal, were the tour guides who had told me privately in 1990 that if they had cancer, they'd choose Keller's clinic. All three later sent supporting letters to the court, and Frank had agreed to testify for the defense.

"So Betty Lee and Andrew McNaughton set you up in a hospital in Rosarito," I got back to the scene of the raid.

"Not exactly," Jimmy said. "It was Dr. Block who wound up with the big hospital on the beach."

"Too bad! What happened?"

"Well, another doctor had a clinic in Rosarito." Jimmy gave the doctor's name, but I'll call him Dr. Garcia. "McNaughton thought Garcia was a good guy and wanted me with him. Garcia treated degenerative diseases, but not very successfully. He had all the equipment and all the money, but he wasn't a very good doctor. That's why he was interested in me, but I didn't trust him. I worked with him for three weeks, but then he doubled the rates on my patients in his hospital. The patients complained, so I left and went to La Quinta."

La Quinta was nearby on the beach. Jimmy rented a cottage there and set up a makeshift clinic. But he didn't last long there either. The FBI had no jurisdiction in Mexico, but they were undeterred by that technicality . . .

Jimmy's son David had come to the La Quinta clinic with his wife for the Easter holidays. On April 19, 1984, David tried to cross the border to tend to some inconsequential business on the American side. The <u>Brownsville Herald</u> reported that day, "Customs agents became suspicious when [David] Keller appeared nervous while crossing the border. He was arrested when his name came up in a computer check."

That was the <u>Herald</u>'s version, but David said no one had even asked him for identification. They seemed to know him by his car. Jimmy was stunned. Why had his son been arrested? And how had they found him? The cottage was well hidden, and few people knew its whereabouts. He thought over the possibilities. On the Tuesday before Easter, Rudnov had made a large Tumorex delivery to the clinic.

I heard more of this story later from Don McBride. Don said he had been visiting in La Quinta with his family the same week. They had come in their 25-foot motor home with their dune buggy, bringing Maxine and a massage table. On Holy Thursday, they returned to take Maxine to the airport; but the woman was nowhere to be seen. What the McBrides did see was a plain white car. "That looks like an FBI car," Don's teenage daughter casually remarked. (The McBrides had friends who were FBI agents.) Then they spotted two American men. Festively decked out in sombreros, sunglasses and Hawaian shirts, they looked suspiciously like undercover FBI. A Mexican state policeman accompanied them.

"It was pretty funny," Don chuckled. "They were running around like Keystone cops. Jimmy was within 100 feet of them in another cottage, but he got away." Don added that he made political trouble for the FBI later: "They had no business down there in Mexico."

Jimmy told the rest. "Someone came flying back and said they were there. About a mile north, I'd rented a beach house from Arlene. I rented it for the phone, which usually took two years to get. The clinic didn't have one. There was nothing in the beach house -- no furniture or electricity or anything -- nothing except Mexican water and the telephone. We said a prayer, and then Junie and I pretended we were lovers. I took off my glasses and shirt. We were laughing and hugging. We walked right by the FBI down the beach to the beach house. By the next morning, I'd arranged over the phone to have a clinic going in Tijuana. I had medicines stored in different places. Before I moved to La Quinta, I'd rented space in the building where Rudnov's doctor associate had his office. I called the doctor from the beach house phone and referred my patients to him. So I had a clinic running by telephone, while I was hiding out and the FBI were trying to get me. They occupied the clinic illegally for four days. They had a manhunt. They interrogated the patients and terrified them. Some of the patients left and never came back. We stayed in the beach house till Tuesday of the next week. The FBI waited those four days, then they found out that I had the clinic going somewhere else. They were furious. When I called my attorney in San Diego, he said the FBI had called him. They said they had given my picture to the Mexican police with the order, 'Armed and dangerous. Shoot on sight.' Shoot on sight!" Jimmy shook his head. "If you ask me, it's unconstitutional."

"What is?"

"The FBI. It's actually a federal police force."

"Were you armed and dangerous?"

"No. I didn't even have a gun in the clinic. I had one in Baton Rouge, but it was legal there. They gave the order after I escaped from the clinic. My attorney in San Diego said to head for the border and turn myself in, but I was afraid I'd get shot on sight. I called Foglio, my Mexican attorney, and he said to stay put until Monday. By then he'd have my *amparo* in place and a demand out against the FBI agents. I'd had an *amparo* already, but Foglio must have let it lapse. Later, he told me he'd heard that the FBI had paid the Mexican police $40,000 to help get me."

"You're kidding! The FBI paid $40,000 to have you shot on sight?"

"I don't know that for a fact," Jimmy conceded, "but that was the rumor; and it made me plenty nervous, I can tell you. One thing I didn't want to do was to get caught by the Mexican police. I'd heard too many stories about Mexican jails."

I nodded, having heard some myself.

"In the end," Jimmy said, "Foglio took me to the Mexican federal police. It was the state police who had been after me. We went with about eighty affidavits, telling what I was doing and how people were getting well. Foglio knew the chief of the Mexican federal police, and the guy spoke perfect English. He read the affidavits and was impressed. The chief said, 'I know what this is all about. Don't worry about a thing.' Foglio told me that if the chief said something, he meant it -- and he didn't take bribes. 'Don't worry,' Foglio said. 'Enjoy Mexico.' A few days later, Foglio said everything was taken care of. The chief had gotten on the phone to the head of the FBI in San Diego and told him to leave me alone. He said if anyone else came over and hassled me, they'd lock him up. And that was the last time we ever saw FBI agents in Tijuana."

I wondered what had happened to Maxine. Jimmy said she'd had a premonition of trouble and had gone back with someone else. "I tried to talk her out of it," he said, shaking his head. "She'd have been a lot better off staying in Mexico."

Along with the Texas state indictment issued against Jimmy in March of 1984, a civil suit was filed in Salt Lake City, enjoining Maxine from using the telephone. She was ordered not to give out Jimmy's phone number, relay calls to him, or talk to him. When patients called, she sometimes broke down and cried; but she told them she could not give out his number.

"She cooperated completely," Jimmy observed, "and they rewarded her with a jail sentence. I was stopped cold. The patients felt abandoned. People were dying and looking for medicine and wanting to get treated. Old patients wanted to come. But nobody knew how to find us. Howard Smith said he looked for me for two months before he found me. Then when he did, I was suspicious and afraid to let him come."

Later, I read in a letter from author Sally Wolper that people had come to see Jimmy from all over the world, "including a Tibetan monk who searched for him for over a year."

"Did you ever treat Howard Smith?" I asked.

"I did, and he's doing well. He was the man who brought me the research on CSA -- chondroiton sulfate. It was a study done at Loma Linda University in the seventies. I doubt you could find it in the library though. It was suppressed. I don't even know where my copy is now. I had it in the clinic in Tijuana."

He slumped in his chair. "Everything in my clinic is gone -- all my remedies and research and files and equipment. I had some great machines. There was one we called the 'sweep' machine that I had made up specially. It went around every eight seconds putting out a vibration. I had a Kirlian camera that measured energy fields. I had a machine that transferred the radiant qualities of one substance into another. It didn't have a name or a manufacturer. I just came across these things and tried them out, and if they worked, I used them."

"What did the CSA study show?" I asked.

"That it can reverse heart disease. The arteries get clogged up as people age, and CSA opens them up. It cleans them out amazingly well. I gave it to all my cancer patients. It helped in arthritis too. It was one of the ingredients in Sulconar, which works better on heart patients than anything I've ever seen. I'd give two shots of Sulconar intra-muscularly to angina patients with crushing chest pains, and they'd be walking around pain-free. The real Sulconar came from Argentina. It was a combination of CSA and live cells from the inner heart and arteries of animal fetuses. You can't get it anymore though, even in Mexico. There's a product with the same name, but it's a fake."

I added "Sulconar" to my list of remedies, and wondered how many others he had forgotten to mention. "So what happened after you were raided in Rosarito?" I asked.

"Well, in May of '84, there was a big expose of my clinic on national TV. It was Peter Jennings on the ABC evening news. They showed an old, decrepit part of Rosarito, which is actually a beautiful resort city. I saw my old Digitron on the screen. Altogether I was exposed on national TV four times, and probably a hundred times on local TV in the Valley."

I smiled. "Some people will do anything for publicity."

Jimmy laughed. "The funny thing was, whenever we got exposed, we did seem to get more patients -- but that was later. In May of '84, I was down to one patient. I thought I'd never get the clinic going again. The FBI was doing all this interviewing, telling people we'd abandoned them and defrauded them; and I couldn't contact the patients, so they probably believed it." He cocked his head and paused for effect. "So guess what I did."

"What?"

"I sued the network that did the expose. I sued them for $15 million. I said they slandered me; they didn't give me a chance to rebut; they didn't do any investigation."

I smiled. "They call people like you vexatious litigants."

Jimmy laughed. "But it worked!"

He rummaged through his papers and produced a copy of the complaint he had filed against the network and Dr. Marley. The complaint alleged that when Dr. Marley had been asked, "What are the statistics of this clinic?", the doctor had replied, "Nil. Everyone that I have talked to that has received Tumorex is dead." Attached to it were the affidavits of surviving and satisfied patients.

"The network apologized," Jimmy said. "Then they made a very favorable documentary. They got six or seven testimonials. It was great publicity for about a year. Then they quit showing it. I called the guy and asked why. He said the FBI had told them the network was going to be indicted along with me, for conspiracy to distribute an unlicensed cancer drug."

So much, I thought, for freedom of speech and the press.

# Chapter 20

## Ferreting Out Witnesses

To get an indictment, the government needed not only "victims of the defendants' fraudulent scheme" but relatives willing to testify about them. The government wasn't sitting back and waiting for complaints. By its own count, the FBI had interviewed over one hundred patients or their relatives in their efforts to build a case.

"Your daughter's dead," an FBI agent said to Melba Call. "Why aren't you on our side?"

Melba retorted, "I didn't think you were supposed to have a side." In a notarized affidavit dated March 25, 1984, Melba wrote:

> . . . Yes, our beloved beautiful daughter died, but not from cancer, rather from the treatments Radiation and Chemotherapy. If she were alive today, she would be shouting from the housetops in an effort to save the lives of cancer victims, and declaring her firm belief in the effectiveness of the treatment TUMOREX in the treatment of cancer.
>
> . . . Jimmy Keller was actually opposed to treating Lois Ann and even more opposed to accepting any money, but both Lois Ann and I had such tremendous faith in this 'miracle treatment' that we finally persuaded him to give her the Tumorex treatment, and . . . she and our entire family believe that it did give her an additional six months at least to live.
>
> . . . We believe with all our hearts that [Maxine and Jimmy] should be blessed for their unselfish efforts to help people, not 'nailed to the wall,' so to speak, as it seems is

*going on at the present. Indeed, we and a multitude of others, believe that Tumorex treatments should be legalized. Let the Medical world put it under test and find out for themselves its effectiveness, thereby releasing innocent people from the crucifixion they are now experiencing at the hands of the News Media and the Law, and also let them continue to save lives from this monster CANCER.*

Blaine C____ also talked about his 1984 interview with the FBI in a letter. He wrote:

*I explained to [the agent] that I contacted Maxine and she did not contact me. There was no undue pressure on neither her part nor on Jimmy's part and certainly Jimmy did not promise me anything. . . . The agent wondered why I did not carry some hostility after learning what the medicine was made from and the price that [we] were charged. I told him I felt I got my money's worth by being exposed to a diet that I felt prolonged my life. . . . When he left he said it did not look like I was a hostile witness against these people and I told him absolutely not.*

Blaine wasn't a hostile witness, but his name now featured in one of the counts of the indictment.

"His wife," Jimmy explained.

"I see." Even when the patients were satisfied, the relatives could be disgruntled.

Marvin Sibner, a research scientist who had been a patient, wrote to the court, "the families of those who died sometimes want to lash out and blame instead of dealing with their own feelings of grief."

Sally Greer wrote in 1991 that she had recovered from breast cancer in 1985 as a result of Jimmy's treatments. "[Due] to my health I was told in the past that I would never have children," she said. But now, "with Jimmy's treatments and God's help I have the most precious, beautiful daughter." Oddly, despite this unexpected addition, her family was hostile. "The most miserable part was the ridicule of my family, and their ignoring me because I went to a 'quack' in Mexico instead of having a breast removed. To this day they still pretend nothing ever happened." It was an interesting commentary, I thought, on human nature.

As for the testifying relatives, no doubt they had been persuaded by the government that the defendant was a fraud. It was natural to side with the government, especially if the patient had died -- and we had heard that prospective witnesses had been told that <u>all</u> his patients were dead. The government had also told them that Jimmy's $3,000 treatment consisted of a common amino acid worth only a few dollars a bottle.

"It wasn't true," he said wearily. "The injectable arginine sold in the U.S. is $150 for thirty grams. That's enough for one infusion. My patients got about that much every day. So just the cost of the arginine, if they were getting it conventionally, would have been about what I was charging for the whole treatment; and I was using a lot of other stuff besides arginine."

While the FBI was busy ferreting out witnesses, a frantic Maxine had been equally busy soliciting letters and affidavits on behalf of the clinic. She had collected a huge stack of them. They reinforced Jimmy's contention that he hadn't been promising cures.

"Only God alone can cure cancer and Jimmy is always the first to tell you so," wrote Clifford Thomas of Akron, Ohio. "One thing for sure, Jimmy has never made any claim to cure cancer. He has only tried to help us cope and feel better. . . . I have lung cancer and I do feel much better after my visit with Jimmy. His treatment and diet plan along with daily vitamins to detoxify the body works wonders."

Al Lippman, another research scientist who had been a patient, wrote, "In all my time there, I heard Jimmy Keller repeatedly state over the phone and in the clinic . . . that he could not make any claims or guarantees of a cure whatsoever."

Floyd Conway wrote, "There were no promises of healing, only what we knew of others. The price they were asking was far less than we had already paid to the medical profession and with no good results." Floyd, who had taken a woman named Elma Ripko to Jimmy's clinic, went on to describe the patient's recovery:

> . . . *We took her in a bed in a station wagon. She was hardly able to sit up. Two weeks later she was free from cancer and has been ever since. She now works as an assistant manager of a busy office, some sixty hours a week. She looks fine and feels like her old self after one year. A year ago we did not expect her to live. Now she is the picture of health. What is that worth in dollars? It is priceless!*

While I was in the clinic I saw many others who could
testify to the same restoration of health. I saw Jimmy Keller
take people in who were burned up with radiation. Jimmy
tried to tell them not to spend the money and yet they insisted
so much that he tried to help.

Elma herself wrote, "I owe my life to him through the direction
of God Almighty and I shall be eternally grateful."

Jimmy hadn't been able to follow up on this patient and didn't
know what had become of her. But even if she were now dead, a
year of health beyond the death sentence imposed by her
oncologists seemed worth the trip to Matamoros. No doubt she
was stopping to smell the roses and kiss her grandchildren.

Pearl Gervais, according to the government, had indeed died,
although we didn't know when or how. But if she were a "victim"
of anything, it seemed to be chemotherapy. She wrote in 1984:

. . . After having thirty three cobalt and fifteen
chemotherapy [treatments] here in Green Bay, I was a very
sick person. I would have never lived through this past
Christmas. My appetite was gone completely and my weight
loss was tremendous. I'm sure my prayers were answered when
I heard about Jimmy Keller as I could no longer stand the
horrible treatments here. I was not forced in any way to go to
Matamoros, I and I myself made up my mind to go and in a
hurry as I knew time was running out.

After my very first treatment my appetite returned, I was
so happy I cried. Then I went out to eat for the first time in
months. I was not told that this or these treatments were a sure
cure and I and my husband were certainly treated with loyalty
there by Jimmy and the whole staff. We just loved them all.

As of now I am feeling super, my weight is coming back
very good and my appetite is tremendous. I can do my own
work and my friends tell me how happy they are for me.

I only hope and pray that one day very soon the AMA
will wake up to the fact that we here in America should have
more Jimmy Kellers and get rid of the torturous treatments we
must go through with, and the thousands of dollars we must
spend, and in the end be told to go home to die.

"So how many of your Matamoros patients had already had some kind of conventional treatment?" I asked Jimmy.

"Practically all of them. If you count biopsies, I guess all of them."

"Then they were practically all in the category of having only a '40 to 60 percent chance of success or cure,'" I mused. "And how many people did you treat in Matamoros?"

"About 200."

"That means you could have lost <u>100</u> patients and still have a 50 percent success rate! The government only has eleven 'victims' in its indictment. It's going to take some sleight of hand," I said confidently, "for them to prove their claims!"

Jimmy wasn't so confident. "The FBI is pretty good at sleight of hand," he said.

His assessment proved to be more realistic than mine.

# Chapter 21

## 1985 Trial

Jimmy's mother Beatrice died of a stroke in October of 1984, the same month three of her offspring were indicted on felony charges. On October 23, 1984, a sealed and secret indictment was issued against Jimmy, his brother Ron, and his son David. Also named were Maxine, her husband, and her brother-in-law, along with Junie and a nutritionist named Barbara. Two other defendants, Rudnov and a woman who had worked at the clinic, were named as unindicted co-conspirators: they were given immunity from prosecution in exchange for testifying for the government. But only Rudnov would actually take the stand.

"When did the grand jury meet that returned the indictment?" I asked.

"I don't think one ever did," Jimmy replied.

"That's unconstitutional!" I said. I hadn't actually practiced criminal law, but I had taken the course. The way I remembered it, a grand jury was guaranteed by the Bill of Rights. Its function was to decide whether there was "probable cause" to believe the suspect had committed a crime. Only if the jurors decided in the affirmative was an indictment returned. Then the case went to a trial jury to determine the question of guilt. That was the theory, but I had also read that in practice, grand juries generally rubber-stamped the wishes of the prosecutor. The defendant had no guaranteed right to be present or to rebut. Still, to have no grand jury at all seemed like a flagrant abuse of the Constitution.

"One met in July of '84," Jimmy qualified his remark, "but no indictment was returned then. We had a friend working in federal court who had learned they were meeting. They were ready to indict, when some of my people showed up -- Ronnie and some patients."

Jimmy said his brother was pushing his luck. Ron had just testified in a Senate hearing in Phoenix for Ken Anderson, who was convicted for the same thing Jimmy was being indicted for; and Ron had worked at Jimmy's clinic. Ron was being counseled by a man I'll call Brash, who wound up representing Ron in his lawsuit against Dixon. Brash wasn't a licensed attorney. He had gone to George Gordon's School of Common Law in Boise, Idaho.

"Brash got Ron into more trouble than he got him out of," Jimmy said wryly. "He was recommended by Rudnov. Later, we suspected he was working for Rudnov more than for us. Brash told Ron he should try to get subpoenaed to testify, and Ron rushed out and did it. In those days, we thought we just had to tell our stories and everybody would be on our side. Ron had to call the U.S. Attorney about ten times before he got through, and then he got referred to Dixon. It was the U.S. Attorney who should have been in charge of the grand jury, acting impartially on behalf of the people; but it was actually Dixon acting for the FBI. Dixon wasn't too friendly, but he told Ron that if he came down, he might get to testify; so Ron paid his own way down. My people had to force their way in, but two of them managed to take the stand. Ronnie testified how he'd seen patients getting well. He also presented a statement in English and Spanish showing that the grand jury was improperly impaneled and instructed."

The other witness who testified, Jimmy said, was Bonnie Cayer. I had read her story in a letter to the court. She was the wife of a California attorney and the grandmother of Wesley Smith, the two-year-old Jimmy had successfully treated for a brain tumor. Bonnie described Wesley's remarkable recovery. She also told about her own case. She had had vaginal bleeding and pain and was rapidly losing weight. She was biopsied, then told by three different doctors that she had cancer of the uterus and needed a hysterectomy. Having seen Wesley's recovery, however, she opted for Jimmy's clinic. The treatments stopped her bleeding and she returned to normal. A year later, when she testified before the grand jury, she was fine.

"She's still fine," Jimmy said. "She's been helping me line up witnesses. She's a gracious, wonderful friend who's done yeoman service for me."

I nodded. "So what did the grand jury decide?"

"They wouldn't return the indictment. The grand jury was dismissed."

"Amazing."

"It was. But the next day, Ron went with Brash into Dixon's office and served him with the lawsuit for searching Ron's house without a warrant. Dixon was furious. He said something about 'your phony fraud brother.' Ron backed Dixon up against the wall with his finger and said Dixon was the phony fraud."

"I see what you mean about pushing his luck!"

Jimmy nodded. "Ronnie's a little milder now. He says he's been humbled. What really got Dixon riled up was when Ron got a lien on his assets and his bank account. You know what happened. Dixon retaliated by naming Ron in the indictment. That got him out of the way all right. He didn't have a job anymore, and he had to go into hiding. He wound up joining me in Mexico. He couldn't prosecute a lawsuit from there. All he got out of the deal was that it turned him into a fugitive."

I shook my head. "But how did Dixon get an indictment if the grand jury was dismissed?"

"Good question. We never heard anything more about a grand jury. We just heard that Maxine had been arrested. That was about three months later. They would have had to impanel a new grand jury, hear testimony, and indict, all within that time. Our friend at court was watching closely and didn't see any sign of it, and the indictment wasn't signed by any grand jury foreman. If you ask me, Dixon was the grand jury."

"That's unconstitutional!" I reiterated my professional opinion.

Jimmy nodded. "Too bad we can't prove it."

We would get some corroboration later, when the government was unable to produce a copy of the transcript of the 1984 grand jury proceedings on demand. But by then, the issue was moot.

I heard the sequel to this story from Maxine. In October of 1984, she and her husband Eldon were holding a quiet business meeting in their living room with their Mormon neighbors, when three FBI agents and two policemen burst in. Television cameramen were right behind.

Maxine requested time to pray. "You should have thought about that before you got involved in this," came the curt retort. A mortified Maxine, her husband and her brother-in-law were arrested in front of their small Mormon community on the 6 p.m. local news. The suspects were handcuffed and thrown into a waiting car.

Jimmy described Barbara's arrest. It came at a court hearing where she was battling for custody of her children. Her ex-husband had apparently set her up. She was ignominiously hauled away as her children and relatives watched. Custody, needless to say, went to her ex-husband.

Ron escaped arrest. The FBI came looking for him in Denver, where his wife and four children were then living while he stayed in Houston trying to sell their house. But this time, his wife was ready for them. When the FBI pounded on the door, she didn't open it. "Who is it?" she asked through the door.

"The FBI," said the agent, who was accompanied by the local sheriff. "Open the door."

"What do you want?"

"Open the door or we're going to break it down."

When the agent pushed the door in, he was confronting a determined woman poised with a camera in one hand and a tape recorder in the other. She clicked a photo of him shoving his badge at her. "Before you ask any questions," she advised him, "I'm turning my tape recorder on. Do you have a Fourth Amendment warrant, sir?"

"No."

"You're not allowed in my house."

The agent told the sheriff to go in; but the sheriff, looking aggravated, declined.

It was a bold gesture on Ron's wife's part, but it was too late to save their marriage. Ron couldn't live in hiding. He wound up joining Jimmy in Mexico. Several years later, she and their four children joined him. But it didn't work out. The children couldn't speak Spanish, and they weren't learning much in school. She finally took them back to the United States. Ron sent money, and she sent the children for the summer. But later, to his grief, even that tenuous contact came to a halt.

The captured defendants were later released, but for Maxine, Barbara, and Jimmy's son David, it was only on bail to prepare for their defense. The three of them were scheduled for trial on

March 12, 1985. Their ring leader was still "at large," but the earlier conviction of his co-conspirators would set a precedent that could be quite useful to the prosecutor in Jimmy's later trial. Maxine retained an astute young attorney named Mike, who was a family friend. Mike protested that he wasn't a criminal attorney, but Maxine said he was like a son to her. He had practically grown up in her home. Mike's law firm contacted as many of Jimmy's 1983 patients as they could find.

"We did our research in January, February and March of '85," Maxine recalled. "We located 130 or 140 patients. Eighty percent of them were terminal -- Stage III and Stage IV -- and practically all of them had already had conventional treatment. Some people who came only had a week or ten days to live. Some of them were so bad off, Jimmy told them not to come; but they came anyway. It would have been a miracle if any of them were still alive. But 50 percent of them were alive in 1985."

"Really!" I said. "Then the representation of a 50 percent 'success or cure' rate could well have been true."

"I never said 'cure'," Maxine insisted. "I said benefit. I meant they got results. They got out of pain, the tumor went down, they felt better, they had more energy." She sounded distraught. "We put 13 months into research. We had five doctors and several experts coming. We also had 38 patients lined up. They were ready to testify to being at the clinic when people were treated free of charge, and to not being promised a cure. The attorneys' fees came to $142,000. We're still paying off the bill."

Two years in jail and $142,000 in debt: no wonder she sounded distraught, I thought.

It was an expensive trial, but the defense was well prepared. The trial began brilliantly for the defense -- too brilliantly, as it turned out. The government put Rudnov on the stand. He testified that he had provided samples of Tumorex to the FBI, and that it consisted of arginine and water. He also told how he had acquired the formula. Mike then asked him if he had ever represented a cure or success rate for Tumorex. Rudnov said he had not. Out of the presence of the jury, Mike proceeded to play a tape of a speech at a National Health Federation convention in April of 1982, in which Rudnov had made just such representations.

The tape wasn't properly introduced into evidence (if it had been, Mike would have lost the element of surprise), so the judge didn't allow it to be played before the jury. But Rudnov heard it, and so did the court and opposing counsel; and the judge said he would allow Mike to refer to it in his examination. Rudnov then admitted before the jury that he had indeed said that at his own clinic, he was getting "between an 80 and a 90 percent success ratio on the use of Tumorex."

"I would like you to explain to the Court and jury," said Mike, "what the difference is between a cure and a success ratio, sir."

Rudnov responded, "By 'success' we meant, and still do, that the patients -- 85 percent of all of the patients started to show regression of tumors; the pain would leave; they would get their appetite back; they would start having bowel movements, and they would show visible signs of improvement."

The implications were clear. The co-defendants had merely repeated the representations of the manufacturer, who had made the same representations researchers generally make when they refer to the effectiveness of a cancer treatment: regression of tumors, relief of pain, an increased sense of well-being.[55] The defendants had had no intent to defraud.

"We went home that night and celebrated," said Maxine. "We were thrilled."

But the party was premature. The next day, the prosecutor, apparently fearing defeat, hastily moved to ensure convictions by inducing plea bargains. Barbara would get a suspended sentence and Maxine would get a mere slap on the wrist ("probably not more than six months, with 3-1/2 to serve") if they would plead guilty to a lesser crime, misprision of a felony. ("Misprision" means they had knowledge of the crime and did nothing about it.) Eldon and Don, who had worked at the clinic and could have been convicted along with Maxine, would go free. And if the women refused? The prosecutor threatened to arrest their friends and relatives, including Don McBride and Lowell Dayton, for "guilt by association." The prosecutor would also arrest Barbara's 19-year-old son (who had helped around the clinic) and Maxine's elderly and ailing parents (who had sometimes answered the phone in her home) for conspiracy.

Earlier, Maxine and Barbara had been told that if they would cooperate in a scheme to entrap their leader, they would not have to go to jail. They were to tell Jimmy that a wealthy patient was waiting on a boat off Rosarito Beach, where his clinic then was. The patient was too sick to come on land. Could Jimmy come aboard? The FBI would be waiting on the boat. It must have been a tempting offer, but both women loyally refused. The plea bargain, however, was harder to turn down. Their friends and relatives were at stake. "Maxine cried and cried," Eldon recalled. "'It's better to do this,' she said."

At this critical juncture, Mike's wife, who was expecting a baby, had a sudden attack of "placenta previa" (hemorrhage in the last trimester). Mike was unexpectedly called away. In his place he left a young attorney who was new to the firm and who purported to have more experience than he did. The young replacement stood silent, as the two terrified women agreed to plead guilty.

David Keller, who had been depending on the trial preparation of Maxine's attorneys, wound up continuing the trial alone and representing himself. The prosecutor had attempted to get him to plea bargain too, but David was convinced the government had no case against him and declined the offer. He hadn't had much to do with the clinic. He had just had some time off and was helping out, arranging housing and transportation for the patients; and he hadn't said much of anything to the undercover agents involved in the sting operation. ("He was arrested because he was my son," Jimmy complained.)

The critical testimony at David's trial came from the woman undercover agent. I'll call her Narda Gomez.

"Gomez testified that Maxine and David both told her that their 'son' could be cured by Christmas," Jimmy said. "It was an obvious fabrication. We were planning to close the clinic for the holidays, so new patients were being postponed until January. Their 'son' couldn't have been treated before that. But there was no way to prove it."

Thinking that sting operations are usually tape recorded, David had asked before the trial for all "Brady material" -- any tangible evidence in the possession of the government that might be of use to the defense, including tape recordings. The law required it to be produced on demand, but the government had produced none. In open court, David had then asked Ms. Gomez if the sting operation had been taped, but she had answered in the negative.

It was a point that would be contested, but not until six years later. In the meantime, David was found guilty of a felony. But he still felt he had made the right decision in refusing the plea bargain. When sentence was issued on April 22, 1985, he got only 45 days. Jimmy said the judge had actually commended David on his performance -- then added that he wished he could say as much for the prosecutor.

The plea-bargaining women fared substantially worse. They sat in stunned and disbelieving silence, as the U.S. Attorney stood up and announced that for the heinous crimes they had committed, they should receive the maximum sentence. Maxine was sentenced to 36 months and Barbara was sentenced to 30 months in federal prison.

"Even the maximum time for misprision was then fourteen months," said an anguished Maxine, "and it was later dropped to ten. They promised us even less time than that."

"Why didn't your attorney announce the plea bargains in open court?" I asked.

"I guess he didn't know he was allowed to. He told us to keep quiet and confess to everything. I had to confess that I'd made fraudulent representations to Jackie Turner, and I never even talked to the woman. We were at an NHF Convention the day she said she called. She said I stole $9,000 from her and defrauded her, and I'd never even heard the sound of her voice."

Maxine served 24-1/2 months and Barbara served 18-1/2 months in federal prison in Pleasanton, California. The last five months were in a halfway house: they went out to work during the day and returned to prison at night.

Maxine, a sheltered and religious Mormon, told some shocking prison tales, including rampant sexual escapades at the co-ed prison. She said her Mormon undershirt proved to be a problem. She had to battle to keep it on when she was body-searched each time her husband came to visit. She thought the experience may have been harder on him, however, than on her. He had a nervous breakdown, and wavered between thoughts of suicide and homicide.

Barbara described her experiences in an interview with <u>Los Angeles Times</u> reporter Paul Ciotti. She said she was chained around the waist, handcuffed, and shackled at the ankles. She had hurt her foot in a motorcycle accident, and the shackles were so tight on it that she cried. When she stepped down from the prison bus, a loose bit of chain caught on the grill of the step, causing her to fall over the shoulder of a guard. He kept pulling on the chain, and she crawled to the prison door screaming in pain. Her ankle wasn't x-rayed until two weeks later. The technician said he saw nothing; but Barbara, who could read x-rays, pointed out five fractures. The technician replied that if she made trouble, he would send her to prison in Kentucky.

Barbara also talked about her experiences at the Matamoros clinic. "We worked eighteen hours a day. It was very demanding. We had never run a cancer clinic before. We had to learn everything. People came in, they'd had chemo, they'd had radiation. They were practically glowing in the dark. The treatment didn't work for everybody. Maybe they were too far gone to start with. Maybe it was just their time to die. When you lost one, it was devastating. I'm not ashamed of going to prison, but it's terrible to be an ex-con. Every application asks if you've been convicted of a felony. The hardest part, though, is dealing with the anger of my kids."

By all accounts, the 1985 defendant who fared the best was Rudnov the informer. His history of informing apparently went well beyond this case. There was the incident involving Wickman and Anderson, then the laetrile busts at the border. Jimmy had heard that Rudnov had also informed his way out of an earlier stock broker's scandal. Rudnov seemed to enjoy an immunity that went further than mere protection from past wrongs. In open court, he promised to get out of the Tumorex business; but Jimmy said he had merely moved his business to the Bahamas. A year later, he was back in business in Tijuana. In 1991, when Jimmy stood trial, Rudnov was still making and selling Tumorex, and he was still successfully operating a Tijuana clinic. He was a wealthy and powerful man, rumored to have millions of dollars stashed away in Swiss banks; and he continued to advertise in the United States.

# Chapter 22

## Narrow Escapes

Jimmy remained obsessed with his work, battling against all odds to maintain a viable clinic. The odds were skewed by his fragile position with the law. Muggings, extortions, and attempted abductions hit as regularly as winter weather.

"It's so easy to get along with Mexicans," he said wistfully, "if you don't have the FBI after you. But the police kept using my Texas warrants as an excuse to pick me up. They'd say I'd best do what they said or they'd send me across the border."

The raids couldn't all be blamed on the FBI. Jimmy had also been targeted by his unconventional competitors in Tijuana. "I was the new boy on the block," he explained. "They didn't like me taking their patients." Apparently, there was no spirit of teamwork and cooperation in the dog-eat-dog world of Tijuana medicine.

"Okay," I reviewed the data, "there was the Matamoros sting operation in 1983 and the La Quinta raid in 1984. Then when was the next raid?"

Jimmy had to think. Perhaps it was the fluorescent lights, perhaps it was the lingering terror of his dire predicament, but he complained that his memory was starting to fail. "It was after I moved back into the medical center in Tijuana," he recalled. "Rudnov's doctor associate had his office there. I liked the doctor, but I was getting suspicious of Rudnov and I needed a bigger place, so I decided to move to a building on Television Street. It had a phone, which was a big deal in Tijuana. We didn't have one at the medical center or in Rosarito. I had just gone back to the medical center to get the last few things, when two immigration officers showed up. They took me to the Mexican immigration office and then to the border, and tried to shove me across."

"That doesn't sound like much of a deportation."

"It wasn't. A legal deportation requires at least one hearing. It's a very complicated procedure that can take years. These guys just said, 'Go across, and you can come right back.' But I could see some men waiting across the border. I figured they were FBI agents ready to nab me. I picked up one immigration man on each arm. I had them off the ground. Normally I couldn't have done that, but my adrenalin was running. They looked to the other immigration men for help, but the others wouldn't come. Then they said, 'If you won't go across, we're going to put you in jail in Mexico, because you've been working illegally here.' They took me back to the immigration office, and the head man came in and he talked."

Fortunately, the intrepid Junie was right behind. The woman was fearless. "They didn't pick her up," Jimmy said sentimentally. "She just came along. She talked to the big guy in Spanish. She told him about my *amparo*, and that they shouldn't be able to put me in jail. Then the men said, 'Come with us,' and we started walking. They walked me down toward the holding tank. Junie stuck right with me. She reached into her underwear and pulled out $2,500. I always let her carry it in case we needed it. She gave the money to the men and they let me go. When they got down to the street, they said 'Buena suerte' -- 'good luck'."

Jimmy sighed. "I probably didn't appreciate Junie enough at the time."

"Why do you say that?"

"Well, I didn't think they were really going to push me across -- I thought they were just holding out for money -- and I was kind of aggravated at her. I said, 'Why'd you give them so damn much?' She said, 'What's your life worth?' I had said, 'I want you to keep this, because one day we may need it.' I guess she thought that's what I meant. She said, 'Don't get mad at me. You were the one who told me to hide it in there. It was all in a wad and I couldn't separate it.' I said, 'Okay, I'm not mad at you, I love you, it's not worth worrying about, to hell with it.' And she was right. It was cheap compared to what happened later."

"That's true. So who do you think was behind the raid?"

"Well, my maid was at the medical center the whole day cleaning up. She said a woman who worked for Rudnov was watching my comings and goings from the second floor the whole time. The woman waited there for hours after I left, and when I came back, she left. It wasn't five minutes till the immigration people showed up."

I nodded. "Rudnov. What happened next?"

Jimmy thought a moment. "In 1986, I was picked up by the Mexican federal police; but they wouldn't tell me what the charge was. They just said I was wanted in the United States. It was Junie who rescued me that time too. She got in the car and followed me. They were trying to lose her, and they couldn't." He gazed into the imaginary past. "What a tiger Junie was! She walked so straight and erect. She just emanated power and control of the situation. She stood up to everybody. She was running her mouth in Spanish the whole time, telling them about my *amparo* and so forth. Mexican women aren't like that. The police looked at her like, 'Who the hell is this?' They asked what my freedom was worth and suggested $30,000. Junie said I didn't have the money, and they let me go so I could get it."

Jimmy added as an afterthought, "But it was Alma who actually bailed me out. We weren't married then. She was just helping out at the clinic. She went to the station with Al Lippman, another patient who's fluent in Spanish, and they got the sum down to $13,000."

I detected that a big chunk of this story was missing. How had Jimmy wound up marrying Alma, when he seemed so enamored of Junie? I was tempted to inquire, but I was afraid he would lose the train of thought he was on. He was into raids and narrow escapes. I bided my time and asked instead, "Who do you suppose was behind that raid? Rudnov again?"

Jimmy shook his head. "I think it was Garcia, the doctor I worked with briefly in Rosarito. He was mad because I wouldn't do business with him. The nurse who had worked for us both told me Garcia directed the police to my clinic; and he was there when they pulled me out, watching and laughing. It was Betty Lee who finally got him off my back. I called her and told her what had happened. She said, 'Don't worry, I'll get the pressure off you,' and she did. She called the doctor and told him to lay off, and I never heard from him again. Betty Lee saved me on a number of occasions. She was another tiger! Everybody listened to Betty, because it was important to be in good with the Cancer Control Society and to have her blessings. That didn't mean she recommended you, but she didn't put you down. To be put down by Betty Lee was a very serious thing."

Jimmy scanned his memory bank. "The next time trouble hit was in July of 1987. Everyone else had left the clinic. It was late and I was locking up, when the phone rang and I ran back in. I left the door unlocked. Two men had slipped in and were hiding in the entrance. I didn't know what hit me. It was the smaller guy who attacked. He got me in the head with something that looked like a night stick. I started screaming. He hit me three times, but I wouldn't go down. The bigger guy was standing there with a machete, but for some reason, he froze. All I could figure out was that the Lord had intervened. Finally I dropped my case, and the little guy grabbed it and they ran off. The case was all they stole. It was just a doctor's black case, with syringes and antibiotics and things. But the next day I heard that I'd been beheaded, and that they had my head to show for it."

It was grim humor, but I had to laugh. "Who was spreading the rumor?" I asked.

"I don't know, but I got the feeling it could have been Brash. He was trying to get his own clinic going down there. I was starting to have my doubts about him. I wondered about the night stick too. Maybe the police were involved. They never did show up."

Running a popular Tijuana cancer clinic evidently wasn't the easiest way to make a living. Jimmy was fighting wars on several fronts at once. He said it was Junie who rescued him that time too. He phoned her and she took him, battered and dazed, for medical treatment. The treating physician was his good friend Jorge Zavala, M.D., a professor at the National University. Jimmy regularly referred patients to him for catheters for IVs.

"Zavala said any one of those blows could have killed me." Jimmy laughed. "I said that's the good of being a hard-headed Cajun. You can't hardly kill a Cajun by hitting him on the head."

I laughed too. "It would take a firing squad, at least."

"At least!" Jimmy paused to wipe his glasses and think. "After that, there was another raid by Immigration; but this time they weren't looking for me. It was my office manager, Rosiline Raz."

I knew the name. Ros was one of Jimmy's "angels," a group of grateful patients who had volunteered to help at the clinic or talk at conventions. Others included Bonnie Cayer, Deborah Jones, Libby Hodges, Selma Meyers, and Celeste Keith. They had all volunteered to be witnesses at his trial.

As Ros later told her own story, when she came to Tijuana from England in 1985, she was facing a double mastectomy, radiation and chemotherapy. Even if she underwent those daunting procedures, her oncologist gave her only a year to live. Having little to lose, she opted for the unconventional. When Jimmy's treatments eliminated her symptoms without conventional therapy, she was thrilled. She returned to England, but she was nervous. She feared the disease would come back. She sold her business and returned to Tijuana. For the next year and a half, she worked in the clinic in exchange for treatment.

Ros's employment lasted, Jimmy said, until Mexican immigration officials showed up at the clinic, looking for an English woman who was reported to be working without a permit and proper papers. The officials questioned all the women they could find, listening for a British accent. Jimmy motioned to Ros, who caught enough of the conversation to get the gist. She grabbed the nearest man's arm and told him to walk out of the clinic as if they were together. She got into her car and drove until she was well across the border. And thus ended Ros's valued employment.

"The next raid was in November of 1988. We were pulling into the driveway . . ."

"You and Junie?"

"No, I was with Alma then."

The prisoner didn't offer any explanation, and he had a story on his tongue, so I bit mine and let him proceed.

"A guy jumped out with a pistol," he proceeded. "There was another guy with a sawed-off shotgun standing at the gate. They searched the apartment and finally found my safe. Then they put the pistol to my head and made me open it. They stole the money and were talking about killing me. I said I'd pay $1,000 a month *mordida* -- forever -- and they agreed."

"*Mordida?*"

"It means 'the bite.' Everyone wants a bite of the pie."

"I see."

"The state police started an investigation after that to find out who did it. It was a hairy situation. If the robbers had found out about the investigation before we found out who they were, they would have killed me; and the state police couldn't figure it out. But finally they did."

"Who was it, another competitor?"

"Just ordinary thieves. But one of them turned out to be a helper for the federal police. He was the son of an old maid I'd had. That made the state police afraid. The federal police were very powerful, and the police helper knew he'd been discovered. He must have figured he'd get me before I got him. The next thing we knew, he came with a bunch of federal police for a raid. They said, 'Keller's got all kinda crack in that clinic. He's got crystal, he's got crack in there.'"

"What's crystal?"

"It's a kind of dope."

"Did you have anything that looked like it?"

"No, and everyone knew better. The state police had been guarding us, so they had investigated us completely. They knew we were just running a clinic. In fact, the head of narcotics for the federal police was my lawyer. I owe my life that time to my old body guard. He saw them coming. The police knocked on the door and said, 'We want to know if James Keller is in there.' The guard said, 'Well, I don't know.' Six guys got out of the police van and were knocking on the door, and the guard was holding them off. He wouldn't let anyone in, not even the patients who were coming for treatment. But then a doctor came who worked in the building. The police told the doctor to open the door, and he did. I was hiding in a room in the back all that time. It was abandoned and full of junk. When the police got the door open, they came running through the clinic, beating on doors and taking people. They took my body guard and beat him up, trying to get him to tell them where I was. They asked everybody where I was, but nobody would say. By luck, it just happened that the screen on the window in back of my office was out. The police saw it and said, 'Look! The screen's off! He musta gone out the window! Son of a bitch! He musta got away!' They were furious, and I was still in there.

"Before that, I'd gotten on the phone and called Alma and told her to call the state police. They were scared, but they came. They said to the federal police, 'We're the state police. What are you doing? Do you have orders to do this?' The federal police said, 'Orders? We're superior to you.' They kept arguing back and forth, but eventually the federal police did go back for orders. Then people started banging on the door where I was hiding, saying it was okay to come out. But I was so far back, I couldn't hear them. Finally, somebody broke the lock off and opened the door and said, 'You gotta get outa here.'

"Then I called my Mexican attorney. He wasn't home but his daughter was. She came and picked me up and I stayed at her house. She went to the federal police station and told them what had happened. The chief of the federal police said he never ordered any investigation. Later, she identified the man who was responsible. The feds prosecuted their own people, and they went to jail. That whole thing was hairy, I can tell you. Even after the robbers were in jail, they kept calling us and threatening us, saying, 'We're gonna get you.'"

Jimmy paused to think. "There might have been one murder attempt that was actually successful. It was a guy named Anino who drafted legal papers for me. He was like a machine grinding out paper. He did great interrogatories. At one point, Dixon complained that I was being protected by the Mexican government, and that I was using the courts to harass the FBI! I don't know who bumped him off, but Dixon and Rudnov both had reason to. I sued them both."

"What did you sue them for?"

"I joined in Ron's suit against Dixon, and I sued Rudnov for fraud."

"What was the fraud?"

"The complaint said Rudnov had told me things that I had repeated and that had gotten me sued for fraud. Anino's ambition was to get a million dollars out of Rudnov at least, because of all the damage he had done. Rudnov settled the suit even though he knew I was in Mexico and couldn't prosecute it, he was that scared of the publicity. He didn't pay the whole settlement, but I thought it would be a good defense if I wound up in a lawsuit myself."

"It wouldn't be," I said, raising a professional finger. "An out-of-court settlement is inadmissible as evidence of the truth of the allegations in a complaint. But Rudnov may not have known that."

Jimmy nodded. "Anyway, Anino mysteriously died, and all my records disappeared. Even more mysterious, the records disappeared at the <u>court</u> where he filed the suit!"

"Weird. So what happened to Anino?"

"He left in his car and we never saw him again. About four months later, the Mexican police showed up at Ron's and said they'd heard he knew the guy who fit the description of this dead body. They said about four months ago there'd been an accident, and they described Anino. They said they disposed of the body because they didn't know who he was or where to bring him. Whether somebody paid to take him out, I never knew."

# Chapter 23

## Trouble at Home

Jimmy slumped pensively in his straight-backed chair. His train of thought had slowed to a halt for the time being. I saw my opportunity and changed the subject. "So what happened to Junie?" I asked.

"It's a long story."

"I guess it had to do with Alma."

"Yep." He looked away. When he roused himself from his reverie, he started in with this tale.

Alma had first come as a patient, he said, in May of 1984. She was so sick he had to carry her into the clinic. She had breast cancer that had metastasized to the liver, bones, colon, and lymphatic system. Her liver was enlarged and her abdomen was bloated with fluid. Her eyes were a deep yellow, signaling the late stages of jaundice. She was 35 and near death.

Jimmy had plenty of time to be attentive. May of 1984 was the month he was down to one patient. He worked on Alma devotedly. "It was amazing," he said. "After about three months, she came back to normal. She had no money and wanted to help us in the clinic in exchange -- and what a fantastic help she was! She became the bright light of the clinic, and the patients loved her."

Alma was Mexican but was then living in the United States, separated from her husband and essentially penniless. She and her two children got enough money from her husband to live on, but just barely. They owned a lot of rental property in Los Angeles, but her husband had gotten her to sign away her interest.

Alma was brought up in a very strict fundamentalist religion. "She was so innocent when I met her," Jimmy said wistfully. "She had phobias about movies and dancing and jewelry." He helped her with her phobias, and she opened up. She broke away from her mother's overly strict religion. In its place, she began attending the religious services of a Mexican *curandero*/healer/minister called "Maestro."

"Alma is pretty, you know," Jimmy approached the subject from another angle. "She has one of these perfect hourglass figures. She looks ten or fifteen years younger than she is."

"Which is already ten or fifteen years younger than you are," I pointed out.

"Seventeen."

"Okay, let me guess," I helped him along. "Junie was jealous."

Jimmy looked sideways out of his better eye. "That's probably an understatement. One time she mixed up Alma's IV bottles with dextrose. The sugar could have been fatal if I hadn't caught it in time."

"Wow! You don't think it was an accident?"

"You'd have to know Junie. She didn't make mistakes -- not usually, although she did hit the tissue instead of the vein once in another patient I thought she might have been jealous of. She didn't have any reason to be; this was a married woman, but a pretty one. Junie probably didn't even mean to do it. She just got over-aggressive."

"I see." Junie was obviously a woman not to be tangled with. "So what happened with Alma and the dextrose?"

"Well, I was furious about it, of course." The prisoner's voice trailed off.

"And you let Junie know it," I surmised, "and she got mad and walked out."

Jimmy looked through the cement-block walls and far away. "It was one of the biggest mistakes I ever made, he said. "I lost a lot when I lost Junie . . . "

"Like what?"

"Well, for one thing, Jose Luis Annaya left after she did. He was chancellor of the University of Baja in Tijuana. He made me an honorary professor of medicine there in 1985."

"You were an honorary professor of medicine?" I was impressed.

"It was after I treated him for lung cancer. He had it so bad, they were draining his lungs every third day. He was on his last leg and going out. After I treated him, he was fine. Later he was appointed to the Supreme Court of the State of Baja, so he was an important supporter. But he and Junie were good friends." Jimmy sighed. "Everybody liked Junie."

Having a gender-based interest in such things, I naturally inquired about the wedding. Jimmy said it wasn't actually planned. In 1989, the father of an influential friend of Jimmy's Mexican attorney had fallen seriously ill and needed treatment. But the man lived in Michoacan, far to the south in Mexico. Jimmy was afraid to go, for fear he couldn't save the old man. But he was even more afraid to say no. Jimmy and Alma were put on an aircraft and were met by a four-star general.

When the patient responded to the treatment and got better, Jimmy breathed a sigh of relief. The man's delighted relatives threw a grand celebration. "You've been wanting to get married," they said in the back-slapping mood of a Latin party. "We're going to bring the judge in." And they did. The best man was the chief of the local federal police.

It was too sudden to suit Alma. "She was mad because it was our wedding, we should have been going places, long honeymoon and all," Jimmy recalled. "But all I could think about was getting back to the people at the clinic."

It would set the tone for their marriage. At first, he said, they were very happy. But soon, Alma started complaining that his patients were taking all his energy. She criticized him for working so much that he never had time to take her anywhere. She said he was a workoholic.

"I wanted to take her places and please her," Jimmy maintained. "I just didn't feel I could get away. What most people don't realize is what a heavy responsibility it is taking care of terminal patients. They could die on you at any time."

Then he confided that their marriage hadn't been so good the year before his arrest as it was at first. Alma was a hot-blooded woman with a tendency to be suspicious and jealous. During the long hours he was at the clinic, Alma's imagination had free reign.

"I was faithful to her," he insisted, "but you'd never convince her of it. If I went home and I went to sleep instead of making love, she would be offended that I didn't have interest in her, that I must have been thinking of somebody else, that maybe when she was gone I did something with somebody else. Really! And she would beat me, I mean physically, with her fists -- to wake me up, because I'd have gone to sleep. I used to get up early, and a lot of times I was tired. I'd get up at 4 a.m. to make up the serums for the day. It wasn't that I wasn't interested in her. I just fell asleep."

Jimmy seemed to be attracted to tigress types. "She hit you so it hurt?" I asked.

"She did! I asked her why she did it. She said it was because she loved me so much. I said if she loved me any more, I'd be dead! When we started having problems, I said, 'Sweetheart, try to make this thing go. It's a pressure, because I'm on eggshells in that clinic. I'm scared you'll jump all over me. I can't hug a lady when she comes in. I'm used to hugging everyone who comes in. That's part of how I do things.' You know, it's all right if I hug old ladies and it's all right if I hug men, but when pretty ladies come in and I hug them, I've got trouble on my hands."

Jimmy stopped to clean his glasses, which were steaming up more than usual. "There was another complication," he said.

"What was that?"

"Alma had political influence."

He explained that her father had died of cancer, alone in Guadalajara, without communicating with her mother. When Alma finally found her father's relatives in 1986, they turned out to be well-off and influential. She was also a Mexican citizen, who could head Jimmy's Mexican corporation and protect him from the *federales*. When she started feeling neglected, she accused him of using her for those purposes.

"I guess it probably looked that way," he conceded, "but I didn't really need the help. I had my *amparo*, and I had other Mexican friends. I realized later that Alma's power was a two-edged sword. It was behind me when she was; but if she were to turn against me, she was powerful enough to do me in."

I wasn't sure what he meant by that, but I detected another twist in the web of intrigue behind this case.

Matters on the home front hit an all-time low, Jimmy said, about a year before he was kidnapped, when his first wife came for treatment. Her second husband had died, and Jimmy had been sending her money. He would say he loved her on the phone. He said that to everyone, even men; but Alma envisioned the worst. She told Jimmy categorically that he could not treat his ex.

He said he couldn't say no. She was the mother of his children and his friend.

Alma said there were other clinics.

Jimmy said he couldn't rely on them.

Alma left in a huff. She was gone for a week, and it took a long time to smooth things over after she came back. She spent more and more of her time with a patient who was one of Jimmy's closest friends. Like Alma, he helped out at the clinic in lieu of payment, and he spent a lot of time there. I had heard him speak on the Cancer Control Society tour. He was tall, handsome, and quite a bit closer to Alma's age than Jimmy was. I'll call him Durk.

As Durk told his own story, when he first came to Jimmy's clinic in 1987, he had non-Hodgkins' lymphoma that had metastasized to the bone marrow. His physician had recommended chemotherapy, but the doctor conceded it would suppress his immune system. The result would almost certainly be leukemia.

"I can't tell you what to do," said the doctor, "but I can tell you the only thing that we can do for you right now, today, is make you feel worse than you already do."

Durk and his wife investigated and prayed, and decided to try Jimmy's clinic. Amazingly, the cancer went into remission and stayed that way, with the help of regular boosters from Jimmy's serum.

Durk had his own business, but Jimmy said it was on the verge of bankruptcy. Durk's insurance covered the initial treatments, but after it ran out, Jimmy wound up treating him free of charge. Durk made up for it by contributing to the clinic with his enthusiasm and support. He became an avid advocate, talking at conventions, to tour groups, and on Jimmy's 1988 video of patient testimonials. "He's a super salesman," Jimmy said. "He's smooth."

The year before Jimmy was kidnaped, Durk spent a lot of time in Tijuana. He lived in San Diego, but he wasn't getting on well with his wife. He would spend the weekend with Jimmy and Alma. Durk would come into the clinic late on Saturday for treatment. Alma would come in after that.

Alma, meanwhile, was spending a lot of time in Southern California. She grew up there after the age of 13, and she had two teenaged children living there. On her frequent trips north, she had to go alone. Jimmy couldn't cross the border because of the indictment.

"Watch out for Alma and Durk," Jimmy's Mexican assistant Juan had once warned him. But Jimmy had brushed it off. He could hardly believe they were consorting behind his back. He had saved both their lives.

# Chapter 24

## Kidnapped

In the late 1980s, Jimmy lost the protection not only of Junie but of another tigress, Betty Lee Morales. After she died suddenly in an auto accident, his competitor Dr. Block told a mutual friend, "Keller's finished. Betty Lee's not going to send him patients anymore. He'd better join up with me or he's going to go out of business."

Jimmy declined the offer, yet his popularity continued to grow. Lorraine Rosenthal, co-founder of the Cancer Control Society, wrote to the district court in Brownsville in 1991:

> When Jimmy Keller had his St. Jude Clinic in Tijuana, Mexico, 1000's of patients were helped. I heard about this through the phone, letters, person to person contacts and through others. Jimmy was helping more patients than the other Clinics in Tijuana.
>
> About every 2 or 3 months we sponsored Bus Trips to the Clinics. When we got off at the St. Jude presentation we were always greeted by a whole table full of patients ready to tell their recovery stories. There was always lots of excitement and we were all thrilled with what we heard and saw.

At the 19th Annual Cancer Control Convention in Pasadena in 1990, 26 of 30 patients giving testimonials had been treated at the St. Jude Clinic.

"I didn't try to get patients to testify at those conventions," Jimmy complained. "I told them to stay home. I was being accused that the whole convention was mine. The other clinics had two or three patients. I had thirty or forty."

He raised his better eyebrow. "There really was a reason why they came after us. We probably had the best program for cancer that ever existed on the planet. The major problem we always had was government interference. It's the main thing that stands in the way of solving the cancer problem. The idea that the government can take care of you is a false policy. I've never seen anything that government did efficiently. We've already got forty or fifty viable cancer treatments, and some of them are really good. The research has already been done. The biggest obstacle is just the FDA."

I looked at my watch. Jimmy was getting that glazed look in his eye that signaled a detour into politics.

"Without the private industry it taxes," he forged obliviously ahead, "government would be nothing. We did what the government claims it does for people. We took care of people who couldn't take care of themselves. We took charity cases, but we never held a tin cup out to anyone. And under my program, the patients lived. I did it without taxing anyone, only because I thought it was the right thing to do. My clinic was totally self-sufficient, and we always had enough money to meet our expenses and go on. We had more than enough. I didn't mean to make a lot of money. It just happened, because my methods were so successful."

He said that in Matamoros, for people who could afford to pay, his fees ranged from $1,800 to $3,000 for a ten-day to three-week course of treatment. In Tijuana, they went up to $4,500, but they were still substantially less than his competitors.' His costs were so high that it was 1986 before he turned an actual profit. Yet by 1990, he had built up a considerable fund. He wasn't sure how much it was. He'd been too busy to count. He just turned it over to Alma or squirreled it away.

"So how much would you guess?" I asked.

"I'd guess it was over a million dollars."

Jimmy's assets weren't reflected in his lifestyle. Paul M. Hamilton, a Los Angeles chiropractor who visited the St. Jude Clinic over 200 times as an observer, wrote in a later letter to the court:

> . . . *Jimmy did not drive around in a brand new car. It was six or seven years older than the current models. Sometimes it did not run too well and he did not have the money free to fix it immediately. He used his money to feed back into his clinic. He did not dress lavishly . . . . His clinic was fixed up to*

*a reasonable state but located in a depressed area which most persons who entered the building the first day were shocked until they became aware of the love and caring available to them there. . . . There are numbers of individuals I met at Jimmy's clinic that were there at no charge. And some were there several weeks at very little or no cost.*

Jimmy didn't flaunt his savings, but somebody knew about them . . .

"The next time trouble hit," he said, "was December 4, 1990, the day after I turned 57. Alma coaxed me into the car. 'Come on,' she said, 'I want to show you something. We're just taking a little ride.' I had told her never to leave the house without someone to watch it, but this time she said the maid had to come along; we wouldn't be long. It turned out to be a surprise birthday party, a gala affair in a restaurant with a dance floor. There were forty or fifty people there, all Mexicans. It went late, to 3:00 or 4:00 in the morning. When we got home, the house had been burglarized. More than $200,000 was gone."

"$200,000?! Why were you keeping that kind of money in the house?"

"I was trying to buy a new clinic, and the guy who owned it didn't want it all in checks. He wanted a big chunk in cash. I had put the money in the safe not long before."

The police said it was an inside job. Nothing besides the safe had been disturbed. The burglar apparently went straight for the safe and pried it open with a crowbar. To get to it, two doors had to be opened, requiring two separate keys. The house was protected with alarms, which were set with remote controls. Jimmy normally didn't leave the house without setting them, but all three remotes had disappeared mysteriously the week before. They reappeared just as mysteriously the week after.

According to the police, there were only two possibilities -- the maid and Alma. The police checked out the maid and said she didn't do it. But Jimmy just couldn't believe it was Alma. He suspected the police themselves -- two state police who guarded his house and were friends. They usually came around together, but at the party, there was only one.

"Did the maid know you had money in the safe?" I asked.

"She probably did. But only Alma," Jimmy conceded, " knew how much it was."

Alma wanted to report the burglary to the police, but Jimmy said he was nervous. They might be reporting to the very people who did it. Then a month after the robbery, a *compadre* of Alma's cousin became the chief of the federal police. Alma said they could report to him, and Jimmy agreed. The chief wound up sending them to the headquarters of the same state police Jimmy feared. It was there that they first saw the liaison officer between the San Diego and Tijuana state police.

"He's a big guy, kind of dark complected, speaks Spanish like a native," Jimmy said. After that, they'd notice this officer skulking around. He seemed to be trailing them.

The last time Jimmy saw him was on March 18, 1991, less than a month later. At 9 a.m. that day, four rough-looking, Spanish-speaking men entered the clinic. One man said he had cancer. Then another man pulled a gun. Jimmy looked up in surprise from the patient he was examining as they lunged for him. Patients and employees fought to defend him. The abductors hauled Jimmy outside and shoved him up against a fence. His brother Ron, who was helping at the clinic, hit one of the men, but the abductors prevailed. Jimmy was thrown into a waiting van.

Ron got away. He evidently wasn't recognized. Jimmy heard later that before the men had come to his clinic, they had gone to Century 21 Mexico in Rosarito, where Ron had been working as a real estate agent. They had a picture of Ron, but it was with a beard; and by luck he had shaved it off a couple of days earlier. He escaped but they took his working papers, so he couldn't go back to Century 21. Jimmy said it was the third career Ron had lost to the cancer industry.

Jimmy was taken to Mexican immigration headquarters. He showed them his *amparo* and his immigration papers, but it was several hours before the officers would say the papers were in order. Then they told him to wait, and they left. He was there from the middle of the morning until late that night. Finally, six other men came in. They weren't wearing uniforms. They were in dungarees and blue work shirts. The one he recognized was the liaison officer between the San Diego and Tijuana state police. They grabbed Jimmy and walked him across the border to San Ysidro, into the building with the holding tank in it. An American unlocked the tank and said, 'Go in.' He seemed to know Jimmy was coming. It was an hour or two before the FBI came and got him.

Jimmy was arraigned in San Ysidro on twelve counts of conspiracy to commit wire fraud. His first court hearing was on March 21 in San Diego.

"The government said I 'fled indictment,'" he recalled, "but I'd already been out of the country for nearly a year before the indictment was issued. They also said I was legally deported, but they didn't produce any immigration papers -- they just had a warrant for my arrest -- and there was never any deportation hearing. But the judge still denied bail."

"Didn't you have an attorney?"

"I did. He was a San Diego man Durk showed up with. Durk lives in San Diego and was the first of my people to get to the jail."

"So what did the attorney say at the hearing?"

Jimmy shrugged despondently. "Not much."

Durk, it turned out, had also retained Jimmy's local Brownsville counsel. I'll call this attorney Black. Black had then suggested Silversmith for lead counsel. Silversmith had assured Jimmy's relatives he would be well taken care of. Jim Jr. was flown from San Antonio to Brownsville in a private plane. (Jim Jr. was in charge of the funds -- Jimmy's, his family's, and donations from patients and supporters.) Silversmith, Ginsburg and Black had all met with their new client to close the deal. Jimmy was totally sold on the team.

"Silversmith hasn't been around since," he said.

"Not at all?"

"Well, he sends an associate sometimes, but it's not the same. I don't feel like my lead counsel knows the facts or the issues."

The Kellers paid $150,000 to Silversmith up front, along with $25,000 to Ginsburg and $25,000 to Black. Durk's San Diego attorney was also paid $33,000, though for what wasn't clear. In the end, the Kellers paid over half a million dollars to attorneys.

"Little Jim heard that the rumor was that I had a million dollars sitting in Mexico for attorneys' fees," Jimmy said. "I did have some money saved up, but it was for buying a proper clinic."

The day after he was captured, the apartments where his patients were staying were peppered with leaflets from Rudnov's clinic. The leaflets declared that Rudnov had the same therapies Jimmy had; and since Jimmy was no longer available, Rudnov would be pleased to furnish them in his place.

"He contacted every patient," Jimmy said. "He must have gotten my patient list somehow."

"So he knew about the kidnapping?"

"He must have."

"Then you think he instigated it?"

"I doubt it. I doubt he was powerful enough to overcome an *amparo*. Mexican officials have a healthy respect for Mexican jails."

Jimmy added after thinking about it, "There had been a change in power then in Baja. That may have changed the political climate. The old party was the PRI. When they were in, they protected the Tijuana clinics. But the PAN had gotten in. They're influenced by U.S. medical interests. They've promised to shut down any cancer clinics that don't recommend radiation and follow U.S. ways. But even with the backing of the U.S. government, I doubt Mexican officials would violate an *amparo*."

"Maybe the men who took you across the border weren't Mexicans," I said.

"Then who were they?"

"Bill thinks they were Mexican/American DEA agents."

"DEA agents! That would make sense! Why does he think that?"

"I don't know. Some kind of private investigation. He says he has it on good authority."

Jimmy turned this idea over in his mind. "Alma said she waited a long time at the border with the Mexican federal police after I was taken across. She intended to have the men who abducted me arrested because they had violated my *amparo*. But they never came back across the border. They must have been Americans! But what about the officers who first picked me up? They were Mexicans . . ."

Before the *federales* could act on the violated *amparo*, Alma had to complain about the kidnapping and make a formal demand. But she said she was afraid and wouldn't do it. In fact, Jimmy mused, Alma had been acting peculiar ever since the FBI paid a visit to her home in San Diego in the spring of 1990. Her children said the FBI frightened the boy who worked for them so badly that he left and never came back. Alma insisted the agents hadn't spoken to her directly, but Jimmy wondered. It would be hard for her to avoid the meeting if they had wanted it, and she wouldn't be hard to intimidate. She was the head of his Mexican corporation. Her children could be in jeopardy . . .

# Chapter 25

## Five Million Dollar Bail

If the straight-backed wooden chairs furnished by the Cameron County Department of Corrections weren't much for comfort, I rationalized that they were good for posture. But Jimmy wasn't taking advantage of that feature of his. He was slumping wearily in it. "I've got another problem," he said.

"What's that?"

He confided that he had hidden funds in various caches known only to himself. But when he had revealed them so that the money could be used for his defense, much of it couldn't be found. Could it have been stolen? He had taken elaborate pains to conceal it well. Without it, he would have trouble financing his trial.

"Who did you reveal the hiding places to?" I asked.

"To Durk."

I nodded, while Jimmy shook his head. We were probably both thinking the same thing.

"Durk never has had any money, as long as I've known him," Jimmy said. "His business was about a million dollars in debt and about to go under."

I didn't necessarily believe in conspiracy theories, but I could see one shaping up. It went something like this: the medical/industrial complex had used its political clout to organize a quackbusting campaign in Congress. The FBI had been induced to rout out "the most notorious quack in the country" -- who happened to be Jimmy -- and make an example of him. The FBI had intimidated his wife, who had gotten scared and decided his handsome friend was a safer bet than Jimmy himself. The friend had then capitalized on the situation to get out of the overwhelming debts in which he had become hopelessly mired, retaining counsel appropriate to his own ends.

It wasn't the best time for stock market advice, but I had to ask why Jimmy hadn't put his money in some prudent long-term investments.

"I suppose I should have," he said. "I should have been putting it in Swiss banks like Rudnov did. But I didn't have time to worry about investments. I usually had about 35 lives in my hands at once. If I lost one, it was a catastrophe."

"Too bad you couldn't get out on bail and make your own financial arrangements," I mused. The constitutional provision for release on a reasonable bail was intended to allow a defendant time to prepare for his defense. He could hover over his attorneys and steer them around any rapids that threatened to plunge his barrel over the falls. "So what happened at the hearing to reconsider denial of your bail?"

"Well, I'd already been in jail for two months before anything happened at all. But finally in May, there was a hearing. And at first, I thought the judge was leaning my way. Silversmith was arguing that only capital offenses are grounds for denying bail -- treason or murder."

"That's a pretty good argument," I said.

"It was. But then the judge asked if the government had tried any legal means to get me out of Mexico, and they said they had. The judge said, 'Show me some documentation,' and called a recess. An hour and a half later, the government came back with two telexes." Jimmy rummaged through his papers and pulled out two documents. "The second one is totally phony . . ."

The first telex was dated 11/28/86 and was from the FBI in San Diego to the FBI in San Antonio, Texas, responding to a telex dated 7/24/86 from San Antonio. The subject was the status of the San Diego office's efforts to get Keller. The San Diego FBI said Keller's whereabouts were known, but he was protected by an *amparo*. Under the Mexican constitution, he couldn't be detained without specific complaints in Tijuana and a hearing in Mexico. Despite diligent effort, the FBI had been unable to find anyone willing to complain, "even though it is apparent that the KELLERs advertise their United States fugitive status." The telex concluded, "One additional attempt will be made to . . . obtain license numbers which may lead to a possible complaining witness."

"They were spying on my patients," Jimmy said cynically, "and tracking them down through their license numbers, and still they couldn't find anyone willing to complain."

The second telex was from the San Antonio FBI to the San Diego FBI and was dated 1/7/87. It read:

> For information of San Diego, on 11/18/86, [Rudnov], key witness against and competitor with the KELLER operation advised he ahd [sic] been able to convince a Mexican Federal Judge through his (the judge's) girlfriend that KELLER should be arrested. The judge subsequently ordered Mexican Immigration to arrest KELLER. They went into the clinic and arrested all three fugitives and placed them in the Immigration Detention Facility. Bond was set at $60,000 United States Currency.
>
> The fugitives were to be deported on or about 11/26/86, unless they came up with the bond. On 11/26/86, DAVID KELLER, JAMES' son and co-defendant in this case, appeared before the court and produced the $60,000 in United States Currency. The fugitives were then released.
>
> [Rudnov] advised that the judge told him that when KELLER resumed his operation he would again be arrested and his bond forfeited. He would then be required to post another $60,000 bond. As of 12/12/86, KELLER had not resumed his business and [Rudnov] speculated that he took his regular Christmans [sic] break at this time to let the heat die down before resuming.

The signature line was left blank, but FBI agent Dixon's name was hand-printed at the bottom.

"That telex is obviously phony," Jimmy reiterated. "How could I have jumped bond, when I was practicing in Mexico every day in plain view? And they wouldn't have set bail in U.S. dollars. It's illegal to do government business in Mexico in anything but pesos. Then there's the part about David. He can testify he never left Louisiana. He was on probation from the 1985 trial and couldn't leave the country."

I had to agree that the document looked suspicious. There was nothing to validate it: no arrest warrant, no order, no bond, no government seal. Nothing was signed under penalty of perjury. "Did you point all that out at the hearing?" I asked.

"I tried to, but I couldn't get Silversmith's attention. He was too busy with his own theory. He jumped up and said the telex showed Rudnov had been conspiring with the government to have me arrested and put out of business. The judge did set bail, but at five million dollars cash. It might as well have been five trillion. I couldn't even post a bond."

I agreed. "Outrageous!"

I went over my notes and realized I had run out of questions. I was "up to speed" on the facts. I searched for an upbeat note on which to end the interview. "Anyway," I said, trying to sound optimistic, "maybe we won't have to go to trial. We think we have a good shot at prevailing on a motion to dismiss. But I need to get back to California so I can get to work on it."

We exchanged farewells. I smiled and waved and tried to look confident, as the sliding bars swallowed the prisoner up.

Back in California, before I could get to work on the motion, urgent family matters demanded my attention. A trip to Magic Mountain had been promised but not yet delivered. Grandma lived in the vicinity but couldn't deal with whiplash, and Cliff got seasick. Meanwhile, the kids were clamoring for thrills.

After satisfying my duties on the home front, I hit the law library and drafted a tentative motion. Then I paid a visit to the medical library and the public library, to check out the non-legal issues on my list.

One was Jimmy's controversial contention that biopsies can spread cancer. I was surprised to find it corroborated in medical studies. Even needle biopsies, I read, have been known to spread the disease.[56]

Another was the highly controversial contention that radiation and chemotherapy, while shrinking tumors, don't necessarily increase survival. Again, I was surprised to find it corroborated in medical studies . . .

> According to biostatician Dr. Ulrich Abel, writing in 1990, reduction of tumor mass does not prolong expected survival. In fact, it can cause the cancer to return more aggressively, since killing off most of the cancer mass allows drug-resistant cell lines to grow.[57] An article in the British Medical Journal concurred. It observed that while tumor shrinkage is the usual way to measure the efficacy of chemotherapy, "radiological

shrinkage of solid tumours . . . often has little or no survival benefit . . . . Unfortunately, few studies have compared chemotherapy with supportive care alone."[58]

One of the few studies that had made this comparison was conducted by Dr. Hardin Jones, professor of medical physics and physiology at the University of California, Berkeley. He told an ACS panel:

> My studies have proven conclusively that untreated cancer victims actually live up to four times longer than treated individuals. For a typical type of cancer, people who refused treatment lived for an average of 12-1/2 years. Those who accepted surgery and other kinds of treatment lived an average of only three years. . . . I attribute this to the traumatic effect of surgery on the body's natural defense mechanism. The body has a natural defense against every type of cancer.[59]

Dr. Jones was speaking twenty years ago, but more recent data were lacking, because studies comparing treated and untreated patients were no longer being done. To fail to treat potentially curable patients with "proven" methods is now considered unethical. Most drug studies merely compare the effects of two treatment regimens, both more or less equally toxic, on the size of tumor growth.[60]

To pass the "effectiveness" test, the FDA requires substantial evidence not that drugs save lives but only that they are effective for their intended uses. Cancer drugs are considered "effective" if they merely shrink tumors.[61] A 1984 review of 80 studies of chemotherapy for breast cancer found that 76 of them had looked only at tumor shrinkage, not at effects on survival or quality of life; and three of the remaining four had found no survival advantage for the drugs.[62] Other reviews reached equally disquieting conclusions.[63]

As for surgery and radiation, they were grandfathered in before the FDA's "effectiveness" requirement. For surgery, large-scale controlled trials haven't been conducted proving a survival benefit as compared to no treatment at all; and for radiation given after surgery, large-scale randomized controlled trials haven't shown a survival benefit as compared to surgery alone.[64] *Radiation is given to shrink tumors in critical situations (e.g., when the tumor is pressing on an artery, airway, vital organ, or nerve), but the long-term effect can actually be to shorten survival.*[65] *A 1987 review of eight trials from around the world found that the risk of death after ten years for women who had not gotten radiation after their breast surgeries was 26 percent* <u>lower</u> *than for women who had gotten it.*[66]

"The majority of cancers," wrote Dr. John Cairns of Harvard in 1985, "cannot be cured by radiation because the dose of X rays required to kill all the cancer cells would also kill the patient."[67]

With chemotherapy, progress has been made in treating certain cancers; but the drugs haven't done much to prolong survival from the big killers -- cancers of the breast, colon and lung.[68] According to Dr. Cairns, chemotherapy prevents death in only 2 to 5 percent of cancer cases. The chance the drugs themselves will kill the patient is about the same: somewhere between 2.5 percent and 5 percent.[69] In a 1991 study in which chemotherapy was compared to no treatment in 250 women with metastatic breast cancer, the drugs not only did not improve survival but significantly decreased the quality of life.[70]

With <u>early</u> breast cancer, on the other hand, a modest survival benefit has been found. A 1992 British review of 31 randomized trials involving 11,000 women found a slight increase in overall survival after 10 years for patients given "polychemotherapy" (more than one drug for more than one month). The women's chances of being alive 10 years later, however, were still only 51.3 percent with the drugs, versus 45 percent without them -- a mere 6.3 percent survival benefit. And this grim prognosis was for women with breast cancer in the early, "treatable" stages.[71] Despite these very modest benefits, the National Cancer Institute has recommended chemotherapy for all breast cancer patients, whether or not they have visible signs of cancer after surgery. The theory is that projected over thousands of women, a significant number of lives will be saved.[72] The problem -- especially for the 93.7 percent who aren't benefitted -- is the drugs' crushing side effects. Virtually all chemotherapeutic drugs are toxic and immunosuppressive. Being unable to distinguish between cancerous and normal cells, they wind up killing both. Most also cause secondary cancers, which can show up many years after "successful" chemotherapy.[73]

On Jimmy's theory, the formation of secondary tumors might be the direct result of shrinkage of the protective capsule. Without this protective shell, the cancer is allowed to escape and spread. In any case, the way I read the statistics, it wouldn't be hard to beat the track record of chemotherapy. If a non-toxic treatment could show a mere 6.3 percent survival benefit for patients with early breast cancer -- or <u>any</u> survival benefit for patients with metastasized breast cancer -- the therapy would be matching the effectiveness of chemotherapy, without the drugs' ominous side effects.

Jimmy was convinced he had beaten both those records. He said he had treated a number of women with metastasized breast cancer who were still alive after five years, the official cutoff for "cure." If we had to go to trial, I would have an opportunity to meet some of these women, who had volunteered to be witnesses.

While I was at the library, I also looked up Wesley Irons, M.D., Tumorex's purported developer. I learned that he had indeed been involved in studying arginine and its effects on tumors in the forties.[74] But there was no mention of a cure. Was it fabricated by Rudnov? Or had it been suppressed, as he claimed?

I also looked up the NCAHF, the AMA, and their ilk. What I found was shocking. But to avoid breaking the flow of Jimmy's story further, I'll relegate the fruits of that and some later investigation to Appendix A.

# Chapter 26

## Pretrial Motions

The pretrial hearing on July 15 was our first chance to size up the principal actors scheduled to play in Brownsville in August. Our motion to dismiss was typed and in my briefcase, but it wasn't scheduled for hearing. Bill hadn't yet gotten signed declarations from his expert witnesses, and time requirements for filing and serving had yet to be met. Bill and I were in court only to be formally joined as counsel.

The federal courtroom was august, stately, and imposing -- perhaps too imposing. The American eagle that presided over it somehow struck me as more threatening than protective. I realized my childhood vision of the American dream was slipping away.

I turned my attention to the players. U.S. Attorney Meier looked to be in his late thirties. He was fair-haired and not bad-looking, but if he had any personality, he refrained from displaying it in court. Other than an unnerving habit of clenching his jaw, the only emotion that showed on his face was a chilling contempt.

Lead defense counsel Silversmith, by contrast, was disarming, courteous, and humble. He had courtroom charm. He looked to be in his mid-forties and was handsome and athletic, a man who apparently had time to incorporate regular exercise into his busy schedule.

Sitting next to him was an associate I'll call Sylvia. She was what my mother would call heavyset, suggesting she did not have time for regular exercise. But she seemed to adore her employer, and to be enthusiastic about her work.

Flanking the defense table was Black, the local Brownsville attorney originally retained by Durk. Jimmy called him the "typical jailhouse crony." His only role on the team seemed to be to visit the jail and relay messages. He didn't look like he got much exercise either. A narrow-shouldered man with a limp handshake, he had the disconcerting habit of hushing his own client with a wave of his hand.

The judge was sixty-ish and of Mexican heritage. Los Angeles Times reporter Paul Ciotti later wrote that he had Lyndon Johnson ears. I viewed this description with frank admiration. By then I couldn't remember the ears of either the judge or LBJ. If I were going to give up lawyering for writing, I admonished myself, I must start paying closer attention to visual detail.

The judge's demeanor, on the other hand, we studied closely. My initial impression was that he was unyielding and impatient with counsel, but kind to the jury in a grandfatherly way. Bill said he wasn't a model of open-mindedness, but Bill had prevailed in front of worse.

Silversmith's pretrial motions raised two points. The first was that the federal search warrant through which the government had gotten its evidence was improperly obtained. The original search was conducted on a health inspection warrant, though its admitted purpose was criminal. Under the "Fruit of the Poisonous Tree Doctrine," any evidence which is the direct result or immediate product of illegal conduct on the part of a government official is inadmissible against the victim of the illegal conduct. The rule is a constitutional one that falls under the due process requirement of the Fourteenth Amendment. Silversmith's brief argued:

> *As Agent [Dixon] testified, the Texas Attorney General 'correctly described' that the State investigators were 'working closely with the FBI' in conducting these searches in the 'hope that enough evidence of federal criminal violations had been gathered so that the FBI can pursue Keller and his bunch.' FBI Agent [Dixon] even prepared the handwritten return on the State evidentiary search warrant . . . . Almost thirty years ago the Supreme Court noted . . . 'The deliberate use by the Government of an administrative warrant for the purpose of gathering evidence in a criminal case must meet stern resistance by the courts.'*

Silversmith's other pretrial motion was to suppress the testimony of the undercover agents who had posed as the parents of a child with leukemia. At the 1985 trial, the government had denied that the sting operation had been tape recorded; but it had now admitted otherwise. Not only had the operation been taped; the government had admitted the tape was intentionally destroyed. Silversmith's brief argued:

> [A]t the previous trial, the Government failed to ever disclose the existence of these tape recordings or their destruction, and [undercover agent Gomez] who accompanied and participated in this 'joint operation' with the FBI agents, failed to disclose such information, despite having been specifically questioned about same.'

Federal rules required the production of these tape recordings if they existed.

According to the government's brief in opposition, "The tape was destroyed because it was felt that the taping . . . violated Mexican law." But even the judge seemed to doubt this justification and to be disturbed by the revelation. He told Silversmith he would be allowed to comment on the tape's destruction in any way he wanted to at trial.

The judge made no ruling, however, on the motions. He took them under submission. That meant he would think about them.

Silversmith then asked the judge if he could delicately approach "a difficult subject dealing with when we actually start the trial."

"How delicately?" asked the judge.

"On my knees, Your Honor?" Silversmith explained that he had a conflict and couldn't start the trial before August 19. "The Court seems somewhat flexible about giving us the month of August. We will finish it well within that. If we could start on the 19th that will help me, Your Honor."

Meier and the judge discussed another long trial that had to be fit into the court's crowded calendar. "One of them is going to go in August and one in September," said the judge.

"We are going to go in August," Silversmith assured him. "All we would like to do is do it on the 19th."

The judge had apparently allotted the whole month of August for the trial, but it was now being limited to two weeks because

Silversmith wasn't available before the 19th. The problem was a common one among attorneys trying to juggle heavy caseloads, but it meant the defense was going to have only a week to make its case. That was going to add an extra element of tension, I thought. Could we enlighten a border town jury on the subtleties of vibrational medicine in a week?

Just as the judge was about to leave the bench, Silversmith managed to get in a last point. He had asked earlier in the hearing to see the U.S. regulation that the government said required it to destroy its own tapes if they violated Mexican law. The rule the government now produced, Silversmith pointed out, actually required the reverse: tapes once made must <u>not</u> be destroyed.

It was a brilliant score for the defense. The government's own good faith had finally been put in doubt. Or so it seemed at the time.

After the pretrial hearing, the defense attorneys all met at Black's Brownsville law office for lunch. The decor was Southern and elegant, but the atmosphere was cool. Over take-out sandwiches and Cokes, Bill and I groped awkwardly for something to say. I got the feeling we weren't welcome additions to the defense team.

I asked Silversmith whether jurisdiction might not be challenged on the basis of the defendant's illegal kidnapping.

He laughed. "Where have you been?"

"Abroad," I said timidly.

"The fact that a defendant has been kidnapped by the government is no longer grounds for contesting jurisdiction," Silversmith assured me. Apparently, the civil rights of the accused had been progressively eroded in the name of the government's high-profile War on Drugs. Manuel Noriega was the case-in-chief.

After surviving that first testy meeting with our co-counsel, I dropped by the jail. The decor was less elegant, but the reception by the defendant could generally be counted on to be warm. On that occasion, however, Jimmy was adrift in his own dark thoughts. He was thinking about his son David.

"The testimony of Narda Gomez was the only thing that convicted David," Jimmy moaned, "and the woman lied on the stand! David already appealed his case and lost. He was a convicted felon at 29. It ruined his marriage and his life. The only reason he did his own defense was that he thought there was no way he could get convicted. He wasn't even working for me in Matamoros. He had just come down on vacation. All he did was move some furniture around and pick some people up at the airport. He handled himself really well at the trial too. But what could he do against falsified evidence?"

"That is too bad," I commiserated, "but there is a bright side. The government has admitted it intentionally destroyed evidence -- and it was the only hard evidence in the case of the representations you were making to patients!"

Jimmy brightened as he pursued this line of thought. Not only did the tape's destruction prove bad faith on the part of the government; it proved he hadn't made the representations charged against him. Otherwise, the government would surely have preserved the evidence, particularly when statute required it.

Then another implication struck him: Maxine's phone conversation with undercover agent Gomez must also have been taped. The government doesn't conduct sting operations without coming away with evidence. Maxine wasn't even in Mexico, so there was no reason for the tape's destruction -- unless the government hadn't succeeded in entrapping her into making the representations they wanted her to make.

I was excited myself. The matter of the mysteriously destroyed tape could be a turning point at trial.

A week after the pretrial hearing, on July 22, 1991, the Ninth Circuit Court of Appeals ruled that jurisdiction could in fact be challenged on the basis of an illegal kidnapping. The Ninth Circuit affirmed the 1990 holding of U.S. v. Verdugo-Urquidez, in which the U.S. District Court in San Diego had held that if a defendant is kidnapped from Mexico in violation of an extradition treaty, and if the Mexican government objects, U.S. courts may not exercise jurisdiction over him. The San Diego District Court was the court that had first exercised jurisdiction over Jimmy. He didn't have a formal protest from the Mexican government, but he was convinced he could get one. Bill and I decided to add another ground to our motion to dismiss: the court lacked jurisdiction over the defendant because he had been brought before it illegally. Alma's cousin Pepe would work on getting a formal protest from the Mexican government, while I redrafted the motion.

My family had been scheduled to return on July 20 to Kenya by way of Asia, our only shot at an around-the-world excursion.

Instead, my husband and children went home by way of Europe. I hadn't meant to be away from them so long, but there wasn't much I could do about it now. I rationalized that they had never seen Paris. I had been there before.

Taking my cue from Bill, I started our motion to dismiss with a long introduction intended to "educate the judge" -- on the facts of the case, the popularity of Jimmy's clinic, and the viability of the non-traditional health care movement. There was the thorny detail of the missing evidence -- the official protest from the Mexican government and the signed declarations from Bill's experts -- but I maneuvered around it by wording the brief to say that supporting evidence would be produced at the hearing.

When the motion was written, I faced the thornier detail of persuading Silversmith to file it. I flew to San Antonio, where he had his office, and had dinner with his personable associate Sylvia.

In the Developing World, restaurants start to fill up around 9:00 p.m., but in San Antonio at that hour we had the establishment to ourselves. The menu choices left in the kitchen were slim. We talked as we picked over them. Sylvia confided that Silversmith was the smartest man she had ever met. She said he could function on only two hours' sleep, and so could she. Apparently, they were juggling an enormous number of cases.

She was enthusiastic about the motion -- so enthusiastic that I briefly entertained thoughts of being invited to help their team prepare the defense's case. But I soon sensed that her employer did not share her enthusiasm. I breathed a sigh of relief when he agreed to file the handiwork I had already prepared.

The next matter on the calendar was the selection of jurors in Brownsville. I wasn't an active participant in the proceedings, but Jimmy seemed to want me there. I got the sense on the phone that he had things to discuss that couldn't be said through that medium.

# Chapter 27

## Jury Selection

The prospective jurors did not inspire confidence. There was some doubt about how well most of them spoke English. They were generally sullen and expressionless, and looked like they would rather be somewhere else. But I rationalized that this was probably normal. Few people really <u>wanted</u> to perform the civic duty of sitting on a jury.

After jury selection, Silversmith met with his client in the little attorney/client cages in the marshal's office. It was a rare opportunity for Jimmy to discuss the issues face-to-face with his lead counsel. Unfortunately, there was no meeting of the minds. If Silversmith was humble and ingratiating in court, in private he proved a hard man for his client to talk to. Black shushed the prisoner with a wave of his hand, while Silversmith said, "You're not listening!"

The dispute was over trial tactics. Jimmy wanted to establish that his remedies worked. Silversmith wanted to show merely that Jimmy believed that they worked. If he believed the truth of his own representations, he could hardly be guilty of fraud, since "knowledge of falsity" is an essential element of the crime. Jimmy's concern was that this wouldn't be enough to establish his innocence. If his methods didn't work, he probably should have realized it. He would at least have been negligent in not finding out. But Silversmith wasn't looking for feedback. He had already made up his mind.

If communication was bad between Jimmy and his lead counsel, between Silversmith and Bill (who was still in California) it was practically non-existent. To be a successful trial attorney required unflappable confidence, and both men were successful trial attorneys. They had egos to match. The two stags soon locked horns. Bill, who was Silversmith's senior by perhaps two decades, declined to be at the younger man's beck and call, particularly when each beckoning meant spending the better part of two days on a plane between Texas and California. Bill quietly prepared the medical aspects of the case, while Silversmith's office complained that he hadn't returned their calls.

As usual, I spent my spare time in Brownsville at the jail, armed with my laptop computer. Not that there was anything compelling about the place, but I could hardly say no. To hear Jimmy tell it, you'd think the whole case turned on my watchful eye. Nobody else of consequence paid much attention to my ideas, but the defendant knew how to be appreciative and make one feel needed.

"So what's the news?" I asked.

Jimmy confided that he was worried about his witnesses. He had heard reports that some of them were being badgered and threatened. Silversmith's investigator had been assigned the task of interviewing them, but the investigator had been nerve-grindingly slow. The FBI was getting to them first. Some of the defense's key witnesses were now afraid to testify.

"Like who?"

"Well, like Chickley T_____ for one. This guy had the most fantastic recovery! He had a huge melanoma. When he showed up at my clinic in 1982, he said they had diagnosed it all over him -- in his liver, in his brain, on his scalp. He'd had radiation treatment, but all it did was to increase his tumors -- by a factor of four in twenty-four hours. He was a big guy, 6'8" or so, but he wasn't able to eat. He was losing weight at the rate of five pounds a day. I told him I'd try to help, but I told Junie he wasn't long for this world."

"And you saved him."

Jimmy nodded. "I was as surprised as anyone. When I started the serum on him, he said he felt bubbling all over. Then he started getting better. After that, he was on fire. He was mad. He started promoting my treatments to anyone who would listen. He put out fliers, he went into hospitals, he spoke at meetings. In 1983, he tried to testify at the injunction hearing. He was mad at the whole medical profession. They weren't feeling too kindly

toward him either. The oncologist in New Iberia called him up
and said, 'Who in the hell do you think you are, sending my
patients to a quack?'"

Chickley had evidently been threatened before. In 1984, he
told Jimmy he'd been pulled off a lonely country road at night
and was beaten by five or six hefty plainclothesmen. His tires and
upholstery had been slashed. He was instructed to say no more
about Jimmy's therapies.

Chickley later modified this story. He said he'd been pulled
over only for a broken tail light. The men had identified themselves
as officers, and had searched his car for drugs -- nothing more. It
all sounded suspicious to Jimmy: a broken tail light isn't legal
grounds for searching for drugs. But whatever happened,
Chickley's ardor suddenly cooled.

When Silversmith's investigator finally made it to Louisiana
to interview prospective witnesses in 1991, he arrived without
authorization forms for the release of medical records. He had to
make another trip with the forms; and by then, the FBI had already
paid the witness a visit. Chickley was so intimidated that he would
authorize the release of his records for only a limited time period
-- so limited that the defense couldn't prove he'd even had cancer.

"If the dog had the bravery Chickley had," Jimmy said with
grim humor, "the rabbit would chase the dog."

Another witness he felt he had lost to FBI arm-twisting was a
man named Ferris, the husband of Chickley's cousin Peggy. The
government had scared Ferris and Chickley at the same time.
Jimmy said he had successfully treated Ferris for prostate cancer
in 1983. When the FBI interviewed him in 1984, Ferris minced
no words in telling them what he thought of their agency. For
years afterwards, all three of his businesses had then been audited
by the IRS -- a very expensive proposition for Ferris. He said he
couldn't afford to testify in 1991.

When I heard this story, I thought it highly unlikely that the
two incidents were linked. But later, I read something that made
me wonder . . .

> It was an excerpt from a congressional sub-committee
> investigation of charges of a medical conspiracy to suppress
> alternative therapies. A police chief was asked, "A detective
> assigned to a case where maybe they had a wiretap surveillance
> could, over a cup of coffee in the morning, pass information

*along to someone in another agency?" The chief responded,
"Probably would, yes."*[75]

At least, Ferris' wife Peggy hadn't been intimidated, or so Jimmy
had heard. She had told her husband she was going to testify even if
he stayed home. But not everyone was that brave. May R. had avoided
the issue by having her phone disconnected . . .

Frustrated with the lack of action by his lead counsel, Jimmy
had wound up lining up most of his own witnesses by calling
them from the communal phone on the jailhouse wall. When he
had first called May, she had agreed to testify for the defense. But
when Bonnie Cayer called her later, May was nervous. "I can't
talk," she said. "My phone is bugged. The FBI called me three
times asking about Jimmy." The next time Bonnie called, May's
phone was no longer in service. Silversmith's investigator later
went to Florida to track her down; but when he found her, she
told him she could not testify for the defense.

What May's testimony might have been was suggested in a
letter she wrote in February of 1984. She said that when she arrived
at Jimmy's clinic in June of 1983, cancer had already spread
throughout her body. Surgery had been recommended, but she'd
had thirteen surgeries in the previous eight years. She was ready
to try something new. "I arrived in Mexico a very miserable
person," she wrote, "and left feeling, for the first time in years,
full of the joy of life. My blood test returned normal and upon a
physical exam [my doctor] could find no evidence of the cancer."

Then there was Carolyn Penton. Jimmy considered her one
of his most dramatic cases. She wrote in a 1984 letter to the court
that she'd had leukemia, and that her doctor had given her only
ten days to live. Jimmy had treated her when only three of those
days were left. She attested:

> *I could not walk or even think for myself to make a decision.
> My son and uncle had to carry me due to the fact I couldn't
> walk. On the fourth treatment of Tumorax [sic] I was able to
> walk by myself and the great pain had left also. . . . I was
> cured of cancer. After I had completed my Tumorax treatments,
> I had my test made to see if I still had the cancer. My test was
> just great. The doctor would not believe this and had the test
> made again.*

"I told her I couldn't help her," Jimmy recalled, "but her uncle wanted me to try. He was the mayor of Mandeville, a well-to-do city near New Orleans. He said he'd sign papers saying I wouldn't be liable if anything went wrong. Her doctors wanted to put her in the hospital, but he was afraid they'd put her lights out. She'd already had 57 chemotherapy treatments. They said if she had any more, it would kill her; and she was too weak for a bone marrow transplant. Leukemia, you know, is actually cancer of the bone marrow. Her uncle said he had talked to a number of people who had been almost dead, who had gotten better at my clinic. He wanted to give her that chance.

"Her veins were so bad, I could hardly get a needle in. Every day I went through the ritual of praying for a vein, and every day the Lord did the impossible and gave one. After a couple of days she started getting better. In a week she was walking around, and in four or five weeks she was back to normal. Her doctor was so amazed she was still alive that he did bone marrow tests on her. Her bone marrow had been wiped out before I treated her. But afterwards, the tests showed it was perfect."

"And she's still alive?"

"She is," Jimmy said, "and cancer-free. But the FBI got there before Silversmith's investigator did. She'd been in a car accident and was in the hospital strung up in traction at the time. They said it wouldn't be in the best interests of the government if she testified for the defense. After that, she told me she couldn't come."

"Too bad! What about subpoenaing her medical records from the doctor who did the bone marrow tests?"

"I already asked Silversmith to do it." Jimmy added wearily, "But that doesn't mean much." He didn't seem to have much confidence in his lead counsel, but I chalked it up to jailhouse paranoia. Silversmith was a luminary in his field . . .

Having no further invitations for work, in early August I went back to Kenya, where my family was showing signs of neglect. The trial glared ominously from my calendar, where it was penciled in for Monday, August 19. The trial date was only 2-1/2 weeks after I got home, but we were reasonably certain it would be delayed. Silversmith had brought a motion for change of venue, aimed at changing the location and the judge. The grounds were that prospective Brownsville jury members had already been prejudiced by unfavorable local publicity. There was also our motion to dismiss to be considered. Bill and I planned to wait for the outcomes of these two motions before boarding planes from our respective distances.

Jimmy, meanwhile, was left to cogitate alone in his jail cell. As trial loomed ever nearer, he kept getting the throat-clutching feeling that the defense was unprepared. He had hardly had an opportunity to talk to Silversmith about the facts and issues of the case. He got more frantic as the filing of the motion to dismiss kept getting delayed. The Federal Rules allowed it to be filed at any time, but the closer trial loomed, the less likely the motion was to be considered. Trial judges generally preferred sitting back and watching a show.

Jimmy was so unhappy with his lead counsel that at the last minute of the hour, he paid $10,000 to another attorney to look over the file with a view to stepping in on the case. This man, whom I'll call O'Brien, had already been retained to represent one of the defense witnesses, but he had been busy with another case. Whether he could come "up to speed" in time to take over this one was unclear.

Silversmith, for his part, was equally unhappy with Bill, who wasn't returning his calls and didn't seem to be cooperating. Silversmith said he couldn't go to trial without a physician attorney to handle the medical aspects of the case. He wanted Ginsburg brought back in. Silversmith gave as his reason for not filing the motion to dismiss that he was waiting for the protest from the Mexican government and the signed declarations from Bill. The protest was Alma's department, but she said she was afraid. Jimmy didn't get word that Alma's cousin Pepe had gotten the document until shortly before trial was to proceed.

I heard the rest of this story later from Jimmy's Uncle Harold, a New Yorker otherwise known as "Jimmy's bulldog." Uncle Harold and Aunt Lou had set up residence in Brownsville during the months preceding the trial, to aid Jimmy in whatever needed to be done. One function of this family liaison was to set up conference calls. The arrangement allowed Jimmy, who could only call locally, to line up his own witnesses when his attorneys seemed to be dragging their feet.

As Harold told it, Silversmith sent the motion to dismiss to Brownsville on August 16, only one business day before trial was scheduled to begin. But for some reason, Jimmy's local attorney Black had declined to file it. The job was left to the bulldog. The papers were on a flight that was scheduled to arrive only shortly before the courthouse was to close at 5 p.m. ("I don't think they really wanted it to get filed," Harold drily remarked.) He did not say at what speed he was traveling, but he did say he arrived at the courthouse at 4:50. "Yankees get things done," he quipped.

When Jimmy heard this story later, he had an affectionate quip of his own. "Harold was in the family twenty years before they called him a Yankee," Jimmy said. "Before that, they called him a Damn Yankee."

Even with the motion on file, Jimmy's anxiety level was at record highs. The weekend before trial was scheduled, Alma couldn't be reached, and neither could Durk. "It was very strange about Alma," Jimmy observed later, "because at that time she always let my father know where she was."

Jimmy's local attorney Black was also unavailable that critical weekend. He was reported to be in California. Were the three of them meeting with each other? If so, what could they be discussing? The prisoner's imagination ran wild.

Then he learned that Pepe hadn't gotten a formal protest from the Mexican government at all. He only had Jimmy's up-to-date immigration papers and similar documents. The trapped defendant had been anxious for months, but now he was terrified. His case seemed to be eroding from within.

# PART THREE

## TRIAL BY JURY

*Whin' th' case is all over, the jury'll pitch th' tistimony out iv the window, an' consider three questions: "Did Lootgert look as though he'd kill his wife? Did his wife look as though she ought to be kilt? Isn't it time we wint to supper?"*

-- Finley Peter Dunne,
<u>Mr. Dooley in Peace and War</u> (1898)

# Chapter 28

## Case for the Prosecution

Our living room in Nairobi was wrapped in bars, but they were the kind that keep people out. Through the wrap-around windows, I watched roses dance in the breeze to the accompaniment of an enormous number of birds. I wondered idly if birds sang for any biological reason, or if their symphony were designed merely for entertainment. My thoughts inevitably reverted to the Cameron County Jail, where there were no birds and no roses. I remembered the time I had brought in a flower and had been reprimanded for it. It was an unprofessional gesture I would know better than to repeat. I was already suspect for spending so much time there. Few attorneys took so much interest in their cases. I had never taken so much interest in one myself, but my earlier cases were all about money. The ghosts of hosts of cancer victims seemed to hover over this one.

I was killing time bird-watching while waiting for a phone call. I was guardedly optimistic. If Silversmith's motion for change of venue were granted, the trial would be delayed. That would give the defendant time to prepare his lead counsel. It would also give the judge time to read our motion to dismiss. If the motion to dismiss were granted, it would summarily dispose of the case. And if it weren't granted, Jimmy hoped to get the trial moved to Houston. A big-city jury was liable to be more enlightened about unconventional medical treatments than one from a remote place like Brownsville.

I was therefore quite disappointed, when Jimmy's brother Ray finally called, to hear that the trial had already started. A change of venue had been granted, but only to McAllen, a mere fifty miles from Brownsville. The local citizenry had been exposed to the same unfavorable publicity, and the judge would be the same. The other pretrial motions had apparently been denied without comment. Trial was to proceed in McAllen on Tuesday, August 20. The judge was allotting only two weeks on his calendar for it, counting August 19, when he heard Silversmith's motion for change of venue. That left 4-1/2 days for the government's case and 4-1/2 days for the defendant's. Silversmith was still lead counsel. O'Brien hadn't had time to "come up to speed" on the case.

By the time Bill and I got to McAllen, it was already Thursday, August 22. I had spent Tuesday and Wednesday on a plane from Kenya, while Bill had managed to miss his Tuesday flight from California. He said he had phoned ahead to Jimmy's family. But either Silversmith never got the message, or he wasn't confident of Bill's contribution, because when Bill arrived, Ginsburg was already there.

Bill took a seat at the counsel table along with Ginsburg, Black, Silversmith and Sylvia.

"The defense table is already more crowded than the government's," Silversmith said to me. "Why don't you sit in the front row of the audience?"

I slipped onto a bench being warmed by Maxine's attorney Mike and <u>Los Angeles Times</u> reporter Paul Ciotti. The three of us got to be good friends. The two men were practical, objective and low-key, stable voices of reason at a time when emotions were running high. We had lunch together at the courthouse and dinner at the Green Tree Hotel, where the defense attorneys and witnesses were being lodged.

We watched the entrance of the jury with keen interest, but there wasn't much to be told from their faces. The only juror who showed any emotion was a tall white man with a mustache and receding chin, who wound up dominating the jury box. Throughout the trial, he would display exaggerated reactions to the testimony and exchange smirking glances with the woman prosecutor who was Meier's assistant.

The rest of the jury appeared to be primarily what one observer described as "Mexican shop girls."

"They don't look intelligent," someone else remarked ominously. "If that's who it's dependent on, I'm really worried."

"The ignorance level in this area goes off the scale," said a local resident. "You have to almost sit down and draw a picture to communicate."

Remarks about the jurors' intelligence I took as mere unwarranted prejudice, but I <u>was</u> worried about their language skills. It didn't take much English to sit on a jury. Even if their English were adequate, it was going to take some education and diligence to understand the issues in this case. I had trouble understanding them myself, and I had studied them carefully. Would the jurors take the time to read anything? Or would they simply be swayed by emotion -- the anger of the relatives, the hostility of the prosecutor, the smirks of his assistant?

There seemed to be a chill in the courtroom. I glanced over at the prosecutor. U.S. Attorney Meier exhibited the forbidding mien of a Nazi storm trooper. He kept clenching his jaw. One thing to be said for him: he had determination. He had a job to do and he looked ready to do it, by whatever means. I was also struck, as he methodically laid out his case, by his disdainful confidence in the face of opponents who were evidently older and more experienced than he was.

The theme of Meier's case was that the defendant had defrauded cancer victims into paying for a worthless treatment. Fraudulent intent was an essential element of the crime. The government had to prove not only that the treatment was worthless but that Keller knew it all along. Meier claimed that Keller had falsely told patients that he had high cure rates and that they were cured or improved upon finishing the treatment, when he knew in fact that his patients were dying like flies.

The courtroom seemed to get colder and more hostile through the parade of testifying relatives. They were clearly angry. They had been persuaded by the government that they had been duped into believing a worthless amino acid could cure cancer. They uniformly testified that they or the patient had contacted Maxine, who talked up Keller's treatment. She represented that it had a percentage cure rate for patients without prior conventional treatment that was said (depending on the witness) to range from 80 to 99 percent; while for previously treated patients, it ranged from 40 to 65 percent. The relatives testified that they had accompanied the patients to the clinic in Mexico, where Jimmy had used either or both the Digitron "D" Spectrometer and a pendulum to diagnose the disease. There was testimony that he had used a sock for a tourniquet ("a dirty sock"), and that he had taken the patients' pictures with a polaroid camera and told them he intended to use the pictures to treat the patients in their absence. The testimony provoked a mocking and amused exchange of eyeball-rolling between the tall chinless white male juror and the woman assistant prosecutor.

Nearly all of the decedents had had prior unsuccessful conventional treatment and had been pronounced terminal before they came to Keller's clinic. The way I saw it, that put them in the "40 to 65 percent success" category. If Jimmy could produce ten patients he had saved to match the ten who had died, he should have been home free. But no one pointed that out to the jury. The relatives all testified that they understood that their deceased loved ones had essentially been promised a cure. Government experts later acknowledged that desperate patients and their relatives tend to hear what they want to hear.

The witnesses said the treatment consisted of daily injections of Tumorex, vitamin and mineral supplements, a strict diet, lymphatic massages, and colonic irrigations. At the conclusion of the ten-day or two-week treatment, Jimmy used the Digitron again and stated that the patients had "zeroed out" on it. This was either said or understood to mean they were cancer free. There were reports that the patients had felt better and that their tumors had shrunk. But in ten of the eleven cases, the patients had gone home and, sooner or later, had died. The eleventh patient, a man named Kevin P., was alive and well. His complaint was that he had had to resort to chemotherapy after Jimmy's treatment.

Two witnesses testified that they thought the defendant hadn't really lost his ear to cancer. One suggested he may even have cut it off himself. Strange, I thought, that two witnesses would come up with this bizarre theory independently.

Then the government introduced a taped speech in which Jimmy had said that he'd had cancer surgery at M. D. Anderson Hospital in Houston. The tape was followed by testimony by the custodian of records at M. D. Anderson, who said there was no record of any such surgery. The implication was that Jimmy had lied in his taped speech; and that, indeed, he may never have had cancer.

The lay witnesses included Jackie Turner, the sole complainant named in the original state court indictment. On the stand, she was grief-stricken over the loss of her husband. But Jimmy's father Guy reported hearing her in the cafeteria after her testimony, "cutting up and laughing with the other witnesses, and asking Mr. Dixon when they would get their money."

A particularly disturbing case involved a two-year-old girl I'll call Jessica. According to the testimony of her parents and her doctors, Jessica had suffered "a slight head injury in an auto accident" on December 14, 1982. On December 15, she was taken to a pediatrician because she was vomiting. The doctor then sent her to Salt Lake City, where a brain tumor was discovered. On December 16, the tumor was removed and was found to be malignant. The hole was so large that a metal plate had to be inserted in her skull. Neither her mother nor her doctors wanted to put the girl through surgery again. "She had gotten meningitis and she had staph infection," said her mother. "She was so sick."

The neurosurgeon testified that he had assured the parents that Jessica "would likely die from the tumor. That I had removed all of the visible tumor, but that it would almost certainly recur." The mother, however, said she was not aware of the gravity of the situation until she took the child back later to the pediatrician. "I took her in for a cold, just for a cold. And, you know, he told me that she was going to die."

True to the neurosurgeon's predictions, a month after the surgery, the tumor had already regrown. It was the alarming size of a baseball and was pressing painfully on the plate. The neurosurgeon then recommended radiation. But he admitted in a note to the pediatrician that it would do no good and, in fact, would probably make the child worse. He justified his recommendation only by saying, "I think radiation therapy is a reasonable alternative <u>to allow the parents the sensation that they are helping the child</u>." Apparently, false hope was better than no hope at all.

The parents finally took Jessica to Jimmy. On the second day, her swelling was gone and so was her pain. Her condition, said her mother, was "Excellent. She was doing real good." Like Bonnie Cayer's grandson Wesley Smith, Jessica went swimming and chased the ducks. She stayed at the clinic for three weeks instead of the usual two at no extra charge; and when she went home, she seemed fine. But a week later, her pediatrician admitted her to the hospital for dehydration; and there, she suddenly died.

When Jimmy was informed of the tragedy, he refunded part of the parents' money. Jessica's mother responded with a note stating that she would "never be able to thank God and all of you for the three weeks of health and happiness we had together." But this sentiment was apparently forgotten when the mother took the stand eight years later. "[T]hey were horrible times," she testified. "I don't think that I can ever forgive myself for putting her through something that she didn't have to go through." She said Jessica hated injections and carrot juice and enemas. The chinless white male juror shook his head and glared disapprovingly at the defendant.

The last lay witness was Chickley T____. I could only see Jimmy from the back, but I gleaned from the way his shoulders fell that he was crushed. The government had managed to turn one of his best cases into evidence against him.

Chickley testified that he had gone to Jimmy for treatment for melanoma in 1981. He had paid $2,500 for the treatment, but he maintained he didn't really have cancer. He just feared he might, because seventeen of his family members had had it. He told Jimmy he had it because otherwise Jimmy might not have given him the Tumorex.

Jimmy whispered in Silversmith's ear. Silversmith then asked Chickley if he'd ever told anyone that he'd had cancer or had been helped by Jimmy's treatments. Silversmith started naming names. Chickley looked nervous. For each name, he said he couldn't remember.

The judge finally asked, "Did you tell anybody that Jim Keller had cured you from cancer?"

Chickley said, "I don't remember. I might have, I might not. I don't remember."

Paul and I exchanged glances. Why would Chickley tell people he'd had cancer and had been cured of it, if he hadn't? And why would he pay $2,500 for a treatment for something he didn't have, and invent a story to make sure he got the treatment?

Chickley was followed by University of Arizona pharmacologist Dr. Dorr, an expert who testified at the 1985 trial about arginine. (The M. D. Anderson doctor who said in 1985 that the NCI had consistently found arginine to have no effect on cancer was not put on the stand. We suspected it was because his testimony would have been too easy to impeach.) Dr. Dorr said he had performed a small study on animals and in cultures, using Tumorex as well as pure L-arginine. Neither, he maintained, had any anti-cancer effect.

Silversmith objected that no chain of custody had been established for Dr. Dorr's sample of Tumorex -- the prosecution hadn't linked it to this case -- but the objection was overruled.

Dr. Dorr later changed his testimony. He conceded that studies have been published in scientific journals demonstrating that arginine may inhibit the formation of tumors. But he staunchly maintained that no published studies indicated the amino acid has any therapeutic effect after a tumor has developed. He also said that there are "no studies in live human beings with L-arginine at all." I hastily passed a note up to Silversmith citing contrary studies, but nothing came of it. Silversmith was evidently saving our research for Bill's experts.

Dr. Dorr later changed his testimony again. He conceded that there were some studies in which oral arginine supplementation had inhibited tumor growth. But he discounted the studies by noting that they were on animals. "[N]one of that has resulted in even a clinical trial," he archly observed. "So apparently the clinicians are not convinced that adding arginine is an effective way to treat cancer."

I was developing a tension headache. The testimony simply wasn't true. Why so few clinical studies had been done could be explained; indeed, it would be explained by the defense experts the next week. But by then, the jurors were liable to remember only that the government had experts and the defense had experts. The rest was splitting hairs. Dr. Dorr's unchallenged contention that arginine was useless as a cancer treatment would hang in the air for days after he took the stand, indelibly coloring the case.

"Now we're going to see some fireworks!" Jimmy's father Guy whispered excitedly. The prosecution was closing the week with the testimony of Narda Gomez, the undercover agent who testified against David Keller in 1985. When David had asked her whether the sting operation had been taped, she had responded in the negative. But at the July 1991 pretrial hearing, the government had finally admitted that she had lied.

We listened to her testimony in high expectation, but no sparks flew. Narda was merely asked to introduce a tape of a presentation given by Jimmy and his patients and supporters. The sting operation wasn't discussed and neither was the destroyed tape, by either the prosecution or the defense.

Even Narda's parents seemed disappointed. They happened to be sitting next to Jimmy's relatives during her testimony. They said they were ashamed of what their daughter had done. The Kellers seemed like such a warm and loving family.

"We are," agreed Jimmy's sister Diane.

# Chapter 29

## Firming Up the Facts

I didn't bump into any other defense attorneys at the jail, but I figured they were too busy preparing the case to take time to consult with their client. I had time to consult but not much influence on the strategy of the defense. My inquiries were directed mainly to casting some light on the murky events of the week. One was the puzzling fact that M. D. Anderson Hospital had had no record of the defendant's surgery.

"That was a low point in the testimony," Jimmy gloomily agreed. "I went to M. D. Anderson for the initial consultation -- my brother worked there, you know -- but they did the actual surgery at the Veteran's Hospital. I was a veteran, and the hospitals were affiliated. It was all one big complex. I just said M. D. Anderson because that's the part people have heard of. It's the head of the cancer industry. It's the biggest tumor center in the world."

Jimmy had another question. "Why didn't Silversmith bring up the destroyed tape?"

"I don't know," I said. "I suppose he had his reasons." But at the time I couldn't think of any, so I changed the subject. "At least Chickley's credibility should be easy to demolish . . ."

"It should," Jimmy agreed. "Silversmith just has to put the witnesses on who heard his testimonials."

"So what did you think of Dr. Dorr's arginine study?"

"It's easy to make a study come out negative," Jimmy responded. You just don't follow the right protocol or use the right amounts. It doesn't disprove the studies that came out the other way. But did you hear him admit that arginine prevents tumors? If they know that's true, why isn't it front page news? You can bet it would be if arginine were a patented pharmaceutical. But you know who we should have challenged on the stand?"

"Who?" I asked.

"Marie S_____."

"She must have taken the stand before I got to McAllen. What did she say?"

"Marie said Maxine and I both gave her husband a 99 percent cure rate. That was ridiculous. Her husband had had surgery and radiation. Why would we give him a better rate than we gave everyone else? And why would we <u>both</u> give him that rate -- in different conversations? Marie said her husband's surgery had made him impotent -- and he was still a young man. They told him they 'got it all,' but the cancer came back. Then they told him it was terminal, and they went on and wiped out his immune system with radiation. They said there wasn't anything more they could do for him. Would we give him a 99 percent chance of cure after all that? Really! There has to be something left for my serum to work with!"

Jimmy sighed. "There was another thing Marie said. I told Silversmith about it, and that it would be easy to demolish her testimony. But he just let it all go into the record."

"What was that?"

"She said she brought her husband to Matamoros in late February of '83, because somebody at Maxine's phone number told her I was moving there. She couldn't even remember if it was Maxine. But it was an impossible conversation no matter who it was, because I didn't have any intention of leaving Baton Rouge until I was enjoined in March. I had just built an addition on the house."

"So why do you suppose she said it?"

"I'll tell you why. The truth is, Marie never even talked to Maxine. She talked to Iris Klampert, who is one of my witnesses. But Iris was just a patient. She wasn't in on the 'conspiracy.' The government couldn't establish wire fraud if Marie told the truth, so they had to have her say it was Maxine."

"Devious," I agreed.

"You know who else we should have challenged on the stand?"

"Who?"

"Margaret W_____. She said Maxine told her over the phone that if her mother hadn't had any treatment at all, there was an 80 percent chance she could be cured. Margaret admitted the conversation was taped; in fact it was the only one that was taped. But the government didn't introduce the tape into evidence. They just let her say what she remembered about it. I saw a transcript of the tape when it was produced in discovery. I don't remember exactly what it said, but I'm sure Maxine didn't promise any cure."

"You're kidding! There was a tape and a transcript? I think the government was supposed to introduce them into evidence!" I tried to remember what I knew about the Best Evidence Rule. "At least Silversmith could have. He could have used them for impeachment. We should look for the tape!"

"We should," Jimmy agreed.

"So what did you think of Kevin P_____'s testimony?" I asked. "He had the same kind of cancer Durk had -- non-Hodgkin's lymphoma. Why did he have to get chemotherapy after your treatment, when Durk didn't?"

"Good question. Durk was actually in worse shape than Kevin was. His cancer had metastasized to the bone marrow, which is usually fatal; and all he got was my serum. But Durk came back regularly for boosters. The problem for Kevin was that he couldn't get the boosters. It was after the FBI cut me off from my patients. You notice that when he first went back to his doctor after I treated him, the doctor said he didn't need chemotherapy. It was only later that he got the drugs. He could have been getting my boosters instead."

"I see. And what did you think about baby Jessica? That whole case was peculiar! Tragic, but peculiar. How could she have gotten a bump on her head in a car accident and developed a big malignant tumor there, in a single day? Maybe it wasn't really a tumor -- or maybe it came from some old injury nobody was talking about . . ."

"It was a tumor," Jimmy assured me. "I saw it. But you can't develop a malignant tumor in a day -- or a week. When that child left Matamoros, it was gone. I kept her an extra week just to make sure. You can't get a new tumor and be dead within a week. Something else must have been going on."

I broached another delicate subject. "Why was it that you had to give a two-year-old enemas?"

"That was another low point," Jimmy said wearily. "They weren't actually enemas. They were acidophilus implants. We did give enemas for cleansing the bowels, but these were 'retention enemas.' They kept the flora in the intestines right so everything worked right. They were only about two ounces each, for an adult; and for a child, they were less than a tablespoon. All the patients were instructed on how to do them; and once they started on them, they could see why. The acidophilus kept the flora from going alkaline and putrifying. I had studies on humans showing they worked on cancer of the colon and intestines. One study involved 200 patients. In some patients, acidophilus alone produced total remissions. Some other Tijuana clinics added acidophilus implants to their protocols later, but I was already doing them in Baton Rouge."

I wondered about something else. Why were Jessica's parents so upset with Jimmy for giving her shots that had made her better, when nobody had thought to sue the surgeon who had cut a big hole in her skull, knowing it almost certainly would do no good? The surgeon had also admitted that radiation would give false hope only, yet he had recommended it in writing. The main difference between the surgeon's "false hope" and Jimmy's seemed to be that conventional therapy, though far more painful and damaging, was accepted and unconventional therapy wasn't.

"You know why they didn't sue the surgeon," Jimmy said, arching an eyebrow.

I nodded. "Because they would have been thrown out of court." The oncologist was merely doing what the law required, following standard practice in the community. If the parents were going to vent their anger and recover some money, it had to be against Jimmy.

I had another question. "What caused Jessica's mother to change her mind about your treatments, when she seemed so grateful at the time?"

"I don't know." Jimmy slumped despondently. "This whole thing has been like a nightmare, a bad movie, where absolutely everything goes wrong." He dug into his ragged collection of papers and pulled out two clippings. "Look at these!"

One was an article from the Brownsville Herald, telling of a Mexican citizen who had been let out on $750,000 bail. His wife had reported his death and was attempting to get the bail money back.

"My guess is he's alive and well and living in Mexico," Jimmy said. "Why are foreign citizens being released on bail, and I'm considered a 'serious risk of flight'?"

The other clipping told of a man arrested for a serious drug offense, who had been let out on a bail of $10,000 cash. He was ordered to come back later for a surveillance bracelet, but he had conveniently failed to keep his appointment.

"Check out the magistrate," Jimmy said. "It's the same one who denied bail altogether in my case."

"What's interesting in your case, though, is that the judge actually did set bail later," I said.

"Sure, at $5 million cash."

"Exactly — it was unreasonable. The order should have been appealable on the spot."

I had looked at the Bail Reform Act at the courthouse library. It provided that the amount set for bail must be reasonable and not intended to result in detention. Five million dollars was an unreasonable financial condition clearly intended to result in detention. I had also looked at the Federal Rules of Appellate Procedure. The way I read them, the defendant's five million dollar bail was subject to immediate appeal to the Fifth Circuit. "Did Silversmith ever file an appeal with the Court of Appeals?" I asked.

The defendant slumped further in his chair. "I asked him to. But if he did it, nobody told me about it."

Jimmy said he was disturbed about something else. He had heard that when Silversmith sought a change of venue, it wasn't to Houston (Jimmy's choice) but to San Antonio, Silversmith's own city. San Antonio wasn't in the same judicial district as Brownsville, so the request was likely to be denied.

"He probably had his reasons," I said, trying to sound reassuring. "He's just too busy to share them with us."

I decided to look Silversmith up and ask him some questions. But when I got back to the hotel, I couldn't find him. Silversmith, Sylvia, Ginsburg, and Black had all disappeared for the weekend. Black had left word that he would be entertaining Ginsburg at his home on an island off the coast.

We learned later from a friend of Paul's that Silversmith was at a convention in Phoenix, giving an acceptance speech for an award as trial lawyer of the year. Jimmy had indeed picked a luminary in the field. Too bad, I thought, that Jimmy's stellar attorney had to gear up for a newsworthy speech in Phoenix the same weekend he was supposed to be preparing a defense in Brownsville.

In his speech to his attorney audience, Silversmith reportedly said that to be effective in your cross-examination, you have to get down and dirty and wallow with the cockroaches. Paul commented drily that we hadn't seen much wallowing in this case.

Bill, meanwhile, was storming around the hotel in a general state of outrage. The testimony of the government witnesses was so uniform, he said, that it sounded like it had been rehearsed. Yet no one had asked the routine question, "Have you discussed your testimony with anyone before taking the stand?" Bill could have asked it, but he wasn't being allowed to say anything in court. The judge was permitting only Silversmith to speak for the defense. What really outraged Bill was that he wasn't going to be able to examine his own expert witnesses. He doubted Silversmith would ask them the right questions.

Bill considered it a glaring omission that the jury hadn't been informed that the government witnesses had all met with the prosecutor before taking the stand. We knew that several months earlier, the government had subpoenaed all its witnesses to come to Brownsville to discuss their testimony. It was what Bill called "firming up the facts." If the witnesses didn't all remember the same facts when they went in, they were likely to by the time they came out. We knew about the sessions because Barbara, Maxine, and Becky Johnson had all been interviewed by Meier and his woman assistant. But all had been rejected as prosecution witnesses after it was clear where their sympathies lay.

Barbara, the nutritionist who had served eighteen months in jail for being an accomplice in Jimmy's conspiratorial scheme, described her encounter with the prosecution in an interview with Paul. She said she had told her interrogators that she had been diagnosed with cancer, and that she had never had a problem after Jimmy treated her.

"It must have been a misdiagnosis," Meier's woman assistant archly responded.

"What does Jimmy have?" Dixon asked Barbara. "Why do all you people love him so much? Does he hypnotize you?"

Barbara said, "No."

"Why did you do it?" he persisted. "I wouldn't go to jail for my wife."

Barbara just looked at him. "I feel sorry for you," she said.

Dixon asked, "Would it surprise you to know that all Keller's patients are now dead?"

He was so assertive that Barbara said she might have believed him, if she hadn't recalled patients she had spoken to recently who were alive and well. When she later spoke to the prosecution witnesses in the courtroom cafeteria, they too maintained that all Jimmy's patients were dead. When Barbara countered that she had just talked to some of his surviving patients, she said the witnesses looked at her very strangely.

I was beginning to understand baby Jessica's mother's testimony. She had maintained on the stand that all Jimmy's patients were dead. But she said it without supporting evidence. Apparently, she was merely repeating what Meier had told her. No doubt, he had also told her Tumorex was a common amino acid worth only a couple of dollars a bottle. When she realized she had been duped into paying for a worthless treatment and subjecting her terminally ill child to it, the anguished mother could easily have been outraged enough to testify for the prosecution.

We learned more about the government's pretrial interviews from Maxine and her husband. Eldon wrote in a later letter to the judge:

> *About two months before the trial Mr. Meier summoned both Maxine and me to his office and interviewed us, during this time Mr. Dixon, in the presence of Mr. Meier, told Maxine about the wonderful recovery of Becky Johnson Nielsen's little girl, he went on and on telling in detail how she had gone home and taken traditional treatment and was completely well. Maxine let him go on and on about it and finally told him that she received a call from Becky within a week after her death that her daughter had passed away due to chicken-pox. . . . Maxine said she caught them in many untruths. . . . In the interview they constantly used the word 'cure' so that the government witnesses were brain-washed just as they tried to brain-wash Maxine. . . . [P]rior to the interview Mr. Meier threatened Maxine and me with keeping us in Brownsville from that day until the trial was over even if it lasted until the middle of September. This was said by him after Maxine told him that we were needed at home to take care of our business and her aging parents and could only stay the minimum amount of time necessary. He said, 'Are you going to cooperate when you come down here?' and Maxine said, 'I am going to tell you*

*the truth if that is what you mean.' Then he said, 'I don't
think you are going to cooperate. . . . I can tell by the tone of
your voice that you are not going to cooperate.' Then he said,
'. . . I won't have you telling people that I threatened you, or
anything like that.' By then, however, he had already threatened
to keep us there and not let us come home until the trial was
over.*

Maxine amplified this story when Paul and I interviewed her.
She said Dixon had asked her, "Would it surprise you to learn
that Chickley never had cancer?"

Maxine replied, "He told me he only had three months to
live."

Dixon said, "Sarah Johnson was a modern miracle. They
forced her to take chemotherapy and radiation and she's still alive."

Maxine replied, "That's interesting, because when her mother
called me in 1985, she said Sarah was dead."

Dixon asked, "Would it surprise you to learn that every patient
Jimmy treated in Matamoros is now dead?"

Maxine replied, "Some of them are my good friends."

Dixon asked, "Would it surprise you to learn that Jimmy Keller
put painkiller in every shot?"

Maxine said, "That is a mighty good painkiller, that lasted
for many weeks."

Dixon said, "The reason Jimmy's serum made the tumors fizz
was that he was spraying hydrogen peroxide on them."

Maxine responded, "I never saw him spraying anything!"

Dixon asked, "How could you be so stupid as to fall for this?"

Maxine said, "I saw things. I saw people's pain go away. I saw
people get results."

She wrote later to the court that when she left the office for a
break, "my head was whirling, I was actually wondering if I could
possibly have been involved in a scam. After that visit I can
understand how you become so confused and frustrated you begin
to wonder what really is right or wrong."

Becky Johnson tape recorded her interview. Meier asked her,
"You don't remember those statements there that the cure rate
was sixty to seventy percent or seventy to eighty percent?"

Becky said she didn't.

Meier's woman assistant asked, "If they didn't make any assurances or say [Sarah] would be cured, and she didn't look that bad, why did you go? . . . . Say you can't remember the exact words. What was your impression?"

Becky replied, "I did not hear anyone promise a cure."

The assistant countered, "You just said you don't remember . . . . We've had victims come in, and they remember a lot more after we start talking to them."

Becky said she felt badgered, as if they were trying to twist her testimony. But it was a subtle pressure, hard to prove in court; and the tape never got introduced into evidence.

# Chapter 30

## Mutiny

While the cats were away, the mice sat around the Green Tree Hotel nervously comparing notes.

Jim Jr. told of something he had overheard Silversmith saying to the court reporter in the men's room. "I don't know what I'm doing," Silversmith conceded. "I'm just going with the flow."

An admiring young attorney from McAllen, who had read about the case and had come to observe, remarked earlier in the week, "Jimmy Keller can't help but win with Silversmith in his corner!" But after he saw the famed litigator in action, the young attorney said he was disappointed. Silversmith didn't seem confident.

I thought he probably wasn't. Silversmith was known as a "quick study," but this wasn't shaping up to be the ordinary quick-study drug case.

Jimmy's father Guy told of something that had happened after the testimony of Narda Gomez, the undercover agent who concealed the destruction of the tape of the sting operation. After Silversmith had failed to challenge her on the point, Guy had been approached by O'Brien, the attorney Jimmy had hoped would take over the case. "I'm leaving," said O'Brien in high agitation. "I can't stand it." He told Guy he thought Jimmy was being sold down the river by his own attorneys.

"I'm talking myself into agreeing with O'Brien," Bill remarked at dinner. "He called me at 1:00 a.m. and said Jimmy was being railroaded."

We were sharing a table with Paul and Deborah Jones, one of Jimmy's "angels," and Bill was in a ranting mood. "Silversmith is supposed to be the hottest attorney in Texas. He don't show me shit! He's board certified. They don't just give those things out. You have to try so many cases and be good. He's supposed to be a fast study. Does he look to you like a fast study? He's asking all the wrong questions. The government witnesses all said Jimmy promised them a cure. Two of them even suggested he had cut off his own ear. They were obviously coached. There's nothing wrong with that, but it should have been brought out in court. Usually if you have twelve people, you get stories from twelve different points of view. You don't get the same story twelve times."

Deborah was nodding attentively, while Paul was busily taking notes.

"There was a recording of Jimmy talking to a prospective client," Bill went on. "It showed his state of mind and how he typically talked to patients. The FBI destroyed the tape. So what are we to deduce from that? Silversmith should have gone into that before the jury, but he let the witness off without a word. If those two things had been brought before the jurors, they might have considered that the government wasn't so disinterested after all.

"Then there was the motion to dismiss. Silversmith didn't file it until the Friday before trial. When you file a motion that late, you really don't expect to get it acted on. All it did was to give away our case."

Paul, who loved a colorful turn of phrase, was quite amused when Bill said, "Silversmith is as nervous as a whore in church. You've got to turn your back on the district attorney, look at him like he's an insect on a pin, say his name with the most exquisite disdain."

Bill gave Deborah a meaningful look. "Jimmy has got to do that too. He's got to get mad. He's got to stand on the desk, or roll up in a fetal position on the floor, and say his attorneys are throwing the case. Then the judge is likely to declare a mistrial."

Deborah looked dubious. "I don't know if Jimmy can do that," she said.

When Jimmy heard Bill's plan, he was dubious too. The tack finally decided on was more conservative. The defense would bring a motion "in limine" (a motion during the trial) to allow Bill and

Ginsburg, the two defense attorney/M.D.'s, to speak in court
along with Silversmith. If the motion were denied, Jimmy would
consider the more drastic approach.

I was drafted to draft the motion. It kept me busy all Sunday
afternoon.

The same afternoon, Sylvia was busy drafting another motion.
She had reappeared along with Silversmith, Ginsburg, and Black in
time to discuss what should be done about a certain prejudicial piece
of reporting. The front page of the local Sunday newspaper featured
an article titled "Keller's Clinic: 'Grasping at straws.'" It began:

> A Polaroid snapshot, a pendulum swinging over the
> patient's head and a dubious cancer-diagnosing machine called
> a 'digitron' were key ingredients in James Gordon Keller's
> alleged cure for cancer. All his patients needed were money
> and faith. Authorities called it 'blind faith.'

The article was accompanied by an enormous picture of Jimmy
in chains. "To this jury," Ginsburg remarked, "a picture is worth
a thousand words. English is their second language." The motion
Sylvia was drafted to draft was for a mistrial.

The same afternoon, the defense attorneys met with several of
Jimmy's patient witnesses. I missed it, being otherwise engaged.
But Dr. Ruth Kerhart, one of the patients, said that when the
attorneys heard the patients' stories, they were "blown away." She
thought it may have been the first time Silversmith's team had
considered that their client's remedies might have been effective.

Too bad, I thought, that the trial was already half over. But
it wasn't too late. I had seen it in the movies: trial attorneys
routinely stayed up all night preparing their witnesses to take the
stand the next day. We had a room full of witnesses eager to tell
their stories. This case, I nervously reassured myself, could still be
turned around.

In court on Monday, August 26, 1991, the first order of
business was to rule on the two motions in limine. The jurors
were questioned to determine whether they had seen the
newspaper. The judge had told them on the first day of trial that
they would not be sequestered, but they were sternly instructed
to avert their eyes from the newspaper and the TV. Seven of
thirteen jurors nevertheless said they had seen the article.

As Jimmy's brother Ray heard it, one juror added, "We've agreed that we saw the picture, but we didn't read the article." What Ray wanted to know was, when did they agree? The jurors had just arrived in the courtroom for the day. They weren't supposed to be talking to each other about the case. Ray pointed out to Silversmith that the juror's statement was grounds for a mistrial.

"You're right," Silversmith responded. "We've got it in the record." In short, the matter would have to wait for appeal.

The final score on the motions was: one granted, one denied. No mistrial was found, but the defense attorney/M.D.'s would be allowed to examine witnesses along with Silversmith. Bill could put his own experts on the stand. Mutiny was averted. The defense's case would proceed as scheduled.

But first, U.S. Attorney Meier had one more witness. He still had to establish two critical elements of his claim -- that the representations concerning cure rates were false, and that Jimmy knew it when they were made. I wondered what Meier had up his sleeve, as he called his last and most important witness to the stand.

FBI agent Dixon strode up in a dark government-style suit and cowboy boots. He testified that he had performed a survey. He had located 103 patients Jimmy had treated in Matamoros in 1983. By 1991, he said, 91 of these 103 had died; and 78 or 79 of them had died by 1985.

Silversmith jumped up. "[T]his is a hearsay recitation of the witness, based upon representations made to him, not based upon any particular expertise . . ."

The adrenalin trickled back into my chest. The defense was finally going on the attack.

"The objection is overruled," said the judge.

Defense attorney Ginsburg made his first vocal appearance as Dixon's cross-examiner. When he opened his mouth, I was struck by how much he not only looked but sounded like Perry Mason. Ginsburg carried on with the attack. He forced Dixon to admit that the dates when the patients in the survey had died and what they had died of were unknown. They may have survived more than five years, the orthodox cut-off for "cure." They may not have died from cancer. Dixon had introduced only nine death certificates into evidence. They included those of Clarence Schwartz and Velma McBride, who had both died from

a stroke; Sarah Johnson, who had died from chicken pox; Marshall
Young, who had died from a gunshot wound.

Marshall's earlier affidavit hadn't been introduced into
evidence, but I had seen it in Jimmy's files. He attested that he'd
had cancer of the prostate and was given only six months to live.
After Jimmy's treatment, he had tests and "was told they could
not find any evidence that I still had cancer." His July 1983 medical
report confirming this statement was attached. Marshall's death
certificate said the gunshot wound was self-inflicted. Jimmy said
he had problems in his personal life.

Dixon was asked where he got the names of Jimmy's
Matamoros patients. He admitted he got three of them from the
files confiscated in the raid the defense contended was illegal.
The rest, he maintained, had come from Maxine's phone records.
But when asked to produce the records, he said they were lost.

Ginsburg was scoring some good points, but he was playing
with a handicap. He had never seen the survey he was trying to
discredit. He asked for a copy in open court, but Meier said it
had already been furnished to the defense a month earlier.
Ginsburg looked perplexed. (He evidently didn't know what the
defense had in its files.) He asked to confer with Silversmith.

"Your Honor," Silversmith stammered, "we didn't -- if that
list was given to us, there is no indication. I am not suggesting
that it wasn't. We had no idea what the list was of until the witness
testified."

Whether the list had actually been furnished was never made
clear, but it was clear that the defense was unprepared to rebut
the evidence. The numbers definitely looked bad. These were
cancer victims. They probably died from cancer.

Dixon testified that he had prepared a poster-sized chart
presenting the results of his survey. Meier sought to have the
chart admitted into evidence, but Ginsburg objected.

"The exhibit, itself, will not be admitted any more than just
an aid," said the judge. Later he reiterated, "It is strictly an aid.
Do not exhibit it to the jury. . . . You may use it as an aid upon
request . . ."

But the jury did see it. How it escaped the judge's earlier order
I wasn't sure, but Dixon not only referred to the exhibit in his
testimony but left it prominently displayed in the courtroom.
With its survey in place, the government confidently rested its
case. The chart with its damning numbers loomed over the jury

for the rest of the trial. Meier continued to insist that the chart established that the representations of cure rates were false, and that Jimmy knew it when they were made.

We were relieved, at least, that we hadn't had to listen to the prosecution's quackbusting experts. Bill had identified five doctors on the government's witness list who were members of the NCAHF, including the doctor Jimmy had embarrassed before the Georgia legislature fifteen years earlier. But none of these experts had been called to the stand.

Or was Meier saving them for rebuttal?

In jail after Dixon's testimony, Jimmy said he had been regularly furnished with copies of documents produced in discovery. He was quite certain he had never seen a copy of Dixon's survey. He didn't believe it had ever been produced. He also didn't believe Dixon's numbers. If all those patients were dead, Jimmy said, no one had told him about it.

"And what happened to the rest of my patients?" he asked gloomily. "They only interviewed half of them. I think they purposely left out the survivors. But how can I prove it without my records or their survey?"

The defense had been taken by surprise. No one had thought to ask Dixon how many of Jimmy's Matamoros patients had died of cancer while the clinic was still in operation. The defendant could hardly have known his alleged rates of "success or cure" were false at the time they were made if no one had yet died. But we couldn't check out those nuances now because we didn't have the survey.

Ray searched the court record for it later, but he couldn't find it. He requested a copy from Meier at his office, but Meier said it was in evidence in the record. Ray countered that it wasn't. Meier said it must have been pulled out, and that he would furnish Ray with a copy; but Ray had never received it. Not only the survey's reliability but its very existence depended on the good faith of the government. The problem was, the government's good faith had never been put in doubt. Its destruction of evidence and priming of witnesses had never been raised before the jury.

Still, I told myself as I demolished a fingernail with my teeth, it was too soon to admit defeat. The defense hadn't yet put on its case. With anxious hope, we waited for the wind to change.

# *Chapter 31*

## *Experts*

It was probably too much to ask for a jury that was still struggling with English to follow the thought processes of Bill's first expert witness, Dr. William Tiller. He was the Stanford Professor of Engineering whose theories of subtle energy fields had been linked to Einstein's. It was the judge rather than the jury who seemed to take an interest in the professor's discussion. Paul colorfully described them in his <u>Los Angeles Times</u> article as "talking like a couple of old codgers sipping root beer on a wooden bench outside the general store."

"Why don't you simplify it?" the judge asked. "Can you take off your professor's hat?"

"It is hard," responded Dr. Tiller, "but I will do my best. It is a burden of the training of one's whole life."

Later, Dr. Tiller apologized to the judge for an exaggerated statement, saying, "I am having fun with you."

"You are having fun with me?" The judge was amused. "I am having fun with you, too."

The judge asked why, if radionics has been researched for seventy years, it hasn't yet come to be accepted. Dr. Tiller replied:

> [P]ractitioners are sure that it works. And I have talked with enough practitioners and seen enough data that I think it works. But the scientific experiments that need to be done to satisfy the FDA, for example, that it works, have not been done. There has never been the funding . . . . The problem [is

*that] we have a mind set and the mind set stops us from being
willing to accept something that seems out of bounds relative
to that mind set.*

Dr. Tiller's ivory-tower aplomb was evident when he faced
the prosecutor in cross-examination. Meier asked whether health
practitioners use radionics machines in the United States. Dr.
Tiller responded, "Sure, some do. . . . Maybe you don't know
about them, but there are some out there you haven't got yet."

Meier's steely eyes flashed. "You think this is a big joke, Doctor?"

"No, it is not a joke."

"Do you think it is a big joke that people get taken for $3,000
apiece and get told they are cured for cancer when they go home
and die?"

Dr. Tiller was equally steely-eyed. "I think you have to also
listen to the people that have been cured. And you will listen to
them. You are going to hear them this week. . . . [Y]ou tried to
set me up in terms of saying, yes, this is a witch doctor, which I
know legally you want to use for your own ends. I just don't want
to fall into that. Okay?"

Then, in a manner that would have made Silversmith proud
if they had been on the same team, Meier got down and dirty
and wallowed with the cockroaches. "Because you have a stake in
this, don't you?" Meier sunk the knife. "You are at the forefront
of this subtle energy movement and you make money off of that.
Bottom line."

It was Meier's stock bottom line. His own witnesses stood to
reap from $3,000 to $10,000 in damages if the government
prevailed, but the cockroach-like questions necessary to put those
facts before the jury had never been asked. Silversmith said it
would have looked bad to attack the bereaved.

Meier then asked Dr. Tiller how he knew Keller's witnesses
were going to testify that they had been cured. Dr. Tiller said he
had heard them talking in the witness room.

"They were talking about the case among themselves?" Meier
was triumphantly indignant. Witnesses weren't supposed to be
exchanging information about the case. The purpose of the rule
was to keep them from shaping their testimony to conform to
what the other witnesses had said.

"No," Dr. Tiller responded. "They were expressing how much
they thought about him. There was no one in there that was

talking about the case, because we didn't have any information. . . .
They are happy with the man."

But the judge was gravely disturbed. He reprimanded
Silversmith for not instructing his witnesses in the rules.

"We did explain that to them, Your Honor," Silversmith meekly
defended himself. "They all have known each other for years."

The damage, however, was done. Most of Jimmy's witnesses
had never even been interviewed by his lead counsel, but they all
seemed to be in cahoots; while the government's witnesses, who
had all met with the prosecutor, seemed never to have talked to
anyone before reciting their uniform testimony on the stand.

After Dr. Tiller, Bill called Professor Lance Bruner of the
University of Kentucky. Dr. Bruner testified that he had gotten
interested in radionics after his wife had been successfully treated
with it for cancer. He also confirmed the use of the pendulum in
medical diagnosis. He called it a "transducer," which provides a
readout or link to read subtle information not otherwise available.
Nuclear resonance imaging and radiation therapies, he said, are
similar in principle. Treatment by radionics involves, not drugs,
but frequencies.

"What we can prove is that it's effective. The means by which
it's effective," Dr. Bruner conceded, "is difficult to prove."

"Can a Polaroid picture act as the witness through which you
transmit vibrations to a patient?" asked Bill.

"Absolutely," said Dr. Bruner. "The picture can also give
diagnostic information. This method is commonly used in other
countries."

While medical radionics is illegal in this country, he said, it's
legal in England, Germany, France, and Scandinavia. In England,
it is actually covered by the National Health Service when used
as an adjunctive therapy. Only in the U.S. is it illegal or considered
substandard.

"Has radionics cured incurable disease?" asked the judge.

"Yes," said the witness. "There are many documented cases
where people considered incurable have survived."

"Could the pendulum tell if someone had been cured of a
disease?" persisted the judge.

"Yes, in the hands of a reliable operator. . . . What makes it
work is the operator."

Dr. Bruner then introduced fifteen books into the record
validating radionics. Stacked up on the ledge of the witness box,

they looked imposing. But I wondered if the jurors would ever lift their covers to look inside.

To counter this expert testimony, the government put on absolutely no evidence of its own. But it probably knew it didn't need to. If the rule of law is that uncontroverted evidence is taken as true, the practical reality was something else. A roll of the eyes and smirk of the lips, indiscreetly passed between the woman prosecutor and the dominant white male juror, were enough to convince the jury that the Digitron was a fraud. It didn't take a Stanford scientist to recognize a quack device.

After the two professors, Dr. Brodie took the stand. It was a courageous gesture. Doctors who had never before had legal problems had been known to get hit with malpractice actions and board proceedings after speaking out in favor of unconventional medicine. Half a dozen M.D.'s who had seen Jimmy's patients before and after treatment had agreed to testify about the impressive results they had seen. But most of them would never appear in court. I knew they existed, but only because they later wrote supporting letters to the judge. We had heard they were under pressure not to come.

Dr. Brodie, however, was not a man to be intimidated. He boldly took the stand for the defense. He said he had used Tumorex on cancer patients over a three-year period and had found it to be highly effective. When asked why he had stopped, he said physicians were being "disciplined" for its use.

But that was as far as he got. The questions necessary to elicit his remarkable arginine stories never got asked. Dr. Brodie hardly got in another word, as Ginsburg, his examiner, used the opportunity to deliver his own lecture about cancer.

"First," said Ginsburg, "let's talk about different kinds of cancer. You are familiar with the term sarcoma, is that correct?"

"Yes, sir," Dr. Brodie obliged.

"That is a form of cancer and a categorization, is it not?"

"That is right."

"You are familiar with the term carcinoma, are you not?"

"Right."

"Another form of cancer?"

"Right."

Twenty-five pages later, measured in terms of trial transcript, Ginsburg was still asking questions like: "Let's talk for a second about something that we call carcinogens. What is a carcinogen, Doctor?"

"A substance which has been shown to cause cancer," Dr. Brodie dutifully responded.

The judge was leaning on his arm, forcing himself to pay attention. I kept waiting to see what Ginsburg was getting at, but I never figured it out. I doubted the jury did either. Apparently, he didn't know Dr. Brodie had anything more interesting to say. Jimmy wanted the doctor to testify about the patients he had seen who had been successfully treated at Jimmy's clinic, and of the doctor's own successful results with Tumorex.

"Now we _are_ going to see some fireworks!" I whispered to Paul as Dr. Irwin Bross took the stand. Dr. Bross was the former National Cancer Institute (NCI) statistician who had charged his own agency with a fraudulent coverup of its dismal results. The government had made this coverup relevant by charging Jimmy with claiming that "the Food and Drug Administration and the American Medical Association did not want a cure for cancer since this would bankrupt the medical profession and the social security system." Jimmy denied having made these claims, but they were in the indictment. That meant the government had put its own good faith in issue.

Dr. Bross had authored some 400 scientific articles, including a 33-page "position paper" he sent to the defense attorneys before the trial. I had read it with keen interest. The doctor said that in response to a Freedom of Information Act request, he had received NCI documents that "revealed an NCI game plan that would lead to genocide" -- the deaths of great masses of Americans by public policies designed to protect private interests. He estimated that cancer deaths for which the government itself was responsible would total a million over the next decade. He supported these shocking charges with statistics. He showed that the NCI had manipulated data in order to justify its continued massive federal funding, and that it had swept under the rug the fact that the growing cancer scourge is largely caused by the government itself or by the big businesses whose lobbies control it. He went so far as to call this coverup "criminal fraud." (The position paper is summarized in Appendix A.)

On the stand, the doctor talked a lot of statistics; but the judge was leaning on his arm again. The statistics were the kind that put people to sleep. Silversmith was limiting his questions to what the NCI's official "Cancer Statistics Review, 1973-1986" said about cancer cases and cancer deaths.

One significant statistic, at least, got into the record. Dr. Bross testified that once cancer has metastasized, or spread from its original site to other areas of the body, all therapies are essentially placebos. Any statistically demonstrable good they do can be ascribed to the "placebo effect" -- the survival factor provided by hope. For most patients with distant metastases, he maintained, "it will take a miracle to save them." Dr. Bross did not personally know the defendant or his therapies -- he was talking about conventional treatment -- but many patients waiting to testify for the defense had recovered from metastasized cancer. The implication was that their recoveries were miracles.[76]

Unfortunately, this significant point was long in coming and buried in statistics, and it never got underscored. It got even further obscured when Silversmith had the doctor introduce a controversial study. Reported in the New England Journal of Medicine in 1991, the study found orthodox and unorthodox treatment to be equally ineffective against metastasized cancer. Survival for both groups averaged a mere fifteen months. The limitations of the study were acknowledged by the researchers: it used patients treated with only one unorthodox treatment, practiced at only one unorthodox facility, which I'll call the L_____ Clinic.

"I told Silversmith that study was no good," Jimmy moaned back at the jail. "If my methods weren't any better than conventional treatment, what was I doing luring cancer patients into spending their money on them? I know my therapies were more effective than the L_____ Clinic's, because in 1984, an ovarian cancer patient came to me after their people hadn't been able to help her. Her tumor went down very quickly with my serum. The L_____ people were impressed and started sending other patients to my clinic. After awhile, all their patients started coming, so they quit mentioning me. But three people who worked at the L_____ Clinic were later my patients."

Jimmy sighed. "I had to fight to get Dr. Bross. He would only talk to an attorney or a doctor, and the attorneys wouldn't call. Then when I finally got him, they took out all his punch lines. He could have shown why the patients were so excited about my treatment. It wasn't because I was hypnotizing them. It was because my treatments were reversing their cancers when nothing else would."

Dr. Bross may have been reticent on the stand, but he came alive at dinner. The evening after he testified, Paul and I cornered him and his wife in the hotel dining room and invited ourselves to join in their repast. The doctor proved to be an astute observer and keen critic, who was not averse to speaking his mind.

He said that the United States is now spending $700 billion a year for health care, and that much of it can be shown statistically not to be cost effective. Autolygous bone marrow transplants, for example, cost $125,000 and don't cure. The most they might extend life is six months.

He revealed that a large-scale Canadian study, reported in the London Times in June of 1991, had confirmed his warnings that breast cancer screening can actually increase the death rate from that disease. He said the researchers hadn't intended to publish their results -- they had decided to sweep them under the rug -- but the news had leaked out. Yet the study had not been reported in the United States. We wondered if the drug industry and the NCI actually had the power to muffle the American press. (The study is summarized in Appendix A.)

Dr. Bross also revealed that the NCI might be implicated in the spread of AIDS. He said a human leukemia virus that had been cultured for five to ten years in an NCI lab had escaped; and when viruses are cultured in the lab, they mutate. In this case, the escaped virus had mutated into something disturbingly like the AIDS virus.

> *Much later, in 1996, Dr. Leonard Horowitz, a Harvard public health researcher, published a book making the same charge. He traced the AIDS virus to the 1960s, when NCI researchers mixed viral genes from different animals to produce leukemia, sarcoma, general wasting, and death, producing the "cancer models" used to begin human vaccine trials.*[77]

I asked Dr. Bross why he hadn't mentioned his shocking NCI statistics on the stand. He said he had been instructed to tone down his testimony. Silversmith thought it would give him greater credibility. We agreed his testimony was credible. It just wasn't very interesting. The fireworks would have to wait for some other witness . . .

# Chapter 32

## More Experts

"Zavala is disappointed," Alma told Jimmy over the phone. "He was all set to come, but Ginsburg said you didn't need him." "What?" Jimmy gasped. "We need him! He's practically my best witness! You've got to get him back!"

Alma agreed to call the doctor; the doctor agreed to come; and when we heard his testimony, we all agreed that Jorge Zavala, M.D., was probably Jimmy's most critical witness. He testified that he was an oncological surgeon and professor at the National University of Mexico, and that he had been Mexico's representative to the International Cancer Congress. He had his own practice, which wasn't affiliated with the St. Jude International Clinic. However, he had examined many of Keller's patients when they had been referred to him for the insertion of catheters for use in injecting remedies. The doctor had seen some 500 of Keller's patients before and after treatment, first when he put the catheters in and later when he took them out. Anywhere from a month to seven months might elapse in between. Dr. Zavala testified in broken English (it was his second language):

> [M]any times when I saw the patients of Jimmy Keller in the first appointment was very ill. Very, very ill, the patients. [At the second appointment] it surprised me a lot sometimes because the mass of the neck or the abdominal, the enlargement of the liver, [was] reduced [in] size. Sometimes the tumor is more soft. By the time [I saw them again], they were in complete remission.

When asked to characterize the patients' response to Keller's treatment, the doctor said, "in general, I think it is good. But sometimes it is excellent, really. . . . Because I think Keller produced remission, complete remission of the disease. Remission means . . . you do a lot of work or follow up by X-rays and you don't have a tumor."

The evidence looked unimpeachable. An independent expert who had surveyed 500 of the defendant's patients had confirmed that Jimmy had produced remarkable remissions. It was equivalent to saying "cure." The problem, again, was that the significance of the testimony never got underscored; and Meier again managed to diffuse it, by getting down with the cockroaches and putting the witness's motives in question. The doctor, he maintained, had made money from Keller's patients.

Dr. Zavala nevertheless struck me as the most compelling witness we had. I asked Jimmy later why he thought Ginsburg had told the doctor not to come.

"I don't know," the prisoner said skeptically, "but as the Cajuns say, 'If he do dat in front of yo' face, just think what he do under the table.'"

I rationalized that it was natural for Jimmy to feel paranoid. He had just spent the last half-year in a cement-block cage. It was up to me to be the voice of reason. "Ginsburg was brought back in at the last minute," I said. "He was probably just unprepared."

I wished he had been a bit more prepared when Becky Johnson took the stand. It was Becky's daughter Sarah who had died of chicken pox after getting chemotherapy. Becky had key testimony to offer. But Ginsburg, her M.D./examiner, was mainly interested in finding out why she had rejected chemotherapy.

"Why in the world did you want to go to alternative therapy," Ginsburg asked Becky, "when you had, I am sure, excellent physicians right there in your home town?"

He was so aggressive in this line of questioning that he reduced his own witness to tears. In an attempt to be sensitive, he followed up by saying, "I certainly don't mean to be mean or challenging. And I certainly don't mean in any way to ask stupid or obvious questions. But is it fair to say you loved your daughter?"

"Well, of course," said Becky. "Yes."

"And you wanted the best for her?"

"Absolutely."

"I still ask you what it was about conventional therapy or alternative therapy that made you so adamant about taking her to alternative therapy and not using available conventional modalities of treatment?"

The witness choked up at this question, prompting Ginsburg to call for water.

What Jimmy had wanted him to ask was, not why Becky had resisted the drugs that precipitated her daughter's death, but why she had finally resorted to them. Maxine said they had been required by court order. Jimmy maintained Becky hadn't been able to locate his clinic because the government's injunction had cut him off from his patients.

"I got that child better," Jimmy insisted. "Becky could have testified to that, but she wasn't asked. Sarah's father testified that the girl screamed when she got injections, but he wasn't even there. She got upset at white coats, because she'd had so much painful treatment. That was one reason I didn't wear one, and why I didn't make the clinic look like a hospital. I had her laughing, and she didn't even notice when the needle went in. Becky could have testified to that -- and she could have weakened the credibility of Dr. Marley, who testified for the government. She could have said Marley refused to give Sarah blood at a time when the girl would have died without it, and that I had to stay up all night locating a Mexican doctor who would."

Jimmy sighed. "Black told me Marley was involved in some kind of insurance fraud, and that Silversmith was going to expose him; but he never did. Why not? Maybe he didn't destroy the bereaved because it would have offended the jury, but there was no reason not to destroy an expert witness. It was Marley who wound up destroying Silversmith, because Silversmith didn't know anything about medicine."

And Ginsburg, I thought, probably knew too much. He had been to medical school, but he worked in a courtroom rather than an operating room. His medical knowledge was largely theoretical. Unlike Jimmy's brother Ron, who had worked in the radiology department at M. D. Anderson, Ginsburg may not have had much occasion to see conventional treatment fail.

One thing to be said for him: Ginsburg cut a dashing figure on the floor. This couldn't exactly be said for Bill. Bill's crumpled second-hand suit hung on stooped shoulders and barely covered his barrel-sized belly. His voice was soft and low-key. He played dumb, asking questions to which he already knew the answers. He let his witnesses speak, limiting his questions to those necessary to allow them to lecture on their specialties. The approach, while lacking in flair, effectively elicited the testimony Bill wanted in the record.

Ginsburg typically began the examination of his own witnesses with the odd question, "You and I have never met, is that correct?" ("I never heard that one before!" remarked the court reporter after the trial.) Bill, on the other hand, prepared his experts like I had seen it in the movies. With Dr. Wallach (who was undoubtedly the best-prepared defense witness), Bill had stayed up all night reading studies and outlining the testimony. The two men had also prepared during the day, which annoyed Silversmith, who thought Bill should be keeping tabs on the trial. But by the time his witness took the stand, Bill knew exactly what the doctor had to say, and what questions needed to be asked to get him to say it. The attorney and his expert played off each other like a Vaudeville act. The testimony was rehearsed, but I had talked to the witness enough to believe it was sincere.

Dr. Wallach testified that he was a comparative pathologist, and that he had performed over 13,000 autopsies -- 3,000 on humans, the rest on animals. He had then gotten into non-traditional therapies. He had spent three years as director of research at Hospital Santa Monica, a popular non-traditional facility in Rosarito Beach, Mexico.

Bill asked why Dr. Wallach had switched from conventional to unconventional medicine. The witness responded by telling the tragic story of his wife's death from cancer. He was convinced she was a victim of chemotherapy. "I was told," he said, "there was a 75 percent chance that they could cure her using chemotherapy. And they killed her within six months with the chemotherapy. The disease didn't kill her."

Bill asked how he knew. Dr. Wallach replied that autopsies are his business. He was trained to determine the cause of death; and in cancer patients, he had observed, "the actual chemotherapeutic agents would kill people more frequently than the cancer did."

The witness then testified that he had successfully used Tumorex on cancer patients at Hospital Santa Monica. Like Jimmy, the hospital had paid the supplier between $300 and $400 for a single vial of the remedy.

Bill asked Dr. Wallach what he thought about Keller's $3,000 charge for a three-week stay.

"I don't know how he can stay in business if they charge $3,000," Dr. Wallach replied. He said that at Hospital Santa Monica, the charge was three times that much.

Bill asked, "Can you characterize for us your observation, your professional opinion, of these patients' response to Tumorex or L-arginine?"

"Well," said the doctor, "at first it is a very remarkable response because you don't expect this. We see patients who come to our facility in air ambulances, semiconscious. And these are ones that you would expect to die within a few days. And in fact, this is why they would come to these facilities, because they have been given the death sentence in the United States, saying that they are going to die in a few days to a week. . . . And we hook them up to these I.V.'s with the L-arginine in it. In many cases, I can't say all, but in a significant number of cases, 65 to 70 percent of them, within a week they are up in the food line in the cafeteria choosing their own food. And the first time I saw that it was unbelievable."

Dr. Wallach said he recommended up to thirty grams of arginine a day for a person with a very aggressive tumor. For prevention, he himself took about five grams a day. He added as an aside that in his opinion, cancer therapy for animals is far superior to that for humans.

"How does it differ, Doctor?" Bill asked ingenuously.

"Well, the main emphasis in the treatment of cancer in animals is, it is heavily weighted to prevention. And because of the callous factors involved and there is no insurance for animals, . . . it was learned very quickly that you could prevent, it would be my estimation, 99 percent of all cancers through preventive nutrition. This is the cheapest way to do it. This is the way the Agriculture Department and the laboratory animal sciences and pet food industries have done it." Arginine, said Dr. Wallach, is routinely put in pet food.

He also discussed the research on L-arginine. "[T]he literature shows that it works in animals and in cell cultures in every known type of cancer, neurological tumors, breast tumors, leukemia. It has a very widespread effect because it is not a chemotherapeutic agent that is directed at the cancer, but it works more on the body and allows the body to maximize its defenses so that the body can deal with the cancer. So that's why it is universally effective." If given early enough, said Dr. Wallach, arginine "will reverse the [cancer] process a hundred percent of the time."

He then referred to a March 1991 article published in the British medical journal <u>Lancet</u>, stating that L-arginine reduces tumor size and prevents tumors. The article discussed arginine's beneficial effects on the immune systems of healthy human volunteers.[78]

When Bill had run out of questions, U.S. Attorney Meier approached the witness box. There was no warmth in the prosecutor's eyes, no smile in his voice, as he began his cross-examination. "Isn't the effectiveness of anything in the treatment of cancer based on how successfully the patients do after they are treated?" Meier asked. "And if the people all die after that treatment, it is not an effective treatment, is it?"

"Well," Dr. Wallach conceded, "if the people all die from any treatment, it is not an effective treatment, that is correct."

The witness had run up against the stone wall of Dixon's survey. If 78 or 79 of 103 patients were dead in 1985, as Dixon maintained, the defendant must not have been getting the high rates of "success or cure" he allegedly claimed.

Bill complained that his next expert, David Steenblock, M.D., was put on the stand practically straight off the plane. There hadn't been much time for preparation.

Dr. Steenblock's testimony echoed Dr. Wallach's: many studies show arginine to be effective against cancer. The witness said he had successfully used it on patients himself, and that he had sent patients to Jimmy whose problems were resolved through its use. In fact, said the doctor, he was jealous of Jimmy's success rate, which was better than his own.

Bill's third expert witness, Daniel Clark, M.D., entered fifteen more studies into the record demonstrating that L-arginine activates the immune system and regresses tumors. Several of the studies were on humans.

The judge asked, "If arginine and all these things are what all of those articles say it is and you interpret them to be, why isn't it more widely used?"

The doctor replied that the literature on arginine actually goes back fifty years, but researchers are very cautious. Double-blind studies take time. Research progresses slowly. Another problem is funding. "[I]n medical research institutions," said Dr. Clark, "most of the research grants are funded by pharmaceutical firms. And part of the problem is . . . that they can't patent natural remedies, [so] there may not be enough money, profit margin in it. . . . I have seen [that] certain substances that showed promise were not further researched because there wouldn't have been a profit margin for them."

The stern glare of the bailiff discouraged any outbursts from the audience, but I felt like applauding. Here at last was the response to Dr. Dorr's contention that arginine hadn't been developed because it wasn't effective. Dr. Clark attested that effective natural remedies can and do exist -- remedies that even the poor can afford without insurance coverage, and that Medicare can afford without going bankrupt -- but they haven't been developed, because their developers can't make the kind of profit margins necessary to fund the studies required for FDA approval. Evidence was finally in the record that arginine worked, not only on mice but on humans. I studied the jurors for some glimmer of acknowledgment, but they were as sullen and expressionless as the day they first filed into the courtroom. Only the chinless white male juror showed any response, and it remained hostile to the defense.

The next doctor to take the stand had imposing credentials. Dr. Bryan Smith Finkle was the pharmacologist/toxicologist who had led the successful development not only of patented human growth hormone but of the cancer drug interferon. He confirmed that there are both animal and human studies in which arginine has regressed cancer. "[T]here are some human studies, [a] study that was done at John Hopkins University and another one that was done at the University of Pennsylvania, [involving] about 36 or 40 patients who had cancer," he said. "[S]ome notable percentage of them showed remission in the treatment of L-arginine."

The judge again asked why, if arginine is so good, more doctors don't use it. Dr. Finkle confirmed that it's a question of economics. FDA approval of a new cancer drug traditionally takes seven to ten years and costs the manufacturer between $80 million and $120 million. Drug companies don't put up that kind of money for unpatentable natural remedies.

The testimony of George Iceberg, M.D., was about a particular case, involving a patient with advanced esophageal carcinoma.

"He had bilateral metastasis, pulmonary metastasis," said the doctor. "He was short of breath, he was cachectic. He was having fairly severe chest pains. Could not swallow nor could he eat at all." The man was in a wheelchair and could not walk. Dr. Iceberg gave him no more than two or three days to live.

The doctor had accompanied the patient to Keller's clinic because he was skeptical: he intended to bring the man home at the first sign of fraud. But the effects of Jimmy's first treatment, he said, were remarkable. "The chest pain subsided. [The patient] was able to swallow. He also had felt quite a bit better."

"Was he able to eat that night?"

"Yes, sir."

"Did you go with him to eat?"

"Yes, sir."

"What did he eat?"

"Lobster with pina colada."

The patient did die, but he survived six weeks longer than expected.

Meier then approached the witness box, jaws clenched. As usual, he looked prepared. His first parry was to suggest that the patient's apparent recovery was due to narcotics. It was a ploy that had worked on less sophisticated witnesses, but Dr. Iceberg was an M.D.

"I doubt he would have been walking if he had narcotics," countered the doctor. "[Patients] are generally more unstable on their feet if they have received a narcotic, especially an intravenous narcotic."

Meier tried another tack. "In the natural course of cancer a patient goes through good periods and bad periods?"

"Yes."

"So while Mr. Keller may have benefited your friend somewhat, he may have had that kind of response without Mr. Keller's intervention?"

Again the doctor failed to take the bait. "I think that response was a little bit too dramatic," he said. "He did have virtually a total occlusion of the esophageal tract. He simply couldn't eat. There would have to have been some intervention of some method in order to make him able to eat. It is an anatomical obstruction."

All else having failed, Meier played his ace: the patient had died. He definitely was not cured.

When I asked Jimmy later about the case, he just shook his head. "Lobster and pina colada!" he groaned. He felt the patient might have survived longer if he had stayed on his diet.

Howard Tobin, M.D., testified about Jimmy's ear. He confirmed that, contrary to the suggestions of two government witnesses, it had been surgically removed. Dr. Tobin said he had performed the surgery at the Veteran's Hospital in Houston, an affiliate of M. D. Anderson. He thought he "got it all," but the odds that this type of cancer would not recur were very slim.

Then he showed slides of the amputated ear. It was a graphic display that evoked sobs from women in the audience. Nose-blowing was also observed in a jury member, although she may merely have had a cold.

It was a poignant moment for the defense; but Meier didn't have to undercut it, because defense attorney Ginsburg did it for him. "Dr. Tobin," Ginsburg asked, "in anticipation of the prosecutor's cross-examination, based on your understanding and feeling about medical ethics, given a terminal cancer patient, do you feel it is unethical or improper to tell a patient that they have been cured when, in fact, you know they haven't been cured?"

Dr. Tobin agreed that it was unethical. The implication was that no matter what Jimmy had suffered, if he had made the alleged misrepresentations, he was guilty of a crime.

Ginsburg, meanwhile, was demanding more money. We didn't hear about it at the time, because Jimmy's family didn't want to upset him. But his brother Ray told him later that Ginsburg had said he wanted $35,000 or he was going to be on the 6 p.m. flight that evening. Ray called it "Ginsburg's holdup." He understood the attorneys had already been paid for taking the case all the way through sentencing. "Don't let the screen door hit you on the way out," Ray wanted to say. But Jimmy's father feared that without Ginsburg, the case would be in jeopardy.

"Another Brownsville lawyer told Ray later that the judge wouldn't have let Ginsburg out of the case for anything less than a death in the family or physical emergency," Jimmy observed after the trial. But nobody told that to his son Jim Jr. or to his father Guy. Jim Jr. put up $10,000 toward Ginsburg's demand, and Guy mortgaged his house to satisfy the rest.

Much later, I asked Guy if he had ever been paid back.

"I got paid back," the pink-cheeked old gentleman replied with a placid smile, "before this case ever got started."

# Chapter 33

## Patient Witnesses

The witness room wound up being so crowded with people waiting to testify for the defense that they had to take turns sitting or lying on the floor. They came, they waited, and they went away, many without taking the stand. But more than twenty patients did succeed in testifying for the defense.

A case that particularly impressed defense attorney Ginsburg (himself an M.D. and a hard man to impress) was that of a woman named Annette (Maxine) Bachich. A slender and attractive 47-year-old redhead, she said she had once been a dancer for the San Francisco Ballet Co. But when she was diagnosed with cancer, she was a rehabilitation therapist at a mental hospital. In February of 1990, her doctor had told her she had inflammatory carcinoma of the left breast in an advanced stage (the third). That meant her prognosis was grim. ("Those cancers don't get better," Jimmy explained later. "They just get worse.")

Annette testified, "It is like your skin is all puckered because the cancer is in the skin, not just a tumor underneath the skin. Because of that being so extensive, I guess, [the doctor] said that I couldn't just have the mastectomy, I would have to have the chemo first to try to shrink the tumor so that it would be safe to do the mastectomy."

She got a second, then a third, then a fourth opinion. All of her doctors agreed -- she needed chemotherapy, then surgery, then more chemotherapy, then radiation. And "because there was so much skin involvement, . . . they couldn't just do a simple modified mastectomy. . . . [T]hey would have to do a grafting off my leg because they wouldn't be able to close the wound when they operated."

Annette bit the bullet and started the chemotherapy. Silversmith, her examiner, asked her how the drugs made her feel.

"You feel -- literally, you feel like you are dying," she said. "I had to work because I didn't have enough money to stay off work all the time. I would just come home and just sit and sit. . . . I couldn't move. I couldn't hardly do anything. And then I would push myself back to work and spend the weekends in bed."

The day before she was scheduled for surgery, she decided to check out Jimmy's clinic. She figured she could make it down to Tijuana and be back in time for her appointment the next day. "I was supposed to be in surgery like 9:00 in the morning," she recalled. "[When] I got [to Jimmy's clinic], I decided I loved Jimmy. I found it right. It just felt good. . . . And I called up the hospital and said, I am not coming in tomorrow morning."

"What happened when Jimmy Keller treated you?" Silversmith asked.

"Well, it felt very good . . . it felt wonderful. After three weeks and three days he said that he had done whatever -- you know, his treatment was finished with me. I went back. I felt great. . . . It wasn't like I just had a lump inside, the whole skin was all puckered up. . . . And so it just all disappeared. It all just got smooth again like a normal breast."

When she went back to her original doctor (who was a woman), Annette said, "My doctor was amazed. In fact, it was funny. Doctors are very reserved. They don't say a lot. But her nurse came in to me and said, the doctor is absolutely amazed. She cannot believe her eyes. She has never seen anything like this."

"Your Honor," Meier hastily interjected, "I would object to double hearsay."

The objection was sustained. It reminded me of the technicality the FDA had used against Harry Hoxsey: patients weren't competent to testify to their own conditions, and what their doctors had told them was inadmissible hearsay.

"Do you think Jimmy Keller is capable of defrauding anybody?" Silversmith asked.

"That is absolutely preposterous," Annette replied. "It is absolutely preposterous."

Her case looked air-tight. I held my breath, as a stern-faced Meier approached the stand. Silversmith's hesitation in attacking the bereaved was obviously not a concern shared by the prosecutor. Like a boxer in the ring, but with substantially more reserve, he looked ready to take down these cancer victims one by one. His first jab was that Annette had had chemotherapy.

She countered that her breast was still dimpled after the chemotherapy, and that her doctor had said she still needed surgery.

Meier's next jab was the biopsy. Annette had had one <u>before</u> she went to Keller's clinic. But had she had one <u>afterwards</u>, to prove she was cancer-free?

Annette admitted that she hadn't had a subsequent biopsy. But she said she'd had another test, the Mayo Clinic CEA. The CEA was negative.

Meier sparred that the CEA was not legally recognized as a diagnostic test. Then he asked if she'd been treated in Matamoros. She said she had not.  "And you don't know what happened in Matamoros?"

"No, sir."

Meier contended that nothing that occurred subsequently in Tijuana was relevant to a fraud arising in 1983.

And that was how it went. One remarkable case after another went down for the count under Meier's bone-chilling examination. A penetrating analysis would have revealed that his points were weak, but not much penetration seemed to be going on. Meier's confident and contemptuous manner projected to the jury that he was winning even when he was losing.

The defense patient/witnesses uniformly testified that they had not been promised a cure or told they were cured; they had benefitted from the treatment; and they did not believe Jimmy was capable of fraud. They made statements like "I can't believe under any circumstances he would ever commit a fraud." "He's the most honest and compassionate man I've ever met." He is "one of the finest human beings I've ever known." They also testified to dramatic remissions.

Arlene Torgesen said she had been diagnosed with metastatic breast cancer in 1981. She was given only three months to live. Ten years after Jimmy's treatment, she was still alive and well.

Astrid Orrell testified that she'd had surgery for breast cancer in 1985. Her doctors said they got it all and that she was cured. A year later, she was told her cancer had metastasized to the bones and she'd be lucky to live two more years. She went to Jimmy's clinic and was alive and well in 1991, five years later.

Allen Nash said that his father George's cancer had also metastasized to the bones, and that a tumor in his spinal cord had paralyzed his legs. George's doctor said the tumor was inoperable and recommended amputating the legs. Instead, George went to Keller's clinic, and walked out on the legs his doctor had recommended amputating. George was still alive eight years later.

Rosiline Raz said she'd been told she had only a year to live, even if she got conventional treatment. She went to Jimmy's clinic and was fine five years later.

Iris Klampert said she'd had cancer six different times in five different places. In 1981, she was told she had only six months to live. In 1982, she got Jimmy's serum. She was alive and well in 1991, nine years later.

All of these patients had been diagnosed with metastasized cancer. That put them in the category for whom Dr. Bross had said it would take "a miracle to save them." Yet all qualified for the American Cancer Society's definition of "cure" -- five years' disease-free survival. Their recoveries were brilliant testimony to the efficacy of Jimmy's treatments.

At least, that's what they were to me. But, no one highlighted those remarkable facts for the jury. What Meier did point out in each case was some defect that disqualified it as a "cure." He had a stock list of possibilities. When all else failed, he said the patient hadn't gotten a biopsy after Jimmy's treatment, so there was no way to know if the cancer was gone.

Meier's parry to Iris Klampert's case was that she had been treated with chemotherapy in 1984. It was this, not Jimmy's treatment, that he said explained her recovery. Iris was too intimidated to object on the stand, and defense counsel remained silent. But on December 12, 1991, she sent a notarized letter to the court stating that when she got back home she had checked her records, which were enclosed. They showed that by 1984 she had moved to California, and that she had never returned to the city where Meier claimed she received the later conventional treatment. She'd had no conventional therapy after she was treated with Jimmy's serum in 1982.

Needless to say, the affidavit came too late to sway the jury.

Meier's rebuttal to the dramatic case of George Nash, the man whose legs Jimmy had saved from amputation, was that at the time of trial eight years later, George's cancer had come out of remission. To George's son Allen, that meant his father needed to go back for boosters, a possibility that was foreclosed because

Jimmy was in jail. But to a disdainful Meier, it meant George was not "cured." He still had cancer.

"It's misleading," Jimmy observed wearily at the jail, "to say George 'still' had cancer. You can't live for eight years with a cancer that's terminal to start with. It's the nature of the disease that it grows geometrically. You can have a recurrence, but you can't have the same cancer all that time and still survive." It was another point, however, that was lost on the jury.

Selma Meyers was in the same predicament as George Nash. Her cancer had recurred, and she could no longer get Jimmy's treatments. A cosmetician by profession, Selma was lovely for a woman of nearly seventy, and she spoke with quiet dignity. She testified that in 1985, she had been told by a tumor board of 42 cancer specialists that her breast cancer had metastasized, and that conventional treatment would do her no good. They gave her only six months to live. Even her own oncologist recommended looking for alternative therapy. She had then found Jimmy, who had kept her alive for nearly five years with regular boosters of his serum.

"Basically," Jimmy commented later about the case, "they told her to go home and die. She was one big mass of tumors inside. It was in the fourth stage. She'd been scheduled for surgery, but they ran more tests and found that the cancer had gone to her bones. They told her nothing more could be done. But I told her she was one of the lucky ones. She hadn't had chemo and radiation and had her immune system destroyed."

The problem was that a new tumor had now developed in her other breast. Her doctors had again told her conventional treatment would do her no good. She had made an appointment at Jimmy's clinic, but before she could get there, the clinic had been closed. In a quiet plea to the jury, she said that her life now rested in their hands.

I glanced around the audience. People who knew the witness were in tears. But in the jury box, only the chinless white male juror showed any reaction; and it was one of skepticism.

When Selma talked about "auric fields" and how finding Jimmy was a "religious experience," this uninhibited juror had nearly laughed out loud. It occurred to me that for all her eloquence, Selma looked and sounded suspiciously like a Hollywood actress. I mentioned to Paul later that the jurors may have thought she was being paid for her performance.

Paul said he was sure she wasn't. When he had interviewed her at the Green Tree Hotel, she had unbuttoned her blouse and showed him the festering tumor on her chest. He was horrified. He said it looked like a raw hamburger patty. He didn't think she was long for this world. I thought we should have let the jury see it. But when I suggested the idea to Silversmith, he said it would be too maudlin. The court would not allow it.

Selma's husband later pleaded her case in a poignant letter to the judge. He wrote:

> *Selma, my 68 year old wife and I have known Jimmy Keller for five years during which time he, with all the serums at his disposal has caused two huge cancerous tumors upon Selma's chest to go completely into remission with no side effects nor loss of dignity.*
>
> *Unfortunately, Selma has developed a third tumor also on her chest which has been steadily and quickly growing at an alarming pace with no known possible way of stopping its growth in that Jimmy has been unavailable to help her since March of 1991 and conventional methods known to us have failed. . . . We believe that Jimmy and his wonderful serums could give her back her vitality, her health and her dignity as he has twice so successfully done.*
>
> *In addition, many of Selma's treatments over the past five years were given to her at no charge, no billing and no harrassment which upon speaking to several other patients of his was not unusual. This is not the type of action of an individual who is attempting to defraud the public.*
>
> *. . . I am pleading not only for Jimmy Keller, not only for my wife Selma whose life depends upon your decision, but for countless others who were labeled by their doctors as terminal and were brave enough to say 'I will not die, I choose to look elsewhere.'*

Olga Quijano made the same sort of plea. She testified that Jimmy had saved her from terminal cancer, but she had relapsed since his incarceration because she could no longer get his treatments. She wrote later to the judge:

> *. . . I am asking you to try to look at his sentencing from my point of view. I feel sentenced along with him. I, and others who now write to you, am alive writing this appeal due to his*

*treatment. My doctor in California had given me 3 months to live in 1989. . . .*

*I don't know if you have ever had the occasion to enter a cancer ward/clinic? I have. Entering St. Jude's was a totally different experience: radiating love and hope, and yes, with people who had been given a 'medical sentence to death,' terminal, yet full of confidence in their personal choice for their physician/healer. . . .*

*I chose treatment in Mexico because it was not offered in my country. . . . Since Jimmy was forcibly taken from Tijuana . . . . I, and very many other satisfied individuals and families who received his care, can no longer receive our treatment of choice.*

Dr. Ruth Kerhart was another patient who stressed the supportive atmosphere at Jimmy's clinic. A clinical psychologist herself, Dr. Kerhart was keenly aware of the role of mental and emotional factors in healing. She attested on the stand that his treatments had caused her metastasized cancer of the cervix, stomach and breast to go into remission at Jimmy's clinic. She later wrote to the court:

*There was a wonderful camaraderie that develops among patients. . . . We were all free to carry our IV's into any room and talk to anyone about anything . . . . It was the most loving, supportive atmosphere I have ever experienced anywhere. We were all commonly united against the enemy -- cancer. . . . We laughed, we cried, we joked, we even sometimes danced. . . . The best analogy I can think of for this situation is soldiers under siege in the trenches fighting the common enemy. Suddenly the everyday things we waste our energy worrying about drop off. All that matters is this moment with our fellow human beings whose goodness and caring is so evident.*

Throughout the passionate testimonials of Jimmy's patient/ witnesses, most of the jury remained impassive. Only the dominate chinless white male juror showed any reaction. Late in the case, the judge finally reprimanded both this man and the woman assistant prosecutor for their blatant responses to the testimony. It struck me then that the jurors weren't supposed to display any emotion. Had the others been secretly moved? It wouldn't be long before we knew . . .

# Chapter 34

## Verdict

On Thursday evening, August 29, 1991, the Silversmith/ Ginsburg/Black team made a rare appearance at the jail. "We think you have to do it," they urged the prisoner.

Jimmy took some convincing. Defendants are not required to take the stand and are typically counseled against it. When they are put on, they are usually coached for days in advance. But in this case the pep talk devoured the time, leaving little for preparing the witness.

The next day, Jimmy dutifully took the stand and, for the better part of the day, simply told his story. Everyone seemed to think he did well. Silversmith said that if the defense lost, "we have no one to blame but ourselves." Ruth Kerhart said, "He didn't attack people when they attacked him. Rather than attack, he would say 'I'm sorry.' He will not aggressively defend himself. He is profoundly self-effacing." Even Jimmy was impressed. He said his memory had been failing him. He attributed his clarity on the stand to fervent prayer the night before.

The problem was that he was winging it. It was suggested later that he could have used some coaching.

The defendant testified that he doesn't believe cancer can be "cured" *per se*, and that he never uses the word. He says only that the disease can be controlled for long periods, if a rigorous diet is maintained and other parts of the program are followed. It was a point about which he felt strongly, but another attorney suggested later that it should have been downplayed. A dozen government witnesses had testified that they understood Jimmy to be promising

cures, and there were more witnesses on the government's side
than on Jimmy's. He had witnesses in the wings who could have
supported his statements, including Don McBride and Lowell
Dayton; but for some reason, they were never put on the stand.

Jimmy admitted he had given percentage survival rates for
Tumorex, but only once. It was in a speech at a National Health
Convention. He said he was merely repeating what Rudnov, the
manufacturer, had said in a similar speech. Jimmy maintained
that the defense had Rudnov's speech on tape. (It was the same
tape Maxine's attorney had played at the 1985 trial out of the
presence of the jury.) The problem was that the defense had never
introduced the tape into evidence.

Jimmy testified that he treated between 180 and 200 patients
at his Matamoros clinic in 1983, and that most of them benefitted
from the treatment. He strongly questioned the accuracy of FBI
agent Dixon's "survey" showing that by 1985, 77 percent of his
patients were dead. But again the evidence he needed to prove
his claims wasn't in the record.

After the defendant's testimony, Silversmith rested his case.
We bench-warmers were a bit alarmed. The defense still had a
room full of witnesses who hadn't taken the stand. Rudnov hadn't
testified. The witnesses who could rebut Chickley's testimony
hadn't been called. Carolyn Penton's medical records hadn't been
produced . . .

Back at the Green Tree Hotel, I tried to look Silversmith up
to inquire about his strategy, but again he had disappeared for
the weekend. We were informed he would be back on Sunday in
time to get Jimmy's input for closing argument, but he never made
it. The defendant didn't see his lead counsel again until Monday,
September 2.

Monday was Labor Day. The jury spent the holiday listening
to closing argument and deliberating on the verdict. Silversmith
and Ginsburg both spoke for the defense. The gist of their
argument was that Jimmy was no more culpable than the
conventional cancer establishment.

"Doctors themselves are not gods," Ginsburg maintained.
"Doctors make mistakes. Medicine is an art as much as a science.
Doctors admit they may be seeding cancer when they do surgery,
radiation and chemotherapy. The medical profession itself is in
doubt. Do we indict doctors for telling patients they got it all,
when the patient then dies? No. We indict the people we don't
understand, who don't fit into our conventional picture.

"Keller has failures and makes mistakes. So do physicians. Keller didn't promise a cure. He promised hope. He acted in good faith. If the jury has a reasonable doubt as to Keller's good faith, it must acquit."

Silversmith observed that a number of the decedents had been told by their oncologists that they "got it all," that there was "no residual tumor," that the patient had "returned to normal," that "we have experienced a good cure rate." In effect, the doctors had promised a cure; yet no one had sued when the patients subsequently died.

Silversmith pointed to instances in the record of conventional misdiagnoses. In one case, bills had actually gone out for conventional treatment allegedly rendered on dates after the patient had died. The cost of a single biopsy, he observed, was as much as Jimmy charged for a whole course of treatment; and a full course of conventional treatment could be fifty times that. Not only were Jimmy's treatments the best deal in town, but when patients couldn't pay, he treated them for free. In at least one case, he even gave a refund. "When was the last time you got a refund from a doctor?" Silversmith asked the jury.

He referred to the testimony of Dr. Finkle, who developed "the most effective cancer treatment known on the face of the earth, Interferon. . . . And what did he tell you about Interferon? . . . . It enhances the immune system. Exactly what the studies found about arginine. . . . Dr. Finkle told us that, in fact, L-arginine . . . inhibits cancerous tumors in human breast cells."

Addressing the issue of intent, Silversith said, "If you were committing a fraud, it would serve little purpose to tell somebody, after they had paid you, that they had been cured. . . . I mean, the guy must have believed it. Just like those doctors obviously did when they gave babies thalidomide."

Thalidomide? I swallowed hard and wished he had chosen another analogy.

Silversmith referred to the study in which orthodox and unorthodox treatment had been found to be equally ineffective against metastasized cancer. He concluded, "It doesn't make any difference and we ain't indicting the doctors."

I swallowed again. Maybe we should be indicting, if not the doctors, at least their immune-system-destroying treatments.

Silversmith closed his remarks to the jury with a parable I later saw used in a movie. It was about "a smart-alec little boy, and a wise old man. The little boy came to the wise old man one morning and said, I have a bird in my hand, old man. Tell me, if you are so wise, whether it is alive or it is dead. The wise old man looked down at the little boy, and realizing the boy had it within his power to make the decision for him, said gently, my son, that little bird's fate is in your hands." Silversmith's voice dropped to a dramatic whisper. "I leave Jimmy Keller in yours."

The defense orations were impassioned, but conventional medicine wasn't on trial. What worried me was that the speakers hadn't nailed down the main issue -- whether the defendant was promising cures he knew he couldn't deliver.

It was too much to hope that Meier's closing argument would suffer from that defect. Like a vulture for a carcass, the prosecutor went for the issues in the indictment and methodically picked them apart. What he lacked in warmth and charm, he had made up for in carefully calculated preparation. For each witness, he had an orderly packet of documents from which he drew; and for closing argument, he referred to neat little cards. The defense sat silent, as the errors so obvious to Jimmy went into the record unopposed.

"Why didn't he bring you black and white evidence," Meier asked the jury, "instead of testimonials of people that he has conned, that he has duped? . . He is an expert at manipulating people . . . . And you got a sample of that when he took the stand. . . . The lies are obvious. . . . [Y]ou can just see what influence he has on people by how they come up here and testify for him against all logic."

The religious fervor of Jimmy's patients had been turned into evidence against him. He must have hypnotized them. It was a cult.

"He didn't bring you one expert that looked at his records to tell you what happened with [his patients]," Meier contended, "because . . . they are not being cured, they are dying, and he knows it. He has known it for awhile."

No mention was made of Jorge Zavala, M.D., the Mexican oncologist who had examined some 500 of Keller's patients before and after treatment and had found a remarkable remission rate. Nor was any mention made of the fact that Jimmy couldn't produce his patients' records because his files had all been confiscated by the FBI.

Meier claimed that the defendant had not put on a single patient who had been "cured." "All these people," he said, "either had chemotherapy, together with Keller's treatments, had chemotherapy before Keller's treatments, or have refused to have biopsies after the treatment."

Sitting through this kind of tortured argument was a gut-wrenching experience. If chemotherapy had worked on the patients, why had they then gone to the trouble and expense of seeking out a "quack" in Mexico? And why would they choose to go through the pain and expense of another biopsy after successful treatment?

The prosecutor then methodically addressed particular cases. One of them was Durk's. "He told you about some type of isotope treatment," said Meier. "And then he went to Keller. He hadn't had a biopsy."

He did get a biopsy, I vigorously objected; but it was only in my mind. Durk had testified that he paid $3,000 for a single biopsy at Stanford -- the equivalent of a full course of treatment at Jimmy's clinic -- and that the subsequent experimental treatment "didn't work, didn't take." His doctors had recommended chemotherapy after that, but Durk had rejected the drugs after he was told there was a 90 percent chance he would get leukemia as a result. He had also testified that his cancer had metastasized to the bone marrow. According to Dr. Bross, it would have taken a miracle to save him. Yet four years later, Durk remained alive and well.

Another miracle cure Meier managed to put in doubt was Wesley Smith's. He was the two-year-old Jimmy had treated in Matamoros for brain cancer. Like baby Jessica, Wesley had gone swimming after that and chased the ducks. The difference was that Wesley was still alive. Don McBride had testified about the case in his affidavit, and Wesley's grandmother Bonnie Cayer had testified about it on the stand. But Bonnie wasn't an eyewitness to the treatment. "Why didn't his parents come here to testify?" Meier asked disdainfully.

The response no one made was that Wesley's father had come to testify. He was one of the witnesses who had waited in the witness room uncalled; and so was Don McBride.

Meier brought up the defense's failure to play the tape on which Rudnov had allegedly represented that Tumorex had an 85 percent cancer success rate. "Where is that tape?" he asked. "Why didn't they offer it into evidence, if it says 85 percent? You can bet they would if they had it. Because it didn't say 85 percent. He [Keller] came up with that figure."

It would have been a fair shot, if Meier hadn't been present in 1985 when Maxine's attorney had played the challenged tape out of the presence of the jury. It was Meier who had conducted the direct examination of Rudnov, his own witness; and it was Meier who had objected to the tape being played before the jury.

By the time the prosecutor methodically discounted the arginine studies introduced by the defense, my stomach was in knots. "[E]very one of those studies was not done on a live human being," he maintained. "There are some [on] human cancer cells done in a Petri dish, but no studies on a live human being."

Studies on live human beings had been introduced by the defense.[79] But the acquiescing nods of the tall white male juror was a fairly clear indication that the jury had either missed or forgotten them.

Over it all loomed the numbers. "We showed you the numbers," said the prosecutor, pointing to the poster-sized exhibit of Dixon's survey. Out of 103, 91 had died; and 78 or 79 of them had died by 1985."

"There's really one issue," Meier concluded. "They've painted Keller as a dreamer, an idealist, who wanted to help people. Mr. Keller is a schemer. Schemers are manipulative and tell people lies. This was a man who said he could cure cancer. But when you look at the facts, the truth is his patients died."

The case closed with the judge's instructions to the jurors. He addressed them with fatherly warmth. He said the defendant was presumed by law to be innocent until proved guilty beyond a reasonable doubt. Lack of reasonable doubt meant you wouldn't hesitate to act on your decision in the most important of personal matters. He stressed that the jury had to find an intent to commit a crime. The defendant could appear to have violated the law, but there would be no crime without the requisite state of mind. The crime had to have been committed "knowingly" and "willfully" -- with the specific intent to do something the law forbids. In this case, the government had the burden of proving that the defendant had acted with the intent to defraud, taking money by false representations. The judge added that the defendant could not be found guilty of anything not alleged in the indictment.

My flagging heart started to beat again. The judge's instructions were favorable to the defendant. Was he hinting he thought Jimmy was innocent?

The jurors retreated to the jury room to deliberate, while the rest of us retreated to the cafeteria for lunch. Apprehensively, we dug in our heels to wait for the verdict. The jury could be at it for days.

After lunch, I visited Jimmy in the cage-like attorney conference room in the marshall's office. Attorney and client were separated by a thick glass pane with tiny holes in it. The light glared off the glass so I couldn't see his eyes, only hear his voice. "I thought it went pretty well," I hedged, trying to sound confident. "At least the jury instructions were favorable."

The prisoner's face was lost in the glare, but I could tell he wasn't buying it. He was nervous, like a cornered animal. He was upset with his lead counsel, who hadn't come to the jail the night before as promised. Jimmy had had to relay the points he wanted raised through third parties, and some key points had gotten screwed up.

"Why didn't he introduce Rudnov's tape?" Jimmy moaned. "And how could he get the wrong injunction?"

The injunction Jimmy wanted stressed was the one preventing Maxine from communicating with him after his Matamoros clinic was closed. That was the only time in over a decade of pursuit that the government had been able to find patients willing to complain. It was also the injunction against Maxine that had kept most of Jimmy's Matamoros patients from coming back for boosters. If they had come back, he felt, the ones who were now dead might still be alive. But Silversmith had named the Louisiana injunction, reflecting the shoot-from-the-hip style that characterized the defense's case. "If you're rabbit hunting and your dog's chasing possums," Jimmy said gloomily, "you ain't got a good dog."

"So what did you think of Meier's argument that DMSO shrinks tumors?" I deftly changed the subject. The prosecution's own witnesses had admitted that the patients felt better and their tumors had gotten smaller, but Meier called this response merely a temporary effect of the DMSO.

"If DMSO is so well known to shrink tumors," Jimmy said in a voice of barely-controlled desperation, "why aren't they using it conventionally for that in the U.S.? DMSO is the world's best solvent. It passes right into the cell without harming it. It brings some of the serum with it, but it's the serum that does the treating. The DMSO only helps to get it in."

(Later, I saw this contention echoed in an official publication of the U.S. government.[80])

"The prosecution can take anything you do and make it look bad," Jimmy moaned. "Instead of saying, 'What a miracle!' they point to the ones who died. At least 95 percent of the patients who came to me in 1983 were terminal patients. These were people who were <u>supposed</u> to die. If we had saved just one of them, it would have been a minor miracle; but when there are 35 or 40 of them, it's a major miracle. But Meier says they don't count, because they didn't get a biopsy <u>after</u> treatment to prove they didn't have cancer. <u>Nobody</u> gets a biopsy after treatment. If the tumor's gone, there's nothing left to biopsy. If the tumor's still there, the doctor just keeps on treating it. He's not going to get sued. He's already got his diagnosis. Why didn't anyone bring that up?"

"Maybe they didn't know," I lamely suggested.

"Maybe Meier didn't know either," Jimmy concurred. "Maybe nobody in there knew except me. But nobody ever came around to ask. No clinic in the United States could withstand the kind of scrutiny we went through without winding up with charges against them. The FBI seized my records and cut me off from my patients, and told them I'd deserted and defrauded them; yet ninety percent of their interviews were favorable to us -- and they stopped counting at 103 people. I think they purposely excluded the healthy ones; but we never saw a copy of their survey, and they confiscated my records, so how could I prove it?"

His voice trailed off. "And now all these people who were doing so well are getting sick. They call me in jail and want treatment. I send them down to Mexico, but they don't seem to get any better . . ."

There was a sudden commotion in the marshall's office. A man had rushed in to say the jurors were back. My heart sank. They had been deliberating for only three hours. It should have taken them longer than that just to review the research we had put into evidence.

Back in the courtroom, Meier and his woman sidekick looked smug. She was laughing, as if they already knew the result. The jurors were giggling like school girls in the hall. "Frivolous" was how Silversmith later characterized their attitude. Charles Whitehouse, a defense witness who waited in the witness room uncalled, wrote later:

> *I was there six days and five of those in the witness room and every time the jury came into their room that was next to ours all I could hear from them was a lot of laughing and giggling and it sure didn't seem like they were taking their responsibilities seriously.*

When the jurors had all filed into the courtroom, the judge asked if a foreman had been picked. The chinless white male juror stood up. We weren't surprised at the choice; and neither, apparently, was the judge. Silversmith said later that when the jury had asked for an instruction and this juror had appeared in chambers, the judge commented, "The white boy got it."

A hushed silence fell on the courtroom, as the judge called for the verdict. The clerk began to read. Soft moans and cries broke the silence, as Jimmy was found guilty on all counts.

I could imagine what it felt like to sit through a medieval inquisition. Several people would use that imagery in letters addressed to the court. Arlene Torgesen called Jimmy's harassment by government agencies "something that might have happened in the Middle Ages." Melba Call complained that Jimmy and Maxine had been crucified and "nailed to the wall." Richard Myers drew parallels with Jesus, who "enraged the ancient equivalents of these all-powerful medicrats who will stop at nothing to preserve their healthcare monopolies." John T. Sinette Jr. (a research scientist listed in Who's Who) wrote to the court:

> *[The] failure of orthodox medicine has led to alternative approaches and to bitter antagonism between the two approaches. It reminds one of the religious wars of the middle ages and the current bitter strife in the middle east. . . . [T]he alternative therapies have been developed by highly motivated, imaginative individuals with extremely limited resources. . . . But they have not been allowed to succeed and prosper in this country. They have been harassed, threatened, intimidated, and even arrested and forced to serve prison terms. As a result, nearly all of these innovative practitioners have been forced to flee to foreign countries where greater freedom exists. But even this appears to be no guarantee of freedom. Our medical Gestapo has now succeeded in reaching into Mexico and seizing Jimmy Keller and prosecuting him. It saddens me to see America moving toward totalitarian methods while most of the rest of the world is moving toward true democracy!*

It felt like a funeral; yet like a funeral, we got over it. But we continued to be mystified as to how all twelve jurors had agreed, in a mere three hours, that Jimmy was guilty of intentional fraud.

Olga Quijano, a charming Mexican/American patient who was convinced she had just heard her own death sentence, thought she knew. She said Mexican women are taught at their mothers' knees to feel inferior and subservient to their men. A single white, dominant male could easily lead them to doubt their own insecure judgment. (In fact, I thought, that could be true of any group of young, uneducated women.) Olga added that the jury was out on Labor Day. The women jurors still had dinners to cook for relatives who would be descending for the festivities. When the foreman urged, "Let's get this thing over with and go home," no one would have dared to hold out and keep the others from their holiday labors.

Jimmy commented later that he probably would have been better off with a jury of twelve oncologists. Medical doctors are disqualified from jury panels because they know too much, but they would have known enough to realize how remarkable his results were. They would have been closer to the "jury of his peers" guaranteed by the Constitution -- closer, at least, than the border town jurors who Silversmith said "never got on the train."

After the trial, Paul tried to locate the jury foreman to interview him for his Los Angeles Times article; but the chinless juror was nowhere to be found. He wasn't even listed in the phone book. He seemed to have disappeared from the face of the earth.

There was no way to prove it, but the rumor among the conspiratorially-minded was that he was a government plant.

# Chapter 35

## Preserving the Evidence

The defense had one last shot: appeal. The lay jurors may not have grasped the issues, but surely, we felt, a panel of appellate judges would. Meier had played on the emotions. The appellate court would look at the facts and apply the law.

Bill's concern was a logistical one: the defendant could raise issues on appeal only if they had been raised in the court below. Some of Jimmy's best arguments and evidence hadn't made it into the record. Bill had a solution in mind, but before he could broach his plan, we heard that the prisoner had been transferred back to Brownsville.

Bill and I followed in a car I rented at the airport. The drive took an hour and a half. I was dog tired and depressed. I tried to get my mind off the trial by looking at the scenery. Not much was out there on the vast horizon, but the clouds were interesting and gave it depth. I wondered idly how much of this panorama Jimmy had seen through the bars on the windows of the prison bus.

Bill, however, had more pressing things on his mind than the view. He was bent on getting Silversmith relieved as lead counsel. I wanted to do some research to see what our filing deadlines and options were, but Bill said the first thing we had to do was to become official counsel in the case. The only way Jimmy could present new evidence or raise new issues, either by post-trial motion or on appeal, was to declare that his trial counsel had been incompetent in not raising them; and he could hardly make that claim unless he first discharged his lead counsel.

When we first saw the convict in the Cameron County Jail, he was past depression. His crushed face was listless and indifferent. Bill tried to revive him by going on about how Jimmy seemed to have been sold down the river by his own attorneys. Jimmy's vacant look finally changed to one of exasperation. "We must have had thirty people left in the witness room," he groaned, "when Silversmith said 'I rest my case.' I probably spent $100,000 on witnesses, and the attorneys never even interviewed them!"

"That's right!" Bill fanned his flames. "Silversmith had enough witnesses left for two or three more days. He had witnesses from Matamoros he never called to testify. I was waiting to hear the trial lawyer of the year deliver a smashing summation, but I didn't hear it. When a man of Meier's ability can show up a man of Silversmith's reputation, something is radically wrong. He didn't hammer away at the positive evidence. There are a lot of traditional things you should say. You tell the jury, 'Vote your own conclusions. If you think you are right, stick to your guns. Vote your conscience.' You stress the presumption of innocence. You characterize the weakness of the government's case. Silversmith went through the motions, but I don't think he was trying very hard."

The catatonic prisoner had been revived, but I was confused. "Why <u>would</u> they throw the case?" I asked. "Nobody wants to lose!"

"It's the old 'wink and nod' system," Bill explained impatiently. "You throw me this one, and I'll throw you one that's important to you. There doesn't have to be an actual agreement. Nobody even has to try to lose. They just have to not try too hard to win. Silversmith doesn't specialize in cancer quackery. It's not going to hurt his reputation with drug dealers to lose this case. This is not a big case for him. He gets two million dollars cash for a drug smuggling case. But this is a big case for the government. Throwing it puts him in a position to get a lot of concessions. It's a good career move for him."

Although Bill called me "naive" and "too trusting," I just couldn't see it. But I could see that Jimmy hadn't gotten his money's worth. He probably would have been better off representing himself. He had started out his college career in pre-law, and he was a persuasive speaker. He knew what questions to ask to destroy the prosecution witnesses and to bring out the defense witnesses. Even if he lost, he would still have had his money. He could have hired the best attorneys available on appeal. Anyway, he had to discharge his lead counsel now just to get the missing evidence into the record. So I was ready to go along with Bill's plan: a change of counsel was mandated.

Jimmy went along with it too -- in principle. The problem, he said, was that he was broke. Any money he had left was in Alma's hands, and she wasn't turning it over for attorneys' fees. She felt the attorneys were eating up all the money and weren't doing much good. Whoever took over from here, it seemed, would be doing it for the cause.

If Bill didn't appear to be worried about that nuance, it may have been because he wasn't proposing to take on the case himself. The man he had in mind was O'Brien, Jimmy's earlier tentative substitute lead counsel. It was O'Brien who had first thought Jimmy was being sold out by Silversmith. Wednesday, Bill said he had phoned O'Brien, who had agreed to take the case without money up front.

"What if he changes his mind?" I asked nervously.

"Don't worry," Bill grumbled. "I won't abandon your boy."

The next day, Bill dictated a letter discharging Silversmith and listing the errors and omissions we hoped to get back into the record by post-trial motion. I tried to soften the language, but all I succeeded in doing was to further aggravate Bill. These were trying times, and he was on a short fuse.

When we took the letter to the jail for signing, Jimmy had plunged back into a black despair. The problem turned out to be Alma. That morning he couldn't reach her. He was worried she might be in trouble. Another possibility plagued him in his paranoid cell. He feared she might have run off with Durk and his money. Jimmy's mood obviously rode on his relationship with his wife, but by that time it was apparently less for love than for money. He said she had the last of his savings. She had declared it was her share of the community property. He couldn't prove he had rights to it.

On the phone later to Jimmy's brother Mike, I remarked that Jimmy was too trusting. He let people take advantage of him. Mike said it wasn't the first time. Jimmy had been taken advantage of all his life.

When Bill telephoned my room Friday morning at 3:30 a.m., I wondered what had possessed me to agree to take him to the

airport at that hour. It was raining, and the airport was half an
hour away. "My mother wouldn't have approved of this," I clucked
to myself as I groped for the coffee-maker. But my spirit of
adventure returned after gulping down the brew.

On the half hour ride back from the airport, I pondered the
drastic measures we were taking. Silversmith was used to defending
drug dealers. He was probably just pursuing his usual tactics: cards
close to the chest; hope for some favorable technicalities. He hadn't
aggressively cross-examined the government's witnesses or
developed the defense witnesses, but maybe he didn't know they
had anything more to say. The rule is, "Never ask a question to
which you don't already know the answer." It was Silversmith's
investigator who had interviewed the witnesses, and Jimmy said
the investigator hadn't asked the right questions. Only Jimmy
really knew what those questions were. But he was trapped behind
bars, where he couldn't coordinate his defense. I wondered why
depositions weren't the rule in criminal litigation. In civil litigation,
we routinely deposed everyone in sight. Was it because depositions
are expensive, and criminal litigators, unlike civil litigators, are
generally paid in a lump sum up front?

Anyway, I rationalized, it didn't matter now who was at fault.
The evidence we needed in the record wasn't there. The only
way to get it in was to argue incompetence on the part of defense
counsel; and for that, Jimmy had to first let his counsel go. I
composed a letter to Silversmith in my head, apologizing for this
brazen step and explaining it was nothing personal. But then I
recalled a bit of Southern legal wisdom of Huey P. Long: never
write a letter when you can talk on the phone, never talk on the
phone when you can go to lunch, never go to lunch when you
can wink, never wink when you can nod, never nod when you
can clear your throat. I decided to keep my sentiments to myself,
lest they show up one day in a pleading clip. The letter I did drop
in the mail, with bated breath, was the one discharging Silversmith
as lead counsel.

I was glad my blood pressure was normally low, because it
must have shot up a few dozen milligrams when I later read the
court rules at the courthouse library. I anxiously called Bill after
he got back to California, and told him what I had found: the
post-trial motions were due a week after the verdict, or the
following Monday. We frantically faxed documents back and
forth, and Bill and his loyal paralegal stayed up late Friday working

on the motions. Then we realized we had another logistical problem: how were we going to get them on file with the court? My flight home was on Sunday, when the courthouse would still be closed. Black, Jimmy's local counsel, was out of the question. If we were barely on the team before, we weren't on it at all now.

Then Bill thought of Deborah Jones, one of Jimmy's "angels." She was a stewardess who could fly for free. When Bill called her in Los Angeles on Saturday, Deborah said her business was already suffering from the days she had taken off to be a defense witness . . . but Jimmy had saved her from breast cancer. Graciously, she agreed to fly out on Monday to file the motions with the court.

That settled, I felt better about leaving the shell-shocked prisoner. If all went well, competent appellate counsel would step in and save the day. All I had left on my agenda for Saturday afternoon was to go through the missing evidence Jimmy wanted in the record, and to say good-bye.

# Chapter 36

## The Case That Might Have Been

"Haste makes waste," I could hear my mother saying when I realized I had locked my only set of keys in side the rental car. After I finally conceded that this particular model was coat hanger-proof, I discovered there was only one locksmith in all of Brownsville, and he wasn't responding to his beeper. Just as I was envisioning having the car towed thirty miles to the airport and gloom and despair were settling in, the locksmith finally showed up, a heavyset young man with slicked-back hair driving a beat up old Chevy. He got the door open in about thirty seconds, and took his fee. It was remarkable, I thought, how fast a car could be broken into with the proper tools.

I raced to the jail. Visitng hours would soon be over.

Brainstorming the missing evidence seemed to rouse Jimmy's flagging spirits. I wasn't sure how much good this exercise would do, but it was a convenient escape from the unspoken: what would happen next? The government had confidently predicted he would spend the next ten years behind bars. He was 57 years old and a cancer victim. Could he survive it? We studiously avoided those issues and talked about evidence.

"Okay," he started in with his list, "we really needed Lowell Dayton and Don McBride. They could have testified that I never promised anyone a cure. They were Mormon missionaries together in Mexico, and they're both fluent in Spanish. They were helping me translate. Lowell worked right with me in the clinic. He heard what I said to the patients, and he remembers some of the government witnesses. Don was there too and saw what went on.

They're both wonderful men, the kind of witnesses you have to believe."

"Good," I said, pen poised. "Who else?"

"Charles Whitehouse. He participated in radionics experiments conducted by the navy."

"Really!" I said. "The navy is part of the same government that was calling radionics quackery in your case!"

"Exactly. So why didn't Silversmith put him on?"

"Maybe he thought there wasn't time, and Dr. Tiller and Dr. Bruner had made out a good enough case for radionics."

Jimmy didn't look convinced. "Anyway, Major Gordon Smith was another one we should have put on."

"Right." I had met this witness at the Green Tree Hotel. He was an older, retired gentleman with long, white, Einstein-style hair. (Perhaps, I thought, that was why Silversmith hadn't put him on. I hadn't gotten a chance to meet Dr. Whitehouse, but I had heard Silversmith express some concern about the doctor's rather eccentric appearance.)

Major Smith's potential testimony was suggested in a statement he submitted for the defense. He said he was Chief Executive of the Confederation of Radionic and Radiesthetic Organizations (CRRO) and an executive member of the National Consultations Counsel for Alternative and Complementary Medicine in England. He observed that the Code of Conduct under which CRRO members practice radionics has been accepted by the General Medical Council of the Royal Colleges of Physicians. The organization has included many eminent M.D.'s, including Dr. Charles Elliott, the retired Homeopathic Physician to Her Majesty the Queen.

"And Norman Cavin and Faye Franklin," Jimmy went on.

"Right." The siblings of Carolyn Creighton were a small-scale study supporting Jimmy's contention that prior conventional immunity-destroying treatment substantially reduces the chances of survival from natural immunity-stimulating treatment.

"And Diane Malachino."

"Who's she?"

"She was a patient in Matamoros who had a huge, painful tumor on her breast the size of a lemon. She hadn't had a biopsy, but the tumor was clearly there. You could see it and feel it. When I gave her the serum, it literally shrank before our eyes. The next day it was gone without a trace, and it never came back. It was one of the fastest responses to treatment I've ever seen. I think the tumor responded so well because it hadn't been cut into with a biopsy."

"No biopsy." I jotted this point down. "Maybe that was why Silversmith didn't put her on."

"Okay, but there was another reason we should have put her on."

"What's that?"

"She could have impeached Chickley's statement that he never promoted my clinic. Charles and Al McGowan and Peggy Skinner could have testified to the same thing, but Silversmith never put any of them on."

"That was strange," I agreed. When Silversmith had cross-examined Chickley, he had named these witnesses in a threatening way suggesting impeachment. "So what other facts could they testify to?"

"Well, Charles got chelation in Matamoros when his wife came for boosters for cancer. A lot of her treatment was free. Charles gave Chickley booster shots. Al was their son. He stayed with his mother for sixteen weeks while she was in the hospital in Tijuana after suffering a stroke. Al could have testified that when her tumor was removed, it had shrunk dramatically. Her doctors couldn't believe it. She died later, but it wasn't from cancer. It was from a fall."

(Bill said later that he would have put Al on for another reason: he was a decorated officer in the Marines, the type of credible witness who sways juries.)

"Peggy was Chickley's cousin," Jimmy went on, "but she was loyal to me because I helped her father."

(We heard later that Peggy had never made it to the courthouse, but she told Jimmy she had gotten as far as the airport in McAllen. The defense attorneys were supposed to meet her there; but when she arrived, no one was around. She called them but no one called back, so she finally went home.)

"We needed Lynn Dorsey," Jimmy said. "He was the husband of Brenda Laughlin. I treated her in Baton Rouge and Matamoros, after she'd been given only a few weeks to live. She lived 2-1/2 years longer than expected, and she gave Lynn a baby in that time. I didn't charge her for the treatments, and I sent her free vitamins after she went home. She died later, but it was from pneumonia. Her immune system was shot from cobalt treatments."

"Good. Who else?"

"We needed Guy Smith."

"We did!" Guy was the father of two-year-old Wesley, whose case was challenged because his parents hadn't come to testify. Meanwhile, Guy had waited in the witness room uncalled.

"And Christopher Bird," Jimmy said. "He wrote a book on the medical uses of the pendulum. I paid for him to come all the way from Canada just so he could testify that it's a valid method of diagnosing. He's written several books. He wrote <u>The Secret Life of Plants</u>."[81]

"Great book," I said.

Jimmy nodded. "He could have introduced a German study I had that validated the pendulum as a diagnostic tool. I paid $1,100 to have it translated."

"What happened to the study?"

Jimmy shrugged. "I gave it to Ginsburg and never heard anything more about it."

"Too bad! Who else?"

"Frank Cousineau. He's a tour guide for the Cancer Control Society. He could have testified to the reputation of my clinic, and that the success rates for Tumorex came from Rudnov. In fact, we should have put Rudnov on the stand. He was the government's chief witness in 1985. His testimony was impeached over fifty times. The contradictions alone could have cleared me. All the representations about Tumorex came from him. He made far more money from it than anyone else. He was kept in business by the government. Silversmith should at least have put him on to introduce the tape of the speech where he said Tumorex had an 85 percent success rate."

"We definitely needed the tape," I agreed. "I wonder why it never got introduced?"

"I don't know," Jimmy said cynically, "but I overheard my attorneys say Rudnov had been telephoning Silversmith's office, and that they had agreed he wouldn't have to testify."

"Really! Why would they agree to that?"

"I don't know that either" -- Jimmy arched his good eyebrow -- "but I can imagine a few possibilities."

I raced on, ignoring the implications. "We don't want to forget the recorded evidence -- the missing tapes and medical records."

"Okay, there was the transcript of the tape of the phone conversation with Margaret W_____, the one where she claimed Maxine had promised her husband a cure."

"Right. Did you ever find the transcript?"

"I did." Jimmy dug through his papers and pulled out a document.

"Interesting!" I said after perusing it. According to the transcript, Maxine had responded to a question about "how effective it was" by saying "we're getting 45 to 65 percent" or "80 to 90 percent," depending on whether the patient had prior treatment. Arguably, she was referring to the same "response to treatment" Rudnov had testified to in 1985: tumor shrinkage, relief of pain, improved sense of well-being. In any case, there seemed to be no promise of a cure. The tape was also potential evidence to rebut Chickley's testimony, since Margaret said on it that Chickley had recommended Jimmy to her.

"We also needed the medical records of Carolyn Penton," Jimmy said. "Silversmith evidently subpoenaed them, but they never got produced in court. I think the FBI told the doctor to ignore the subpoena."

"That's contempt of court!"

"Sure. So why didn't Silversmith go after him?"

I shrugged and looked at my watch. My heart sank. It was nearly eight o'clock. Attorney visiting was over. As the guard came for the prisoner, I was suddenly gripped in fear. Would O'Brien save the day? Or would Jimmy spend the next ten years in prison? I wanted to say something upbeat, but nothing credible came to mind.

"Good luck," I said. "Don't worry. Everything will work out." There was no way to phone prisoners in jail, so I said, "I'll write." I smiled bleakly and watched, as the sliding steel bars swallowed the convict up for the last time.

Outside in the starless night, I battled overwhelming depression. I didn't have much faith in our motions, and I wasn't sure about the appeal. I thought of the case of Dr. Halstead. He was a highly credentialed M.D., who had gone so far as to obtain written release forms from his patients attesting he never promised them a cure. By 1991, he had spent eight years in legal battles and seven full months in the courtroom. As a result of that valiant effort, he had been stripped of his medical license, virtually bankrupted by the proceedings, and deprived of $2.5 million in research grants. He had been targeted by what one writer called the "Medical Gestapo." He was a marked man whose fate had been sealed.

On the bright side, Dr. Halstead was still free on bail pending appeal. He might yet prevail. He had the advantage over Jimmy, however, that his favorable testimony was in the record. Jimmy's record contained substantial gaps. It was that defect that we hoped to remedy by post-trial motion before the district court case was closed . . .

Sunday morning before boarding a plane for Kenya, I called Bill in California. My blood pressure must have shot up again, when Bill said he hadn't succeeded in getting O'Brien to sign the motions or the substitution of counsel. I was leaving the convict in the lurch; but I didn't have the kind of plane ticket that could be changed, and my marriage could be on the rocks if I stayed any longer.

Bill said not to worry. He had prepared the motions for Jimmy's own signature. O'Brien or some other attorney could be substituted in later.

Okay, but how were we going to get Jimmy's signature? Deborah Jones had agreed to fly to Brownsville on Monday to file the papers with the court, but visitors who weren't associated with law offices had to stay behind reinforced glass.

Deborah solved the problem herself, by using the ploy of saying she was from a paralegal service.

It was working until Jimmy, who was enormously glad to see her, impulsively reached out and kissed her hand.

Deborah recovered well. "Sir!" she said coyly. "Your reputation as a Southern gentleman precedes you!"

# Chapter 37

## Suitable Counsel

Below our weekend beach house on the Kenya coast, a variety of tropical plants splashed color over the hillside, while the Indian Ocean stretched blue and green to the horizon. My husband had arranged a relaxing four-day weekend at Mombasa. But it was no use. The world in my mind was walled in by cement-block grey and bars. Had either O'Brien or Bill agreed to be attorney of record? The beach house had no phone.

When we got back to Nairobi, I hastily dialed Cherise, who had been keeping in touch with the Kellers from Hollywood by phone. She confirmed what I had feared. Jimmy had been abandoned and betrayed -- "like Job," she said in her Hollywood way. But it wasn't his attorneys she was referring to. It was his wife and his good friend. Jimmy had called Durk and confronted him with his suspected affair with Alma. Durk had failed to deny it, so Jimmy had concluded it was true.

I reached Bill the next day. He said he had heard that Durk was trying to open a clinic in Tijuana, and that he had borrowed $200,000 from Alma for the project. "If he's opening a clinic," Bill commented drily, "it's not going to be as Jimmy's partner. It's not in Durk's best interests for Jimmy to be out of jail."

"What about O'Brien?" I asked nervously. "Is he going to do the appeal?"

"He'll do it, but only if he gets $100,000 up front."

"$100,000?!" It was an impossible sum.

"Don't worry," said Bill. "I have a plan."

His plan was to raise support for Jimmy's defense among the other clinics in Tijuana. The argument Bill planned to use was that Jimmy's clinic was merely the first domino to fall. Non-traditional cancer clinics had sprung up all over Tijuana. They were all a thorn in the side of the cancer establishment, and they all received patients referred by telephone from the United States. (In fact, Jimmy observed, his was the only clinic that did <u>not</u> do this in Tijuana. He got his patients by word-of-mouth. He had learned his lesson in Matamoros.) Bill's argument was that Jimmy's case established legal precedent for holding that telephone referrals from the U.S. can constitute wire fraud. If the holding were not reversed, the Tijuana competitors of the cancer establishment risked being shut down one by one.

I remembered something Maxine's husband had said about his interview with FBI agent Dixon: Dixon revealed that his plan was to destroy all the clinics in Mexico.

The next time I talked to Bill, he said he had approached a number of clinic directors, and that most of them had agreed to contribute to a Keller defense fund. Unfortunately, there was one significant hold-out; and it happened to be Bill's own highly-valued client. Like O'Brien, Bill wound up refusing to take the case without money up front. Whether this was because his highly-valued client had discouraged him, or because he didn't think he'd ever get paid, I never knew. Bill quit returning my calls.

So much, I thought ruefully, for standing behind a competent man. I was suddenly in the unnerving position of being Jimmy's sole remaining active counsel, though 10,000 miles away. I rationalized that it was probably fate. I'd been hiding behind a man too long. I could pull this appeal off by myself. At least I was affordable. I'd gotten $5,000 in fees in the beginning, but after the Kellers went broke I was just working for costs . . .

*By myself? Was I kidding?* I didn't have a clue about local criminal procedures. And what if I had to speak in court? Jimmy, a man of consummate faith, thought I could do it -- at least, I had the advantage over his earlier attorneys that I knew the arguments he wanted made -- but I lacked their Orson Welles intonation and cool confidence in shooting from the hip. My law firm had generally won on paper by summary judgment, over matters of mere money. I had never before been responsible for a man's freedom.

I handled this terrifying prospect maturely, by going into denial. There was other work to be done. I wanted to prepare a brief in support of the motions we had hastily filed to meet the deadline in the court rules. But I faced another logistical problem: how was I going to get the papers on file from Africa? Luckily, a woman who lived near Brownsville had called the Kellers and volunteered her services. Her name was Cindy Olson. She had never met Jimmy, but she had heard of his plight at a health convention in California. People had a way of appearing, I thought, when Jimmy needed them. I hoped this trick of fate would work to fill the current void in his counsel.

I thought of Maxine's attorney Mike, and hastily dialed Utah. "He's not in," said the receptionist. "May I take a message?"

Twenty-four hours later, I had a sixteen-page brief addressed to Cindy in the overnight mail and had just drifted off to blissful sleep, when the phone rang. "What time is it there?" asked the voice on the other end. It was Mike, with urgent news. He said Jimmy could be in dire straits if his counsel didn't get involved in the Presentence Investigation Report (PSI) and have some input into it. Jimmy was facing a possible 55 years, and we knew the government fully expected him to serve ten. Sentencing by the judge, it seemed, was as critical as the verdict by the jury. But Mike had a very crowded calendar. He didn't know if he could step in on the case himself.

It was already Thursday, September 19. The PSI was supposed to be served by the probation officer ten days before sentencing, or on September 27. But my husband was scheduled to be out of the country on two back-to-back business trips. I hadn't planned to go to Brownsville again until September 30. Panic set in.

I dealt with this crisis the way I always did. I had a good hysterical cry on my husband's shoulder. I felt enormously grateful for his support. The man had a way of making mountains look like mole hills.

By Friday afternoon, my fingernails were in a ragged state, but otherwise things seemed to be under control. Mike had provisionally agreed to take the case, at least through sentencing. I had managed to find friends willing to keep the children for the next week, so I could leave for Texas the following Monday to help with the PSI. (The kids said they understood. "Did you get Jimmy out of jail yet?" they would ask with unbounded confidence when I called home.)

By Friday evening, however, my nails were non-existent. Mike had called to say he hadn't been able to clear his calendar until

November. He suggested getting a month's continuance, or doing the hearing myself. I called Bill twice but just got his answering machine.

Then I thought of another attorney I knew in Texas, Rick Jaffe. I had met him in New York before he moved with his family to Houston. It was the location of his principal client, Stanislaw Burzynski, M.D., a well-known cancer therapist who had developed a natural, non-toxic unconventional therapy called antineoplastons. The therapy had been approved by the FDA for clinical trials, but Dr. Burzynski was nevertheless in heated litigation with that agency. I called Rick for advice. He too said he had a busy calendar, but he suggested dinner when I passed through Houston on my way to Brownsville.

A tall, red-bearded man in his late thirties, Rick talked about having studied the Jewish mysteries in Israel before becoming an attorney. He said he liked watching the weather from his seventeenth story office in Houston. He hadn't been happy with the pace of life in New York City. He had more time in Texas for his family. He had two small children.

I nodded and tried to look professional, as I hid my tennis shoes in the shadow of the table cloth at a fashionable restaurant in Houston. I had arrived before my suitcase, which hadn't made it on the plane in London.

Like Mike, Rick suggested a continuance to allow time to educate the judge. "The case needs to be characterized as political," he said. "We should bring in the non-traditional health care movement."

"Exactly!" I concurred. He hadn't gone so far as to say he would take the case, but I liked the sound of the word "we."

From Houston I flew to Harlingen, then rented a car and drove to Brownsville. On the way, I indulged in a new pair of shoes.

Jimmy was glad to have a visitor. He kept punctuating his sentences with the same desperate refrain: "I've got to get out of here!" Conviction had changed the tenor of life behind bars. He said when he had returned to Brownsville after the trial, the jail had been taken over by a drug lord. Inmates and jailors alike seemed to have ganged up against him.

"There's always a big fight in here for the phone," Jimmy complained. "Sometimes I have to stand in line for two hours. Then when I get it, it gets ripped out of my hand. The drug lord doesn't have that problem. The guards <u>bring</u> him the phone every morning!"

Jimmy brightened as he added, "But I've made one interesting friend."

"Who's that?"

"They call him Elvis."

Jimmy described Elvis as a rather handsome young Mexican-American inmate with slicked-back hair. When he had first come to the jail, all the other inmates were terrified. Elvis turned out to be one of the most wanted men in the Valley, sporting an imposing record of murders and rapes. But he had taken a sudden interest in religion, and Jimmy had encouraged him. He had then become Jimmy's fast friend -- and body guard.

In some ways, Jimmy trusted Elvis more than Black, the local Brownsville attorney Durk had retained to represent him. "When I told Black about my problems with the drug lord," Jimmy said, "he rushed back to say hello. I guess they're old friends." Jimmy didn't trust Black for other reasons. The attorney had been on the West Coast the weekend before the trial. It was the same weekend that Alma and Durk, who were also there, couldn't be reached.

Uncertainty deepened Jimmy's depression. He had more and more reason to believe Durk had run off with Alma and his money. But he didn't have proof. Were these terrible thoughts the paranoid delusions of a man who had spent the last seven months behind bars?

He lamented the money his family had spent because Alma hadn't come through. They were already out $70,000, and his father had had to mortgage his house. "It shouldn't have been this way," Jimmy grieved. "The joy of my life was helping my father. When you reach a certain point in life . . ." Then he broke down and cried.

It was in this low mood that, on October 4, 1991, Jimmy met his fourth round of counsel, Rick Jaffe. Rick had agreed to step in on the case after prevailing on a motion for summary judgment, unexpectedly clearing his crowded calendar.

Rick talked strategy; but Jimmy was out of money and he couldn't reach his wife, and he couldn't let his family pay any more. How could he finance more litigation?

"I ran the clinic as ethically as it could be run," he said in a voice that was as low and listless as I'd ever heard him. "I know this is true. But they got me, and that's that."

Rick, however, wasn't talking money. He expected to get paid eventually, but he was willing to step in with practically nothing up front. I breathed a sigh of relief. We had found the man for the job.

"Too bad you didn't find him sooner," Silversmith said later. "I could have worked with Jaffe."

On October 1, 1991, Silversmith filed a response to our motion for a new trial, in which he defended his defense of the case. We all agreed it was the finest piece of work we had seen from his office. Not that there was much fear our motions would prevail. We were mainly building a record for appeal, while Silversmith was building a record against a potential malpractice action -- of which there had, indeed, been some discussion among the Kellers. I read the brief with keen interest, hoping to finally understand Silversmith's elusive strategies.

One was his failure to raise the government's intentional destruction of its tape of the sting operation. Silversmith pointed out, in rather hurt tones, that it was his own pretrial Motion for Disclosure of Electronic or Other Surveillance that had led to the tape's discovery. The court had denied his motion to suppress testimony concerning the sting, but the government had apparently been respectful enough of the issue to let this sleeping dog lie. If the defense had raised the destroyed tape, the government would have felt free to put its two undercover agents on the stand; and government agents are generally convincing to a jury. Their testimony that Jimmy had made fraudulent representations would have been hard to refute. Silversmith had decided to let the government look clean in order to avoid making his client look worse than he already did.

Okay, I thought, we may have to give him that one. Jimmy would have preferred to take the risk, but I could see Silversmith's point. The government was liable to get us coming or going.

Then there was the matter of the uncalled witnesses. Silversmith observed that it was the judge, not he, who had eventually cut off testimony from people who had been patients only in Tijuana. The judge had finally agreed with the government that this testimony was irrelevant to charges of a fraud occurring earlier in Matamoros. It was also the judge who had requested a ten-day limit on the trial. By acquiescing, Silversmith had avoided the caustic testimony of the NCAHF witnesses. If he had called more witnesses, the prosecution could have called more as well.

For particular witnesses, Silversmith also had his reasons. Don McBride, he said, was being saved for rebuttal. He maintained

Jimmy had agreed. Guy Smith was rejected as a witness because
Guy had told Silversmith's investigator he thought the pendulum
was "satanic." Lowell Dayton was rejected because he wasn't
"cured": he'd had to get conventional treatment after Jimmy's.
There were other witnesses Silversmith had his reasons for, and
others yet he never mentioned.

We, being professional advocates, had responses ready for
each of these contentions. Jimmy said he had been told Don
McBride was being saved for rebuttal, not asked; and he hadn't
been told rebuttal would never come. Don said Guy Smith had
told him in the witness room that he intended to testify favorably
for the defense. Silversmith just hadn't talked to the witness.
Lowell Dayton's own explanation for why he'd had to get followup
treatment after Jimmy's was that his treatment in Baton Rouge
had been interrupted by the Louisiana injunction. His more
important testimony involved Jimmy's representations to some
of the government witnesses; but again Silversmith was apparently
unaware of that impeaching testimony, since he hadn't personally
interviewed the witness.

We had notarized affidavits to support our contentions. Lowell
Dayton had written to the court:

> *I spent my entire time in the witness room and was never
> called to testify on behalf of Mr. Keller. I have remained very
> disturbed by this because I felt that I had crucial testimony to
> offer . . . . There are some people whom I am aware appeared
> as prosecution witnesses, and I have had reports of their
> testimonies. I was present when some of them were initially
> counseled and treated. . . . Some who said that they had been
> given guarantees have not told the truth because I was there as
> their witness . . . .*
>
> *I and others there felt frustrated and angry. . . . As witnesses
> we were kept in the dark by the defense attorneys. At no time
> was I approached by any defense attorney to determine what
> testimony I might offer or to inform me when I might expect to
> testify or what questions I might be asked. I have participated
> in other trials, in which I have always been interviewed ahead
> of time; but in this one there was no communication. I do not
> believe that they had done their homework as to the witnesses
> and how to use them properly. Something about the whole
> situation seemed wrong.*

It is my understanding that the prosecution argued in closing that the defense could not produce any of the Baton Rouge and Matamoros patients who had survived and could only produce recent patients from Tijuana. The fact is that there were many survivors from Matamoros who were in the witness room waiting to testify who were never called.

Don McBride wrote in his notarized affidavit:

My wife and I paid <u>all</u> of our own expenses to fly to McCallen, Texas and I sat in the Jury Room the last four days of the Trial, but due to the length of the Trial I was unable to testify and it upset me that he was convicted. . . . Jimmy Keller and these people who work with him are the most dedicated group of people that I have ever met in my life. They have been literally abandoned by medical science here in the United States. . . . It is beyond my comprehension why the FBI and those prosecuting were so intent on Criminal Prosecution of a man who only tried to help those who sought his help.

Dr. Charles Whitehouse was another disgruntled witness who had sent a letter, but it was addressed to the jailed defendant rather than the judge. Dr. Whitehouse wrote:

It saddens me the way the verdict came out. All those good people that came down to testify from the heart. Jimmy I have never seen so many people that had such a great love for you and what you have done for them. It was worth the trip to experience that type of compassion that these people expressed to you and your work. . . . Jimmy as far as radionics is concerned I think your lawyers really mishandled that part. As of this day I have yet to talk to an attorney. The three months they had to prepare for this case we could have given them better methods of approach. . . . Major Gordon Smith from England should have been called to give the historical facts of what happened in England and what they are doing over there now. These people have to take a three year course to become qualified as operators and they do work to some degree with the medical profession. . . . I have slides that show a psychokinetic effect on physical objects and the experiments

*that we did with the U.S. government from tracking the
submarine in the Pacific to breaking an electromagnetic x-ray
beam at great distances. We have valid material on agriculture
experiments to prove that these instruments are not medical
devices but devices of the mind.*

The new defense team diligently examined the evidence,
scrutinized the arguments, and bandied the matter about. In the
end, we concluded it was probably hopeless. Silversmith's
omissions all boiled down to discretionary tactical decisions. We
could see it was going to be an uphill battle arguing incompetence
of counsel on appeal.

In court on October 9, 1991, the defense waited
apprehensively. We had been warned the judge would be annoyed
that Jimmy kept switching attorneys. To our relief, the judge was
kind. He said to Jimmy, "You have a lot of friends -- a lot of
friends. I've been overwhelmed with letters." He followed these
felicitations by ruling that Jimmy's motion for a new trial was
denied.

The judge said he wanted to hear from the defendant himself
as to his choice of counsel. Jimmy asked to confer with his
attorneys. Jimmy, Silversmith, Black, Greenburg, and Jaffe all
trooped out into the hall. When they trooped back in, the
defendant announced that he wanted to be represented by all of
them. The trial team was taken by surprise, but they could hardly
object. They had already been paid up front for taking the case
all the way through sentencing.

"I was thinking survival," Jimmy explained after the hearing.
"The judge said this was one of the best conducted trials he'd
ever sat through. I figured if Silversmith was the bright star of
Texas, I better not come down on him."

The association of counsel would prove to be a nominal one.
Jaffe remained attorney in fact. But at least nobody went away
mad.

# Chapter 38

## Houston

The weather in Nairobi that fall was magnificent. One thing exposure to prison had done was to make me appreciate the jacarandas in bloom and feel the breeze. Offsetting the fine weather were the riots, which were the order of the day in downtown Nairobi. We didn't worry too much about them (they were like the weather: you listened to the reports and stayed home), but legal writing was as good a way as any to keep busy.

The next writing to be done was the Presentence Investigation Report (PSI), Jimmy's last shot at input into sentencing. We were taking the matter seriously. The government and Silversmith's team had both predicted the convict would be behind bars for the next ten years, an ordeal it wasn't clear he would survive.

To do the paperwork, Jimmy had retained a one-time California attorney I'll call Bernice, who had been recommended by Maxine. Maxine said Bernice knew what could be done. That was because she had seen the system from both sides, as a lawyer and as an inmate. Maxine knew her from federal prison in Pleasanton. But the weeks had passed and not much seemed to be happening. Jimmy couldn't telephone from prison outside the United States; but when his brother Ray managed to concoct a phone patch, I detected from the nearly inaudible tone of the convict's voice that his once-indomitable spirit was draining away. So when he asked, I naturally said I'd tackle the PSI myself, with Bernice's guidance on the format.

Bernice then had a brainstorm: we could try to get Jimmy moved to Houston "for the convenience of counsel." We could all meet there and work on the PSI. It was a small victory, but a victory nonetheless, when the judge granted the motion Bernice had proposed. In mid-November, Jimmy was moved to Houston. We women got there on Sunday, November 24.

Instead of dinner that evening as planned, however, Bernice called to say she was going to bed. She wasn't feeling well. I used the time to visit the jail. I was jet-lagged and thinking wistfully of sleep myself, but Jimmy said he had news that couldn't be repeated over the phone. The excitement in his voice raised my adrenalin enough to get me off the couch in the Holiday Inn and into the '76 Mercedes his brother Ray had obligingly left parked in the hotel parking lot. Getting lost in the rain in a part of downtown Houston where it seemed imprudent to ask for directions served to keep my adrenalin up until I found the Houston jail.

The facility wasn't much of an improvement over the Brownsville jail. It had the same heavy atmosphere, the same forbidding aura of evil and gloom. I tried to ignore how sinister it was, as I rummaged in my purse for my Bar card and assumed the competent look of a person who routinely visited clients in rough circumstances.

The attorney conference room consisted of a tiny cubicle divided by bars, with counters and chairs on either side. The bars loomed in duplicate between prisoner and visitor, so our eyes had a tendency to cross while we tried to talk. Jimmy's voice was subdued. He didn't seem well. The months of greasy prison food, cement walls, fluorescent lights and grinding tension had drained his vitality. What the food lacked in nutritional value, it had evidently made up for in calories, because he looked like he had put on weight. He said he sorely missed his supplements. Arginine might be standard stock in health food stores, but you couldn't get it at the prison pharmacy, and there was no convincing the prison doctor that it was essential to the life and well-being of a recovered cancer victim.

"So what's the news?" I asked.

"There still isn't any money for attorneys' fees," Jimmy said. "Alma refuses to pay up. She and Durk keep saying they're broke. But Durk just made an offer on a house in a very nice part of San Diego -- for $750,000!"

"You're kidding."

"Twenty-five percent down in cash -- that's close to $200,000. So where did he get the money? Alma says my money is her money, because she was the head of the corporation and taking the risk. She said it like it was her idea, but it's not the kind of idea she normally gets. Durk must have planted it in her head."

"It does sound like they're involved," I cautiously stated the obvious.

"Alma has always needed someone to take care of her," Jimmy said pensively. "If it's a recent development, I can understand. But what if it's been going on a long time? Maybe they even helped get me arrested. I don't deal well with confrontation . . ."

"I know."

"But I decided I had to find out. All the things that used to work for me -- prayer and meditation and positive thinking -- got stifled in jail. But this time when I prayed, I asked the right question. I asked for the truth, and I got it!"

I wasn't sure what he meant. (He'd had a vision? Heard voices?) I asked, "How?"

"I called up Durk's wife and asked."

"Good plan."

"The way I got her to open up was, I said 'I know about Durk and Alma.' She said, 'You do?' She wasn't going to say anything because she didn't want to hurt me."

"So what did she say?"

"She said that three days after I was arrested, Durk left her. They hadn't been getting along for the last year and a half. She thinks he moved in with Alma. Durk used to tell her how pretty he thought Alma was. Durk would go with Alma to church, a charismatic church. Maestro told them the Lord had brought them together."

Maestro was the *curandero* Alma had taken up with after she broke away from her mother's strict fundamentalist church. I'll call Durk's wife Hannah.

"Hannah says Durk's business is failing," Jimmy said. "It has no employees. She and the kids are starving. They have four kids. She says if she ever sees Alma, she'll kill her. She says Durk and Alma met regularly with Black. I knew it! I wonder if they didn't set up the robbery and the kidnapping and everything."

"It's hard to believe of two people who owe you their lives," I said doubtfully. "I mean I can understand how Alma could have fallen for a younger man who had more time to be attentive, and I can understand how Durk could have fallen for her. But the rest of it . . ."

"Hannah says she has evidence. She xeroxed some documents from Durk's office and gave them to Little Jim. He's coming here on Friday, but he can't bring documents into the jail. Will you meet him and bring them?"

On the phone, Bernice had the voice of a younger woman. She turned out to be 65 and heavyset, with a butch haircut and masculine clothes. On Monday, we staked out a room in Rick's offices where we could tackle the defendant's version of the PSI.

Before we got to work, we bonded with small talk. Bernice confided that she could relate to Jimmy's plight. She felt that she too had been wrongfully convicted (for reasons that are too complicated to go into here). She could also relate to being mutilated by oncologists. Not that she blamed them -- forty years ago there was no other way -- but she knew what it was to lose body parts. She had been a young mother in her twenties when she agreed to exploratory surgery. She came out from under the anesthetic minus both breasts. Not long afterwards, her uterus had gone the way of her bosom.

After exhausting those disturbing topics, we got down to what we were trained for -- generating paper. We began by reviewing the government's PSI. Our first impression was that it looked bad for our side. The government named 92 Matamoros patients who were called "victims" of the defendant's fraudulent scheme, including 76 patients who were listed as deceased in 1991.

Then we studied the list. "Look at this!" I said. "Arlene Torgesen testified for the defense -- they have her down as deceased! Bonnie Cayer, JoAnn Brown -- they testified for the defense! Pearl Gervais, Laura Hebert, Edith Moon, Judith Smeester -- we have supporting letters from these people!" The government seemed to consider anyone who had gone to Jimmy's clinic a victim of his fraudulent scheme. The ones who thought they had been helped were simply deluded. It was the kind of paternalistic argument that had to be rebutted.

Our rebuttal was that patients weren't "victims" if their pains had been relieved or their lives had been extended by the treatment. Over the years, many patients or their relatives had written letters and affidavits expressing their appreciation and describing benefits received. Treatment success, we maintained, included these benefits -- and that was true even if the patients had later died.

Judith Smeester's was a case in point. In 1984, she had written that she had undergone "a modified, radical mastectomy, which was followed by one year of chemotherapy (one year of hell for myself and my family). [I]n September, 1983, I chose to discontinue all cancer treatment. A few months later . . . , I chose to undergo an alternative cancer treatment called 'Tumorex,' . . . administered with a fantastic amount of love and concern. This, like any treatment, carries no promises; but I feel the Tumorex treatment has worked for me. The pain I was experiencing is gone, and the tumor which was so prominent on my chest, has almost disappeared. I feel great! I thank God that I heard about the Universal Health Center, and 'Tumorex.' Also, for the beautiful, caring people I have met since hearing about the Universal Health Center." (The underscorings were hers.)

Judith was now listed, along with many other patients, as deceased. But of what, we asked, were these patients "victims"? We maintained it was more likely to have been their conventional treatments than Jimmy's. It was because they felt victimized by conventional treatment, in fact, that they had been driven to seek alternatives.

Dr. Ruth Kerhart had expressed this feeling vividly in an interview with Paul. She said:

> Doctors have this technological approach. Rape the land, rape bodies -- it's a cowboy mentality. They strip mine women's bodies. When a surgeon says he 'got it all,' he means he cured you; but six years later, you've got metastasized cancer all over the place. Doctors are in bed with insurance companies. My premiums went up from $78 a month to $1,107 a month, with a $5,000 deductible; and alternative treatment isn't covered. The whole health care system is unconscionable. It's a dinosaur. There's a massive grass roots movement for holistic health care. They can't stop it.

When Ruth talked about Jimmy's approach, by contrast, her images bordered on poetry:

> We are dying when we come to him. Ninety-five percent of patients who go to Mexican clinics have tried everything else that traditional medicine has to offer. They have given up. They are at the line. . . . We know we are headed for death and all of a sudden we are going in the other direction. . . . Jimmy is very calm and he listens very attentively. You feel comforted by the

*way he is just present. You feel intensely cared about. He empowers people. He lets them know that their healing has a great deal to do with them.*

Oncologists, I reflected, seemed to feel it was their duty to assure their patients that they would <u>not</u> get well -- that they had only weeks or months to live. The dutiful patients were liable to accept the suggestion and proceed Voodoo-like to their deaths. Jimmy reprogrammed these hopeless patients with positive affirmations that they would survive. A plaque above his mantle said, "I do not have cancer. Therefore I am going to live." One of his favorite tension-relievers was to joke, "You have cancer? Thank God! I thought you had something serious!"

But no amount of positive suggestion could re-build an immune system that had already been destroyed by radiation and chemotherapy. When his patients died as a result, the blame fell on him for fraudulently planting the suggestion that they were cured.

# Chapter 39

## Thanksgiving

I spent Thanksgiving in jail. Bernice had gone back to California, and Rick was on the East Coast with his family. My job over the four-day weekend was to call Maxine and every patient and relative we could track down who might have evidence for the defense. But for the holiday, I thought I'd visit the oppressed.

Through the glass door of the attorney conference cubicle, I could see animated wives chatting with their incarcerated husbands, and mothers chatting with their sons. They seemed to take it all in stride. It was a way of life for them, and it was a day for counting your blessings.

When Jimmy was escorted into the conference room, he was carrying a paper. After his usual cordial Southern greetings, he slipped it under the bars. "Look at this!" he said.

I scrutinized the document. It was a package insert to a drug called "R-Gene 10," a patented version of L-arginine in injectable form.

"This says injectable arginine is FDA-approved as a test for pituitary function," he explained. "The pituitary is considered to be functioning normally if growth hormone is released on its injection!"

I hadn't a clue what he was talking about. I remembered what Bill had said: a remedy that has been FDA-approved for some purpose can be used for any purpose a doctor deems appropriate. "So injectable arginine can legally be used to treat cancer?" I guessed Jimmy's point.

"That too."

"What were you thinking of?"

"I was thinking that growth hormone is the most fantastic rejuvenator ever known! Studies have been done on it in Europe. Everyone is looking at it as the fountain of youth. And according to this, L-arginine causes a large secretion of it. It's actually better to give the precursor and let the body make its own hormone. Then you can't get too much."

I had to smile as I pictured the convict in his jail cell, poring over the package insert to a drug. The language was obscure and the print was fine, and the man wore glasses that were practically half an inch thick. Still, he took an interest in these things. The mind ran free . . . .

Then I studied the insert. What it revealed was indeed interesting. L-arginine was the safer, more economical precursor to a high-priced "wonder drug." I had read that the FDA was trying to make amino acids, along with herbs and high-potency vitamins, prescription drugs.[82] Was it because the natural, unpatentable precursors were competing with much higher-priced synthetics?

I realized I was thinking like a conspiratorialist . . .

> Later I read that, suspiciously, proponents of removing amino acids from the over-the-counter market were attempting to lock in "use" patents for these same amino acids. (A "use" patent patents a particular application rather than the substance itself.)[83] I also read that FDA approval had been granted for the patented version of human growth hormone, a "youth" drug from which manufacturers stand to gross about $14,000 per patient per year. Besides its exorbitant price, the problem with the drug was that it could have serious side effects.[84] L-arginine, by contrast, was safe, effective, and inexpensive. Research had shown that it stimulates growth hormone release, aiding healing of wounds and immunity from disease; decreases cholesterol levels and atherogenesis (degenerative changes in the arteries), in both animals and humans; increases the weight of the thymus, a gland essential for immunity; and actually stimulates wound healing better than an injection of growth hormone.[85]

After we had exhausted that topic, conversation reverted to the PSI. I shared a bit of gossip I had heard in a phone interview.

My informant was a woman who had occupied the Brownsville motel room adjoining baby Jessica's in 1983. She described the child's seemingly miraculous recovery -- how Jessica had run around chasing the ducks. Then she told of something that had gravely disturbed her at the time. She had seen Jessica's father, a "strict disciplinarian," hit his daughter so hard on the bottom that the child flew into the air. What was alarming, said the woman, was that Jessica's tumor was of the type that the sheer weight of it could have killed her. (This witness would later tell the same story in a letter lodged with the court.)

Jimmy didn't seem too surprised. "I think child abuse could have had something to do with the little girl's death," he said. "I heard her father really knocked her around."

At the time of trial, Jessica's parents were no longer married; but why we didn't know. The child abuse theory was mere conjecture. The issues, I thought, would have been interesting to explore in a pretrial deposition. But it was all water under the bridge now.

When we ran out of legal business, I asked Jimmy to tell me some stories -- the ones he had said "you wouldn't believe."

"Okay," he obliged after a moment's thought, "there was a twelve-year-old girl I treated in Rosarito Beach. She was from Boston and she had cancer in her jaw. Her doctors wanted to remove part of her jaw, but the surgery would have made a freak out of her and her mother wouldn't let them do it. When the girl came in, she was in pain and her jaw and gums were swollen. I started treating her, and within three weeks you couldn't tell she'd ever been sick. Her cheek and gums went back to normal. But the authorities in Massachusetts had a court order and a warrant out for the arrest of the mother. They were furious because she'd gone to Mexico. I was afraid they'd do the surgery anyway, and I told her not to go back. But the mother said, 'How can they? There's no tumor.' I said they could. I'd heard of it happening before. But the mother was afraid of losing her job if she didn't go back. I said why didn't she leave the girl with me? But she was sure that when they saw there was no tumor, they'd forget the whole thing. They went back and sure enough, the authorities arrested the mother and put her in jail. By the time she got out on bond, her daughter was already in the hospital and they were doing the surgery. They took out half her jaw. They already had a written diagnosis. The mother had a nervous breakdown."

"Wow," I said. "That's hard to believe!"

"I told you you wouldn't believe it."

"You're right. I asked. Tell me another one."

"Okay, here's one you can ask Little Jim about -- or Ryan." Jimmy explained that Ryan was his grandson. The boy had gotten a tumor in his groin when he was six or seven years old. Jim Jr., who was then divorced from his first wife and had custody of their children, had brought Ryan to Mexico. "I gave him the serum, and the tumor shrank from the size of a lemon to almost nothing," Jimmy said. "It was just a lymph gland that had gotten swollen. Ryan went out riding horses after that, and went swimming at the beach."

But Ryan's mother, who wanted to regain custody of her children, found out and complained to the health department. She filed papers to try to get the children away from Jim Jr. The grounds were medical neglect: he hadn't allowed a biopsy on the lump.

"State officials pulled Ryan out of his bed at night," Jimmy said, "and put him in the charity hospital. Little Jim said he had insurance and could afford better, but they wouldn't move the boy. They already had the court order. They tried to biopsy what was left of the lump, but of course they couldn't get anything. They poked around with a big needle, while Ryan screamed and screamed. It took several people to hold him down. They kept him for three days as a prisoner. Little Jim went to court for custody after that, and he won."

Then Jimmy told the tragic tale of a teenaged girl he had treated for a vaginal tumor in Baton Rouge in 1982. The tumor had shrunk substantially, when the health department nabbed the girl on the way to school. "They'd gotten a court order because the mother wasn't taking proper care of her daughter," Jimmy said. "She was taking her daughter to a quack. They cut into the remains of the tumor to biopsy it, and the girl died in the hospital a week later."

He told several more stories of the same sort. A year earlier, I would have been shocked and appalled, and I might not have believed them. But I had become accustomed, even jaded and numbed, to such tales, having read them in patient letters, in books, even in the media.[86] I had come around to accepting that these things could happen.

Friday, Jimmy's oldest son came to the Holiday Inn with a huge notebook full of documents. A congenial Southerner with a sense of humor that didn't get much play in these troubled times, Jim Jr. expressed his concerns about his father. I asked about his son Ryan. He confirmed the story his father had told. When he left, I duly delivered the notebook to the jail.

The tiny glassed-in conference room reminded me of an aquarium, as Jimmy peered with goldfish eyes through his Coke-bottle-bottom lenses at the documents. The gist of what they revealed was that Durk had invested heavily in a notorious Nigerian scam. We surmised that he had "borrowed" Jimmy's money for the purpose, probably intending to pay it back from the proceeds with no one being the wiser. But the Nigerian scam had fallen through. We imagined desperate straits leading to desperate measures thereafter.

"I think his motivation was sheer survival," Jimmy mused. "Durk has been hopelessly in debt all the time I've known him. He talked big, acted like a successful businessman, when really he was tottering on bankruptcy." To illustrate his point, Jimmy drew on his copious collection of Civil War stories. "During the Civil War, soldiers would come out of the trenches at night and trade goods with each other across enemy lines. The next day, they shot each other. They did it for survival."

The prisoner lapsed into brooding thought. "They probably figured I'd only be in jail a short time, long enough for them to get the formula, then I'd get out."

"The formula?"

"To my serum. It was keeping them alive."

"I see! They couldn't run off together without it."

Jimmy nodded. "I never even told Alma how I made it. Not that I didn't trust her, but it was proprietary. It was a jungle out there in Tijuana. My serum was my competitive edge. Anyway, there wasn't just one formula. It was different for different people and at different times. You had to tune in. It was an art. But after I got arrested, everyone was saying, 'What are we going to do?' They could have guessed I would tell someone the basic formula, and Durk was my good friend. I did tell him, and he and Juan started making the serum for the patients."

That could explain it, I agreed. No matter how well-meaning Jimmy might have been, he had put Durk and Alma in the untenable position of being totally dependent on him for their well-being. His serum wasn't something they could purchase at the drugstore. They were trapped and had to break free, by hook or by crook.

Jimmy found receipts in the notebook showing that Durk had gotten $85,000 from Juan's operation of Jimmy's clinic using Jimmy's serum. Durk had also gotten thirty or forty thousand dollars from insurance from the residue from Jimmy's old patients. There were huge bills for past treatments to Selma Meyers, a patient Jimmy hadn't charged because she'd had no money. There was a bill to one patient for $210 for six Mannitol. "That's unconscionable," Jimmy said. "They should have been five dollars each."

He added pensively, "Alma always did want to run the clinic more like a business. She wanted to cut out the free people."

"Didn't you treat her for free?"

"I did," he said, but he wasn't thinking about ironies. "No one could have gotten me but Alma. The Mexican police are really afraid to violate an *amparo*. But Alma could tell them nothing would happen, because of her friend with the federales - - or because she wouldn't file a complaint, which she never did. I think she probably was loyal until the FBI came looking for her in San Diego. Then she got scared. She had children to worry about. It was me or the children. She made the obvious choice. She feels really guilty about it now. She cries enough on the phone. A number of patients have died since I've been in jail, and they can't get the clinic going without me."

It was further evidence, I thought, that Jimmy's success wasn't just from his serum. The patients needed his "wholistic" approach to the body's total needs at the time. I thought of Olga Quijano. While Jimmy was treating her, she was fine. But after he was jailed, she got Juan's version of Jimmy's serum and was plummeting downhill. Jimmy said what she really needed was love -- and to have her acupuncture meridians unblocked, and whatever else muscle testing might have come up with if he could have checked her.

Olga actually tried to get into the jail to have Jimmy muscle test her and make some recommendations. But rules were rules. The guards had made the desperate woman, like everyone else, stay behind reinforced glass.

# Chapter 40

## Family Ties

Jimmy's brother Ray's house, where I was invited to stay after his family got back from vacation, was a pleasant change from the isolation of the Holiday Inn. The living room was usually invaded by children, largely because it featured a giant-screened TV that was usually on. The kitchen, which harbored the telephone, saw nearly as much action. The lengthiest calls were from Jimmy, who talked for hours.

Bernice also called from California. She said she had spoken to a senior DEA agent, who reported that a directive had gone out to all DEA agents stating no kidnapping incidents would be tolerated thereafter. The directive was dated before March 18, 1991, the day Jimmy was kidnapped.

Ray also put in a call to Hannah. He asked where her husband had been the night of the birthday party robbery. Hannah said Durk had told her he was going to the party. But when Ray relayed this information to Jimmy, Jimmy said Durk wasn't there.

Other calls were from supporters. The Kellers were out of money, but they still had friends. The task of soliciting for the Jimmy Keller defense fund had fallen on Ray's shoulders. They were solid shoulders (he ran a karate school at night, along with a printing business during the day), but the task was still a heavy one. His wife Debbie contributed to the cause. She said she could relate to it: her first husband, who worked as a carpet-layer, had died of cancer when he was still quite young.

All Jimmy could do in return was to say thank you, but this he did in profusion. He started and ended every conversation with "I love you." He did that with everyone, but as between the men, I thought it was nice. Not many brothers were that expressive of their feelings. Perhaps they might have been if they had found themselves in similar straits, since crises tend to bring families together; but the Kellers still seemed remarkable for their solidarity. They were all going down together fighting Jimmy's cause.

Hannah later had more to reveal about her husband. She talked to Jimmy and then to Paul. She said Durk had been a good man until he ran into financial problems. But lately, all he could think about was money.

Once when she had been in his office, she overheard a conversation between him and a patient named Mike Johnson. Mike had come to Jimmy's clinic near death. Jimmy had treated him and had turned his condition around. Mike had then moved to Washington, where Jimmy would send him serum. But after Jimmy was arrested, Mike's condition got worse. When he called Durk for serum, it was taking all his energy to talk. "I'm very sick," he said, "but I'm broke. This disease has taken all of my money. Can you help me?"

"I can send you five bottles," said Durk. "$200 a bottle. That will be $1,000 COD."

Hannah thought, "You son of a bitch."

She also overheard a conversation between Durk and Selma's brother Marty. Selma hadn't gone to Durk for treatment because she couldn't pay. But when she was near death, Marty called Durk. "Selma is dying," he said. "Can you send her some serum?"

Durk declined. "What difference would it make?"

"He was very cold," Hannah commented. "It wasn't like him." She thought perhaps Alma was slipping him drugs, or Maestro was casting his spells.

Perhaps, I thought. But being a million dollars in debt could explain Durk's profit orientation as well.

I spent the week after Thanksgiving gathering affidavits and tabulating the results of our telephone interviews into a survey. We were able to get information on two-thirds of the patients listed in the government's PSI. Counting the eleven people listed in the indictment (whom we conceded were "unsatisfied"), our survey indicated that 75 percent of the alleged "victims" fell into either the "satisfied" or the "very satisfied" category.

Jimmy thought the 75 percent figure was probably low. There were other satisfied and surviving Matamoros patients, he said, who hadn't been included on the government's list.

Rick was also making some phone calls that week. He was considering another motion for a new trial, to give Jimmy a chance to present the case that hadn't been presented so far. He thought Silversmith had done about as well as could be expected under the circumstances. But he also thought key evidence had been omitted.

First on Rick's list was Dr. Charles Whitehouse. They talked for about an hour. Dr. Whitehouse told Rick how ineptly he thought the witnesses had been handled. He said he could have testified from personal knowledge to the Navy's use of radionics. Rick sounded surprised. "That kind of evidence might have influenced the outcome," he said.

Then Rick called Bill. It was the first time they had talked. Bill told Rick he thought Silversmith had thrown the case. Bill went into Silversmith's failure to raise the meeting between the prosecution and the government witnesses. Again Rick sounded surprised. "I can't believe they never brought that up," he said. "That's the first thing you ask any witness: 'Who did you talk to about this case?' Even when you don't expect it to lead to anything, you ask that."

Then Rick called Dr. Brodie. The doctor had a compelling manner that made Rick give him credence. Dr. Brodie, too, was quite unhappy with how the witnesses had been handled. He said he could have testified about the dramatic Tumorex cases he had seen. But Ginsburg had merely delivered a lecture about cancer and had hardly let the doctor speak.

The next time Rick talked to Silversmith, he mentioned the navy's use of radionics. Silversmith agreed that if he had known about it, he would have put Dr. Whitehouse on the stand. Silversmith said no one had told him.

"He never came around to ask," Jimmy said dourly when I passed that information on to him. "But I did tell him. I told him on the phone, and I told his associate Sylvia."

A conference call between the attorneys and the judge was scheduled for December 10. Rick had intended to have Silversmith join in, but after these disturbing phone interviews, he decided to carry on alone.

At the telephone conference, the judge said that if the defendant wanted to submit affidavits for sentencing, he could.

But the judge did not feel the need or desire to hear more testimony. He had already received some 500 letters and other pieces of literature in the mail. He said he was particularly affected by "letters from the heart."

So were we. More than 350 letters had come to Rick or to Ray for forwarding to the court, and Debbie and I had the task of reviewing and copying them. We sat around the kitchen table exchanging poignant letters and the Kleenex box.

Most of the letters were from people who said Jimmy had saved or improved their lives or the lives of their loved ones, or had made the deaths of their loved ones pain-free. Abby Juneau of Bonita, California, wrote:

> *Jimmy Keller . . . greatly aided my oldest daughter's recovery from acute lymphocytic leukemia (ALL). . . . Because our finances were pretty well shot by the time we got to him he often treated her as a charity case. . . . As a mother who has been from death's door with her child, to the hope of a real future for that same child, I beg the Court for mercy in the sentencing of Mr. Keller.*

Nancy Herchman Johnson of Vernon, Texas, wrote:

> *After the last surgery, the medical physicians gave [my father] 3 months to live which they stated would be so painful that no medication would help. My daddy became frighten[ed]. Not of dying, you see, but of pain. . . . [T]he medical physicians were in shock that he had no pain. My family attributes this lack of pain to Jimmy's treatments. . . . There is no charge for treatment if one is poor and he never turns anyone away. . . . Your Honor, please, for the sake of the people that he has and still was helping set him free. Even if one life is saved, that one life is very special to someone near to it. . . . It chills me to think that my daddy could have died drawing his last breath begging for relief of pain. Please, Your Honor, set Jimmy Keller free so others may, at least, lay loved ones to rest with peaceful remembrance.*

Carolyn Babin of Baton Rouge, Louisiana, wrote:

> *I owe my life to him today. . . . I had bone cancer and also a brain tumor . . . . I told him even though I believed in what he was doing, I did not have the money to have treatment. . . . [H]e did the treatment free of charge. . . . It's been 8 years now, possibly 9 years. . . . I also delivered a healthy baby girl 4 years ago. I never thought I'd get better much less have a new life to bring into the world.*

Other letters were from medical professionals, like Eugene A. Wohrlin, Clinic Director of the Lovelace Medical Center in Corrales, New Mexico, who wrote:

> *When I left [Keller's clinic], my outlook on allopathic medicine as practiced in America completely changed. . . . [M]y mother-in-law [who] came down to Mexico with only 1 year to live per her physician, now is in perfect health. I am a clinic director of two offices (medical) in the Albuquerque, New Mexico area. . . . My experience tells me that my type of organization does well in treating patients when we are talking about trauma or injury cases. When it comes to chronic, degenerative ailments, we, like other similar medical institutions, are still in the dark ages. Drugs do not cure; they merely hide the symptoms of sickness. . . . Jimmy Keller is a humble, compassionate person. He is not in it for the money. His whole reason for existence is to help others. He is unselfish, a genuine healer. . . . The efficacy of his methods is phenomenal.*

Other letters are excerpted in Appendix B.

# Chapter 41

## Court of Last Resort

On December 16, 1991, Jimmy Keller was sentenced. When the judge addressed the defendant, he was remarkably warm. He called Jimmy a "man of compassion." He said, "I agree that you believe in what you were doing." He seemed moved by the letters from patients and supporters. But he wasn't moved enough to set the man free. There were other considerations . . .

"If you're looking from me for endorsement of alternative cancer clinics as something that should be available and legal," said the judge, "I think they are a menace. He's not a doctor. He was giving people substances that had no positive chemical effect whatsoever." Of radionics, the judge said, "I think Santa Claus is more real than that." He added, apparently in deference to the professors, "And that's not to insult anybody who believes in it. They have that right."

I sighed. The stack of radionics books and arginine studies we had so laboriously introduced into evidence had apparently made no impact on the court.

"I [must] let it be known throughout this country that this simply cannot be tolerated," the judge went on. "I also regret that what we do in this country is confinement. But this is a case with very grave [implications]. . . . I learned something from this case. Medical science doesn't have a cure for cancer. But I agree with the jury that Mr. Keller does not have a cure for cancer either." Rick jumped up. "That's not what my motion for a new trial is all about. These letters show he <u>believed</u> he had a treatment that helped cancer." The defendant could not have been guilty of fraud if he believed his own representations.

"I agree with the jury's finding in this," said the judge. "Medical science and alternative medicine don't have a cure for cancer, either one. He may have given comfort that other doctors didn't give. But he didn't cure them. I wish he could. I don't think he caused the death of someone. He may even have prolonged life in some cases. He's a good man. I don't have any problem with that. But I agree with the jury -- he doesn't have a cure. He engaged in fraudulent activity. I think he did some good for a lot of the people. But Mr. Keller's problem is the jury found him guilty of ten counts of defrauding cancer patients."

The judge added, "My recollection is, and I stand to be corrected, . . . ninety people had died, not ten. . . . And if these people had been offered a cure and they died, then obviously the cure was not there. So let's not confine ourselves necessarily to ten people. But I am confining myself only to what was adduced at trial." It was an issue to be tested on appeal.

The audience collectively drew in its breath, as the judge announced the sentence: twenty years in federal prison. We all collectively exhaled, when he added that eighteen years were to be suspended. Jimmy was to serve four consecutive 179-day terms, or two years. Nine months had already been served, so only fifteen months were left. Probation was to follow for a period of five years. But if Jimmy violated its terms, he would be facing the full twenty-year sentence. He was also to pay a $20,000 fine. While on probation, he was restricted to the Baton Rouge area. That meant he wouldn't be free to leave the country until January of 1998.

The other probationary terms were rather vague. Jimmy was "to refrain from engaging in any occupation, business or profession bearing a reasonably direct relationship to the conduct that was involved or that constituted this offense." He was also not to "advocate these alternative means or methods that caused this case to come before the Court before anybody." Apparently, freedom of speech was not a right of men on probation.

When Jimmy asked if he would be allowed to take his remedies, the judge said he would. But "if you ever prescribe anything . . . like this L-arginine or whatever it is . . . you may be in violation of law because you may be practicing medicine without a license."

*Therein, I knew from law school, lies an interesting legal query. Medical practice acts make it a crime to "diagnose,*

*prescribe, or treat" any physical condition without a license.
But can you "prescribe" something that isn't a "prescription"
drug? The answer is yes. People who merely recommended
over-the-counter products have been held to be practicing
medicine without a license.*[87] *Under the letter of the law, the
board of medical examiners can arrest mothers for
recommending chicken soup for colds.*

When Paul interviewed U.S. attorney Meier after the hearing,
the prosecutor spoke through clenched teeth. "The Court has
more confidence in his ability to control Mr. Keller than I do,"
said the prosecutor icily.

Sylvia, on the other hand, was warm. She congratulated us on
the result. Apparently, Silversmith's office had anticipated worse.

I never heard how Alma had taken it, but Hannah reported
that when Durk learned that Jimmy had gotten only two years,
he responded by kicking boxes around the office in a rage.

Jimmy's relatives and supporters, if not elated, were at least
relieved. The judge could hardly have let Jimmy off with less than
two years. It was the amount of time that Maxine, a mere
accomplice, had already served. Jimmy's relatives felt he could
survive under those trying conditions for fifteen more months.

Unfortunately, this wasn't true for some of his patients. Selma
Myers passed away the same month Jimmy was sentenced, and
Olga Quijano died early the next year.

We got a followup report later on Alma and Durk. Hannah
said the happy couple were honeymooning in an elegant hotel in
Hawaii.

"Isn't Alma still married to you?" I asked when Jimmy passed
this piece of gossip on to me.

"As far as I know," he said with a rueful laugh.

Later, we heard that Alma and Durk were both seeking
treatment at another clinic for cancer. Just knowing Jimmy's
formula evidently wasn't enough to keep their conditions in
remission.

And after that, we didn't hear anything for several years.
Bernice, who lives in San Diego, tried to locate the couple but
was unsuccessful. Like the chinless jury foreman, they seemed to
have disappeared from the face of the earth.

Compared to the Cameron County Jail, the South Dakota
prison where Jimmy served out the rest of his sentence was a
country club. The Yankton Federal Prison was a converted college

campus reserved for "white collar" criminals. I saw it in the summer of 1992, in transit between Kenya and Honduras, our new post. Besides an appeal brief, Jimmy wanted a Petition for Writ of Habeas Corpus to be filed under his own signature, aimed at shortening his sentence.

The South Dakota landscape was green and rolling, and the temperature that week was perfect. But the woman who managed the motel where I was staying warned that I should sample the winters before passing judgment on the local weather conditions.

After we covered the weather, the manager related the chilling details of her husband's case. She happened to be the wife of one of Jimmy's cell mates. She maintained that he had been convicted on falsified evidence. "Jeopardy assessments" permitted confiscation of the property of suspected tax evaders before the crime had been proven in court. The targeted property in her husband's case, she said, was the family farm.

The visiting area where attorneys could interview prisoners was graced with sunlit windows, vending machines, and padded chairs. Jimmy said prison security was minimal. Rumor had it that one prisoner managed to slip out periodically at night to visit his wife, then slip back in in time for breakfast.

I asked what Jimmy thought of the motel manager's story about her husband. He replied, in hushed tones, that it was probably true. He had heard a number of disturbing stories of convictions based on falsified evidence; and since the convicts had no reason to lie to their fellow captives, he tended to believe them. The police had quotas and weren't always too scrupulous about how they were met. Besides the law providing for jeopardy assessments, there was the tempting incentive allowing for the confiscation of the property of drug dealers. Drugs had been known to be planted in raids just so the raiding agencies could get title to certain desirable pieces of real estate.

After Jimmy described what he wanted in the way of a Petition, I went back to the motel to hammer out a draft. My new doll-sized printer suffered from the inefficiencies of compactness, but it was portable, and it was cute. The arguments the Petition raised, we thought, were irrefutable. We consoled ourselves by thinking that was probably why they were never refuted. The Petition wasn't ruled on until after Jimmy was released, and then it was merely denied as most.

When my family arrived in Honduras, an enormous box was waiting at the embassy post office. The trial transcript ran to a weighty 2,000 pages. I read it perched on a hilltop overlooking Tegucigalpa, nestled in the mountains of Honduras. From that distant perspective, the bitter emotions of the Keller case receded into an intellectual exercise.

As I read, I tallied deaths. I counted only six that had occurred while Jimmy's Matamoros clinic was still in operation; and for five of these, there was no record that he had been informed at the time. The only death he definitely knew about in 1983 was baby Jessica's, the case in which he had given a refund. One death out of nearly 200 patients was an apparent success rate of 99-1/2 percent, and six deaths out of 200 was an actual survival rate of 97 percent. I was excited. We had a leg to stand on.

I looked for Silversmith's query concerning the U.S. regulation requiring the government to destroy its own tapes if they violated Mexican law. The rule the government produced actually required the reverse -- tapes once made must not be destroyed -- or so I remembered it. But this last crucial point wasn't in the pretrial transcript. Had my memory failed? Or had the court reporter already concluded the official proceedings for the day?

I decided it was an expendable argument. By the time I wrote up all the points Jimmy wanted raised and added them to the ones I had in mind, the brief already exceeded the allowed fifty pages. I sent it to Rick, who could be counted on to whittle it down.

I was rather sad to see my literary efforts go. The deleted arguments included prosecutorial misconduct, defense attorney malpractice, and that the "fraudulent" claims were actually true. But Rick wanted to stick with the sure winners. He went with these:

(1) The judge admitted at sentencing that Jimmy believed in what he was doing. If he believed his own representations, he could not have been guilty of intentional fraud.

(2) Testimony established the deaths from cancer of only six out of nearly 200 Matamoros patients during the time Jimmy's clinic was in operation; and during that time, according to the testimony, he was informed of only one of those deaths. As far as Jimmy knew in 1983, then, his therapies were more than 99 percent successful.

(3) The court erroneously refused to require production of the April 1991 grand jury transcript. The defense was legally

entitled to it for impeachment purposes, since it qualified as "Jencks material:" the transcript contained witness testimony that may have contradicted what was said at trial.

It was only a hunch, but the defense wanted to see a copy of this 1991 grand jury transcript. Rick filed a motion with the Fifth Circuit Court of Appeals to compel its production.

Then we waited. By the time the motion was granted, it was November of 1992, over a year after the trial. And by the time the government produced the transcript, it was March of 1993.

Rick's first reaction to what he got was to be disappointed. He had hoped for prior conflicting grand jury testimony by one of the testifying relatives. All the government produced was the testimony of FBI agent Dixon. Rick took it home to look it over.

That evening when he called Jimmy's brother Ray, however, his tone had changed. "He was like a little kid," Ray said. "It was the most enthusiastic he'd been about anything in the case. He kept saying, 'We've got him! We've got him lying about the principal issue in the case!'"

What had fired Rick's enthusiasm was this: before the 1991 grand jury, Dixon had testified that his survey included 93 people, and that only 45 of them had died by 1985.[88] That put the death rate at less than 50 percent. But at the trial four months later, Dixon had testified that his survey included 103 people, and that 78 or 79 of them had already died by that date -- a death rate of 77 percent. There was no way to reconcile the figures, even if Dixon had managed to come up with ten additional "victims" in the intervening four months. Even if all ten had died by 1985, the death toll would still be only 55, not 78 or 79. The discrepancies demonstrated the bad faith of the government and the unreliability of its evidence. They also proved the truth of Jimmy's representations. Fifty percent was the survival rate that he was allegedly quoting to patients with prior conventional treatment, and that Maxine's attorneys had arrived at in 1985. The government's own figures, it seemed, established the innocence of the defendant!

That was how it seemed to the defense. But we'd had enough experience with the court system not to expect instant reversal. With cynical realism, we waited and hoped. Rick's first move was to bring a motion for a new trial before the district court, "based on the incontrovertible and substantial discrepancies between the trial testimony of the key government witness and his unproduced grand jury testimony."

The government submitted no opposition. In theory, the defense should have prevailed. But we weren't really surprised when the motion was summarily denied. We hardly expected the district court to find its own ruling in error. Our real hope was the Fifth Circuit Court of Appeals.

Rick filed the defendant's brief on appeal in August of 1993, nearly two years after the jury's verdict. The brief asked the Fifth Circuit:

> Which set of numbers is accurate, the trial testimony (and the summary exhibit which was in the courtroom for most of the trial), the Grand Jury numbers, the PSI numbers or none of the above? . . . . The survey provided the only proof in the entire case that the Defendant's representations concerning his cure or success rates from his Tumorex based treatment were false. . . . [T]he only number of deaths which is completely reliable and which was proven beyond a reasonable doubt at trial were the nine [patients named in the indictment] and the nine other patients whose death certificates were introduced into evidence (including one patient who died of a gunshot wound). What would have been the verdict if the prosecution only proved beyond a reasonable doubt that 17 out of Keller's 180 to 200 terminal cancer patients died of cancer?

The obvious result would have been a fatal lack of evidence that the defendant's representations were fraudulent. But a less obvious result might also have followed:

> The fact that the government survey was so demonstrably corrupt might have emboldened the defense to take a much more aggressive stance in this case. The defense could have used the survey as the first part of an argument that the government concocted the whole case. Step two could have been the fact that the only irrefutable evidence as to what the Defendant had said to an individual prospective patient at his clinic was the tape which the government had intentionally destroyed.
>
> The defense might also have decided to more aggressively challenge the relatives of the 'victims' by impeaching one or

more of them through the testimony of an eyewitness, and by attempting to prove that the government brought all these witnesses to Brownsville together shortly before the trial to prepare them and make sure their testimony was consistent.

Unfortunately, none of these opportunities was utilized, and it is therefore only speculation as to what might have been different had the Jencks material been provided.

Hopes ran high, as we waited for the government's opposition. Its brief was slim. The government argued:

[E]vidence of Keller's intent to defraud rests not in numbers, but in the fantastical nature of the procedures he claimed cured people of cancer. . . . The fantastical nature of the Digitron D and crystal pendulum defy reality and fly in the face of what a layman perceives as appropriate diagnostic procedures. By their verdict the jury implicitly rejected the expert testimony attesting to these procedures' legitimacy. . . . Keller's use of these procedures raises an inference that he was attempting to wrongfully influence his patients' conduct. This is evidence of an intent to defraud.

To us, it was the rankest myopia and closed-mindedness. The government was saying in effect, "Forget your sophisticated legal arguments. The man was diagnosing with a pendulum. Obviously, he was a quack." No matter what the witnesses testified to or Keller believed, to the government his methods were *per se* "fantastical" and therefore "fraudulent." No authority or evidence was cited. Surely, we thought, we had won.

But we were wrong.

On February 14, 1994, the Fifth Circuit Court of Appeals issued its ruling. It found that the discrepancies in Dixon's numbers were immaterial. It rejected the argument that the defendant had no way of knowing his representations were false, on the ground that "the jury was entitled to conclude that Keller's claims that he could diagnose cancer with a plastic pendulum and a Polaroid photograph were <u>patently</u> false . . ." To the Fifth Circuit, the matter was evidently so obvious that no proof was required; reasonable people could not differ on it.

The district court judge had declared that anyone who "believes" in radionics and radiesthesia "has that right." That right had now been sharply limited by the Fifth Circuit. "Belief" might be permitted, but anyone who tried to put that belief into practice could be found guilty of a patent and actionable fraud.

There was still the court of last resort, the United States Supreme Court. But Jimmy respectfully declined to pursue the option. Partly, it was because he was disillusioned with the court system. But mainly, it was because he was broke.

The mills of the courts had ground slowly -- so slowly that by the time the grand jury transcript was produced, Jimmy had already served his sentence. He was released on January 22, 1993, after spending 22 months in prison.

The occasion was celebrated by a fine crawfish boil at the home of Jim Jr. and his wife Suzanne, marked by general hugging, storytelling and carrying on. The guests included Jimmy's father Guy, his brother Ray and sister-in-law Debbie, his son David and David's wife Faye, his daughter Joyce, his brother Michael and Michael's wife Cita, his sisters Gwen and Diane and their husbands, Uncle Harold and Aunt Lou, Uncle Boone, Uncle Irvin, Uncle Roland, Jimmy's first wife, their seven grandchildren, and their two great grandchildren.

Jimmy also celebrated his release by indulging heavily in a forbidden substance he had craved throughout his jail term. He took 60 capsules (or 30 grams) of arginine, and chased them down with an assortment of vitamins and minerals. He had had various health complaints in jail, but after these therapeutic doses of supplements, he said, "I feel great." He added, "If arginine were toxic, it should have killed me by now."

Absence had increased his fondness for other simple pleasures. He was restricted by the terms of probation, but he was free to indulge in pure food and water and breathe fresh air. He could freely visit his family. He could also visit his first wife, who resides in the area he was restricted to. The couple had a happy reunion, taking up where they had left off nearly thirty years earlier.

On October 24, 1994, Ron Keller was finally arrested on the 1984 Keller indictment. Rick wanted to fight the charge; but the Kellers were already heavily in debt, and by then they had concluded the cause was hopeless. Ron opted instead to plead guilty to one count of conspiracy to commit wire fraud. The prosecutor said the matter could be settled without a trial: "The pressure is off." We wondered who had been applying the pressure when it was on. Ron was sentenced to five years: six months to serve, the rest on probation. I met him after his release, when I passed through Texas in the summer of 1995. He looked tired and he walked with a cane, due to an old ski injury that had been aggravated by sleeping on the floor of the Cameron County Jail. But like all the Keller boys, he had charm.

As for Alma and Durk, it wasn't until 1997 that we learned their fates. Only one death was confirmed by death certificate, but we heard that both of them had died.

For me and for my family, the Keller story remains a source of inspiration. When my husband was transferred from Honduras to Guatemala in 1994, our teenaged children had to adjust to their sixth new school, and sometimes they felt lost and depressed. When they did, I reminded them about Jimmy: how he had once felt such a loss that he was suicidal, yet he had managed to turn his life around. Facing death, he had learned how to live. He had made the remarkable discovery that helping other people could bring him more love and more satisfaction than anything had before.

The risk my children run when they admit to getting depressed is that they will have to listen to inspirational literature. Digging into my collection for an appropriate quote, I found this one from Stewart Edward White, writing in the thirties:

> *Supposing you offered yourself completely and eagerly, joyously spent yourself on something because you wanted to more than anything else in the whole wide world; and while doing it you suddenly found you were receiving something beyond anything you had ever experienced before, so that you didn't know whether you were giving or taking; that would be the beautiful state, the beautiful union, this wonderful thing we are trying to get hold of and are evolving toward.*[89]

# POSTSCRIPT

After the raid on Jimmy's clinic, Cancer Control Society tour guide Frank Cousineau reported that not much was happening in Tijuana anymore. Jimmy's kidnapping and conviction seemed to have blunted the natural cancer treatment craze. A wave of raids followed, including:

* The May 1992 raid of the Kent, Washington, clinic of Jonathan Wright, M.D., by six FBI agents backed by ten local policemen. Wearing flak jackets and with guns drawn, they broke down the door and stormed the clinic SWAT-team style. The stated offense was possession of an imported injectable mixture of B-complex vitamins.[90] Critics maintained the raid was in retaliation for Dr. Wright's successful suit against the FDA for withholding the amino acid tryptophan from the market.[91]

* The June 1992 arrest of Mihai Popescu, a Los Angeles distributor of Gerovital (GH-3). Eight FDA and customs agents entered his house with guns drawn, holding his wife (who was eight months pregnant) and his 83-year-old grandfather at gunpoint for ten hours. The distributor spent more than eight months in jail.[92]

* The November 1992 raid of a Reno clinic that, according to the Nevada Sentinel, resulted in the deaths of at least six patients due to disruption of care.[93]

* The May 1993 raid of Dr. Zerbo's Health Food Store in Livonia, Michigan. Armed U.S. marshals and FDA agents cleaned coenzyme Q-10, selenium, carnitine, and GH-3 off the shelves, and arrested the 78-year-old owner and his daughter. The owner, who has Parkinson's disease, pleaded guilty to "illegal drug trafficking" after being threatened with seven years in prison.

* The May 1993 raid of the San Diego office of Hospital Santa Monica in Tijuana. More than fifty federal agents, with guns drawn, seized $80,000 from the owner's safe and over $300,000 from the company's bank accounts, along with a tractor trailer of business records, patients' charts and computers. The owner was forced into bankruptcy.[94]

* The FDA's March 1995 raid of the Burzynski Cancer Center in Houston, after the CBS-TV Evening News ran a favorable news clip on the clinic the same month. Ironically, the National Cancer Institute had previously granted Dr. Burzynski permission

to conduct Phase II clinical trials on his remedy antineoplastons.[95] The FDA filed criminal charges against Dr. Burzynski that carried a potential prison sentence of 290 years. The charges did not involve bodily harm; in fact expert testimony established that the patients involved would have died without his therapy. His offense was that he had treated patients who were not Texas residents. Using his therapy inside state lines is legal, since the FDA has jurisdiction only over "interstate commerce." In 1997, represented by Rick Jaffe, Dr. Burzynski prevailed.[96]

   * In 1997, Dr. Hulda Clark's Tijuana cancer clinic was closed, after she lost a U.S. lawsuit brought by the manufacturer of a product she allegedly misrepresented in a book. Tijuana, it seems, is no longer "off limits" for the long arm of U.S. law. For certain purposes, NAFTA now gives the U.S. joint jurisdiction with Mexico within 200 miles of their common border.

   On October 24, 1994, the Dietary Supplement Health Act of 1994 was signed into law. It was designed to protect the natural supplements market, but compromises were inevitably made. Critics noted that the FDA can still ban supplements of nutrients and herbs via several loopholes, including controversial safety issues based on anonymous toxicity reports.[97] The loophole also still exists for natural remedies used in the treatment of cancer.

   Meanwhile, cancer incidence and deaths continue to rise. In 1995, American experts predicted that by the end of the century, cancer would have overtaken heart disease as the number one killer.[98] In 1997, the World Health Organization predicted that cancer rates in most countries would double in the next 25 years. Committee for Freedom of Choice founder Michael Culbert wryly observed:

> With between 1,500-1,900 Americans dying per day from cancer by 1993/1994, with more than 5,000 being diagnosed with the disease at the same time and with historic highs in both the fatalities from and incidence of cancer, the notion of a 'proven' cancer remedy provokes as much funereal humor in the unbiased observer as does the hoary Cancer Society concept of 'unproven' methods.[99]

   After Jimmy was convicted of fraudulently claiming that L-arginine can shrink tumors, several studies were published demonstrating the cytotoxic (cancer-killing) and immune-supporting effects of L-arginine in human cancer patients.[100] In

1994, the medical journal <u>Surgery</u> published "the first study showing that L-arginine enhances lymphocyte reactivity . . . and augments natural cytoxicity in patients with previously untreated cancer" -- that is, in patients whose immune systems hadn't already been destroyed with radiation and chemotherapy. The authors observed:

> Immune biologic modifiers in current use, in particular interferon and IL-2, are known to enhance natural cytotoxicity [but] they have achieved limited clinical success, often at considerable expense and with significant treatment-related toxicity. There is, therefore, a need to explore other modalities of treatment. Animal studies suggest that L-arginine may have a role as an enhancer of host defenses. Our studies confirmed this role in patients with breast cancer.[101]

In the cautious language of medical science, these researchers were proposing that L-arginine is cheaper, less toxic, and more effective even than interferon, the drug Silversmith had called "the most effective cancer treatment known on the face of the earth." A full decade after Jimmy was indicted for using arginine to treat human cancers, medical research was finally catching up to his empirical findings.

**\*\*\*\*\*\*\*\*\***

On January 15, 1998, Jimmy was arrested for a second time, for treating cancer patients in violation of his probation order. Whether he will serve the rest of his twenty-year sentence in prison remains to be adjudicated. However, one of his patients has suggested this more useful alternative: he could serve out his time treating volunteer cancer patients under the auspices of the Office of Alternative Medicine of the National Institutes of Health. Jimmy maintains that forty or fifty effective non-toxic cancer treatments are now available, and that some of them are really good. He used them all in Mexico. Their validity needs to be tested in a controlled clinical environment.

But that is an unlikely result. Jimmy is not an M.D. The fate of the protocol he developed through thirty years' work with terminal cancer patients is slated to be determined, once again, in a courtroom.

# APPENDIX A

## WAR ON CANCER --
## OR ON NATURAL CANCER REMEDIES?

*The disturbing facts of this case prompted further research into the
conventional and unconventional approaches to cancer and the relentless
war between them. My sources, which appeared to be well-researched,
are footnoted here along with a summary of their more unsettling data.*

### Conventional Treatment and the Vested Interests

*Surgery, radiation and chemotherapy, the conventional treatments
for cancer, seem to have had shady histories. The following summary is
drawn largely from* The Cancer Industry: Unravelling the Politics *by
Dr. Ralph W. Moss, former assistant director of public affairs at
Memorial Sloan-Kettering Cancer Center (MSKCC):[102]*

Surgery was developed as a cancer treatment in the nineteenth
century, mainly through the work of Dr. J. Marion Sims, founder
of MSKCC's predecessor, Memorial Hospital in New York. One
of the more notorious figures in recent medical history, Dr. Sims
developed his surgical techniques by experimenting on slave
women in the South. His surgeries, which were performed before
the development of anesthesia, were said to have been "little short
of murderous."

When plantation owners finally refused Dr. Sims access to
their slave women, he purchased his own. He bought a healthy
seventeen-year-old girl and proceeded to perform some thirty
operations on her in the space of a few months. Dr. Sims continued
these experiments for four years, then moved to New York. There,
with the support of a wealthy heiress, Mrs. Melissa Phelps Dodge,
he founded Women's Hospital. He was eventually fired, after the
trustees reported that "the lives of all the patients were being
threatened by . . . mysterious experiments." In the meantime,
however, he succeeded in secretly negotiating financial backing

from the Astors, a family whose wealth came from tenements and furs. With this backing, he opened the New York Cancer Hospital, later renamed Memorial Hospital.

Radiation joined Memorial Hospital's cancer armamentarium after another wealthy investor, James Douglas of the Phelps-Dodge Company, discovered large pitchblende deposits on his mining properties. He donated $100,000 to the hospital on condition that Memorial would limit itself to the treatment of cancer, and that it would routinely use radium in its treatments. By 1924, radium therapy was Memorial's largest single source of income.

Control of Memorial Hospital soon went to the Rockefellers, who had taken an interest in the world pharmaceutical business after Standard Oil of New Jersey (Esso), which they dominated, signed a cartel agreement with a huge German drug cartel called I.G. Farben. John D. Rockefeller I contributed heavily to the formation of both Memorial and the American Cancer Society. The Rockefellers' systematic contributions began a year after Standard Oil's vice president, Frank Howard, paid his first visit to the I.G. Farben laboratories, where cancer research was already in full swing.

Later, Howard became chairman of the research committee at Memorial. It was here in the early forties that chemotherapy research began in the United States, headed by Cornelius P. "Dusty" Rhoads, chief of research for the U.S. Chemical Warfare Service. Originating in World War I with the mustard gases used in the trenches, the drugs were tested under the mantle of military secrecy during World War II. The tests were continued openly on cancer patients after the war, resulting in the widely-used neoplastic agents in the mustard, or alkylating group.

## I.G. Farben and the International Drug Cartel

*I.G. Farben, the German drug cartel I heard mentioned on the Cancer Control Society tour in 1990, proved to be one of the arch-villains in the alarming scenarios of conspiratorialists. I read more about it in* World Without Cancer *by G. Edward Griffin, an author who sent a letter to the Brownsville district court in Jimmy's support. The following summary is drawn largely from Griffin's book:*

By the beginning of World War II, according to the U.S. Department of Justice, I.G. Farben had become the largest industrial corporation in Europe, the largest chemical company in the world, and part of the most gigantic and powerful cartel in all history.[103] A cartel is an international grouping of companies bound by anti-competitive agreements designed to defeat the free market forces of capitalism. The I.G. cartel stemmed from the international oil industry. Coal tar or crude oil is the basis of most chemicals, including those used in drugs and explosives. (Ironically, oil refineries are now said by some scientists to cause 30 to 40 percent of all cancers.[104])

I.G. Farben controlled the chemical and drug industries in Germany and produced the poison gas and nerve poisons used by German armies and in German concentration camps. In 1945, General Eisenhower reported that I.G. Farben had stock interests in 613 corporations, and "operated with varying degrees of power in more than 2,000 cartels."[105] I.G. established cartel agreements with hundreds of American companies. Most had no choice but to capitulate after the Rockefeller empire, represented by Standard Oil of New Jersey, had done so. The other giants could not hope to compete with the Rockefeller/I.G. combination. In 1929, I.G. and Standard Oil divided up the chemical and petroleum markets and agreed not to compete with each other. They also formed a jointly-owned company by which they would share in any future chemical developments and patents. A complicated web of cartel agreements with other industry giants followed. Today, the oil monopoly built by William Avery Rockefeller in the nineteenth century and reorganized in 1899 as Standard Oil of New Jersey controls over 322 companies and has cartel agreements with countless others, domestic and foreign.

Although best known for oil, the Rockefeller empire actually got its start in the medical business. William Avery Rockefeller was a wandering nineteenth century purveyor of medical nostroms composed mainly of crude oil and alcohol. He advertised himself as "Doctor William Avery Rockefeller, Celebrated Cancer Specialist," although he had no medical training. That made him another "quack" in the dictionary sense. His biographer wrote, "The man had practically no moral code. . . . He was what was later called a 'slicker,' and he was fond of doing what he could to be sure his sons would be 'slickers' like himself."[106]

The cartel was the stock in trade of William Avery's son, John D. Rockefeller I. John D.'s biographer wrote that he "was definitely convinced that the competitive system under which the world had operated was a mistake. . . . His plan [was to] bring all his rivals in with him. The strong ones he would bring in as partners. The others would come in as stockholders . . . . Those who would not come in would be crushed."[107]

The Rockefeller group's greatest influence was exerted through international finance and investment banking. Much of its power came from the leverage gained by controlling large blocks of stock held as part of the investment portfolios of the financial institutions it controlled. That put the Rockefeller group in control of a wide spectrum of industry. Its influence was particularly heavy in pharmaceuticals.

The directors of the American I.G. Chemical Company included Paul M. Warburg, brother of a director of the parent company in Germany and a chief architect of the Federal Reserve System. The Rockefeller and Andrew Carnegie groups were instrumental in inaugurating not only the Federal Reserve System but the federal income tax. To avoid paying these taxes themselves, they ingeniously arranged to transfer most of their visible assets to foundations, tax-exempt organizations whose stated objectives were philanthropic. Included among their charitable projects were drug research programs, from which the pharmaceutical industry benefitted enormously. Griffin called the scheme "a malicious conspiracy hiding behind the smiling mask of humanitarianism."[108]

Writing just after the Second World War, another commentator warned, "Farben is no mere industrial enterprise conducted by Germans for the extraction of profits at home and abroad. Rather, it is and must be recognized as a cabalistic organization which, through foreign subsidiaries and secret tie -ups, operates a far-flung and highly efficient espionage machine -- the ultimate purpose being world conquest . . . and a world superstate directed by Farben."[109]

Fifty years later, concerns like this are still being voiced. I.G. Farben was technically disbanded following the Nurenberg War Trials for its role in manufacturing the poisonous gas used in German concentration camps. But in fact it merely split into three new companies -- Bayer, Hoescht and BASF -- which remain pharmaceutical giants today. The UN/WHO's Codex Alimentarious (Nutrition Code) Commission is largely controlled by these three I.G. offshoots. The January 1998 <u>Townsend Letter for Doctors</u> reports that this organization is attempting to make radical changes in the rules governing dietary supplements worldwide. The German plan calls for prohibiting the sale of vitamins, minerals, herbs, etc. for therapeutic or preventative use, and the sale of any new dietary supplements unless they go through an expensive CODEX approval process first. The intent seems to be to limit manufacture of nutritional supplements to the pharmaceutical giants. Under the General Agreement on Tariffs and Trade (GATT), CODEX decisions are binding; the World Trade Organization has the power to cripple entire sectors of the economy of a nation that fails to comply with them. The single U.S. delegate to CODEX is an FDA bureaucrat who has voted against the proposal, but with little result. At the last meeting, the vote went 16 to 2 in favor of the German proposal.[110]

## The American Medical Association

*The AMA is a highly-respected professional organization that has undoubtedly done much that is good. But not all of its pursuits seem to have been benevolent ones. Ostensibly a union of doctors, it has been accused of being the mouthpiece of the medical/industrial/ pharmaceutical complex that underwrites its costs. I read . . .*

The AMA was not the first national medical society. The American Institute of Homeopathy preceded it by several years. The favorite treatment of "allopaths" (conventional doctors) was then blood-letting. Homeopaths, who practiced a natural, non-toxic therapy imported from Germany, were stealing patients at an alarming rate. When the homeopaths succeeded in persuading the New York State Legislature to withdraw the power to license from the county medical societies, the allopaths counterattacked by forming clubs dedicated to destroying homeopathy.[111] The AMA was the most active of these quackbusting clubs. It was so effective that where the country had 10,000 homeopaths and 20 homeopathic medical schools at the turn of the twentieth century, by the end of it these figures had dropped to less than 600 homeopaths and no exclusively homeopathic schools.[112]

Real power came to the AMA at the turn of the century, with the development of new methods of treatment that had the potential for reaping huge profits. Anesthesia and anesthetics made surgery a more feasible approach to eradicating disease. Doctors began recommending major operations that required the development of expensive and lucrative hospital systems. The discovery of medical uses for radium added radiation to the therapy regime, causing the price of that toxic mineral to rise tenfold. The thriving patent medicine business developed into the synthetic drug industry, overtaking traditional herbalism, which came to be regarded as primitive and crude. Patentable synthetic drugs provided an economic incentive that was lacking in the common weed business. In a single decade, advertisements for the new pharmaceuticals increased the revenues of the <u>American Medical Association Journal</u> by a factor of five. By promoting the new treatments, the AMA not only helped transform medicine into an industry but gained political power. Soon, it was in a position to change the licensing regulations to exclude other medical schools.

Carnegie, Morgan, and John D. Rockefeller invested heavily in the new medical developments. When the AMA's project to assess the status of American medical education seemed to be floundering, the president of the Carnegie Foundation offered to take it over. The result was the infamous "Flexner Report," published in 1910. The upshot was that half the medical schools in the country were closed down, either because they were substandard or because they refused to accept foundation funds and guidance. The other half were showered with funds, making them vulnerable to foundation control.[113]

A new accreditation program thus rigidly standardized medical education into an allopathic mold, paralleling the policies of more typical cartels. Product standardization frequently characterizes price-fixing conspiracies, which are hard to maintain unless products are homogeneous. According to a Duke University law review article:

> *[T]he AMA-dominated Liaison Committee on Medical Education . . . imposes on medical education a particular professional ideology, deeply rooted in a particular perception of the physician's role in society and antagonistic to education endeavors premised on different perceptions. . . . By limiting educational diversity, professional interests in medicine, as in other professional fields, successfully prevented the emergence of different traditions and of different types of professionals who might have served the consumer better.*[114]

Ironically, the two men primarily responsible for the AMA's stellar rise to power were "quacks" themselves in the dictionary sense: they pretended professionally or publicly to qualifications they did not possess, holding themselves out to be licensed medical doctors when they were not.

"Doc" George H. Simmons, who headed the AMA from 1899 to 1924, practiced a great deal of medicine but seems never to have attended medical school. He was forced to retire as AMA leader after he acquired a mistress, gave his wife heavy doses of narcotics, and attempted to have her framed on a charge of insanity. The highly publicized lawsuit that followed inspired a number of books and movies, the most famous being Gaslight with Charles Boyer and Ingrid Bergman.

"Doc" Simmons was succeeded by "Dr." Morris Fishbein, who has been credited with single-handedly burying more promising cancer cures than any other man in medical history.[115] Fishbein's downfall came when Harry Hoxsey, the principal target of his anti-quackery campaign, defeated him in court. Fishbein admitted in litigation that he had never graduated from medical school, and that he had never practiced medicine a day in his life.[116]

Neither of these notorious AMA leaders was elected by the doctors they represented. Both men derived their power by controlling the AMA's major source of revenue, the prestigious and influential American Medical Association Journal. The editor of the Journal had absolute control over all the publications of the AMA. Dissenters were unable to voice their opposition. One of the AMA's publications was the Index Medicus, which determined what literature was accessible to doctors. The AMA Journal, in turn, got its power from drug advertising. After Fishbein conceived the plan of granting the AMA "Seal of Acceptance" to drug companies that advertised in its pages, the Journal became the most profitable publication in the world.[117]

The conspiratorial and anti-competitive activities of the organization created by these two men were uncovered in a congressional investigation conducted under the direction of Senator Tobey in 1953. Benedict Fitzgerald, Department of Justice special counsel for the project, wrote:

> *The alleged machinations of [its officers] could involve the AMA and others in a conspiracy of alarming proportions . . . . [B]ehind and over all this is the weirdest conglomeration of corrupt motives, intrigues, selfishness, jealousy, obstruction and conspiracy I have ever seen. My investigation to date should convince this Committee that a conspiracy does exist to stop the free flow and*

use of drugs in interstate commerce which allegedly [have] solid
therapeutic value. *Public and private funds have been thrown
around like confetti at a country fair to close up and destroy
clinics, hospitals and science research laboratories which do
not conform to the viewpoint of medical associations. How
long will the American people take this?*[118]

Fitzgerald was precipitously fired and the hearings were closed
down, after Senator Tobey died suddenly and rather mysteriously
of a heart attack. But charges of the AMA's conspiratorial purposes
continued. In 1978, a federal court concluded:

> [T]he AMA has produced a formidable impediment to
> competition in the delivery of health care services to physicians
> in this country. That barrier has served to deprive consumers
> of the free flow of information about the availability of health
> care services, to deter the offering of innovative forms of health
> care and to stifle the rise of almost every type of health care
> delivery that could potentially pose a threat to the income of
> fee-for-services physicians in private practice. The costs to the
> public in terms of less expensive or even, perhaps, more
> improved forms of medical services is great.[119]

## The National Council Against Health Fraud (NCAHF)

*The NCAHF was the organization that had branded Jimmy the
most notorious quack in the country. We suspected it was also behind
the case against him. But what was behind the NCAHF? I read . . .*

The National Council Against Health Fraud was originally
formed in 1977 as the "Southern California Council Against
Health Fraud." It claimed to have no anti-competitive financial
interests. However, it inherited the files, goals and functions of
an earlier AMA campaign against quackery, after the latter was
forced underground by adverse publicity.

The AMA's earlier campaign was carried on through two
committees, one overt and one covert. Its overt Committee on
Quackery was formed in 1963. The anti-competitive mission of
this group was revealed in a later antitrust suit to be the elimination
of the rival profession of chiropractic.[120] The suit dragged on for
years and culminated only in 1987, when a U.S. District Court

found the AMA guilty of a conspiracy in violation of the antitrust laws.

The Coordinating Conference on Health Information (CCHI) was a shadow organization formed by the AMA in 1964 to work for similar anti-competitive ends behind the scenes. The CCHI included representatives from the American Cancer Society, the American Pharmaceutical Association, the Council of Better Business Bureaus, the Arthritis Foundation, the FDA, the FTC, and the U.S. Postal Service. According to its minutes, the CCHI was called a "conference" rather than a "committee" because government agencies are forbidden to participate in outside committees that are not matters of public record. The meetings of the CCHI were held in secret.[121] Opponents charged the CCHI with enlisting the police powers of the federal government to impose restraining orders, fines and prison sentences on independent health practitioners who competed with the drug industry. People were arrested for such practices as giving away booklets that advised the taking of vitamins. It was not alleged that the preparations caused injury or death, only that their manufacturers had not complied with statutory procedures for marketing. Meanwhile, drug manufacturers that could afford the high cost of FDA studies continued to sell drugs with potentially lethal side effects without government interference.

In 1975, the CCHI and the Committee on Quackery were disbanded in response to public demands for a Congressional investigation of their activities. The AMA's campaign then went underground, and an organization called the Lehigh Valley Committee Against Health Fraud was given access to its "quackery" files. The Lehigh group's incorporator wrote in the AMA News in 1975 that the group was backed and funded by professional medical societies, and that it worked "undercover" to achieve what those societies could not achieve openly.[122] The Lehigh group then linked up with the Southern California Council Against Health Fraud, based in Loma Linda, California. Later called the National Council Against Health Fraud, this organization soon became the principal source of data in the media against alternative health care modalities and products in the United States. When an alternative treatment is the subject of a television or radio talk show, a representative from the NCAHF usually appears for the opposition. The goals of the NCAHF and its predecessor AMA organizations are substantially identical to those set out in anti-quackery bills introduced in 1981 and 1982 by Representative Claude Pepper, who was well known for his loyalty to the medical/pharmaceutical complex.[123]

In 1983, the Pharmaceutical Advertising Council (PAC) initiated an agreement with the FDA to jointly finance a "Public Service Anti-Quackery Campaign." The NCAHF took over the AMA's former role as spokesgroup for this campaign, which involved most of the same governmental agencies and private organizations as the CCHI, its AMA-backed predecessor. The difference was that PAC replaced the AMA in funding the new campaign, and PAC and the NCAHF together replaced the AMA as its primary sources of data. The campaign was headed by the president of one of the world's largest medical advertising firms and was jointly financed by the FDA and the drug industry. The upshot was that the agency set up to police the drug industry wound up investigating and prosecuting targets designated by that industry -- i.e., its own competitors.

In 1985, the PAC/FDA campaign conducted a poll to determine what non-drug therapies the public considered most effective. These therapies then became the priority target list for the PAC/FDA anti-quackery campaign. In a free market, ineffective products disappear naturally due to lack of consumer demand. The FDA's policy, however, targeted products that <u>were</u> effective as determined by consumer demand. The FDA's new policy on "Health Fraud" provided, "Regulatory Actions should be considered for products of limited health significance when it appears there is a growing national or substantial regional market for them." Again, these were the products that represented a competitive threat to the drug industry.[124]

Fifteen years earlier, Dr. Miles Robinson, head of a congressional committee investigating allegations of a conspiracy to suppress alternative therapies, wrote:

> [T]he Food and Drug Administration (FDA) is largely controlled by the orthodox medical profession . . . and the industries which FDA was set up to regulate . . . . The slanted publicity arm of FDA endlessly portrays this agency as a white knight attacking food faddism and other alleged quackeries, while behind this facade of publicity FDA secretly dispenses its million dollar favors to industry, and often deprives the public of its health and of its right to know the truth about health.[125]

## The American Cancer Society

*The American Cancer Society (ACS) is another highly respected organization that is known for the selfless work of its volunteers. Yet its roots, too, seem to be murky ones. I read . . .*

The ACS was formed with financial backing from John D. Rockefeller I. It got its power from drug advertising. The ACS became a powerful force in the medical world after it was put under the control of two prominent drug advertisers, Albert Lasker and Elmer Bobst. Lasker was called "the father of modern advertising." He was also called "the father of women's lung cancer" after his successful national advertising campaign to persuade women to smoke in public. Bobst, who headed two pharmaceutical giants, was instrumental in helping Richard Nixon gain the presidency. Nixon, in turn, formally declared the War on Cancer. The War was conceived by Lasker's wife, New York socialite Mary Lasker, who persuaded Congress to fund the attack. The effect was to swell the coffers of the National Cancer Institute, which has interlocking directorships and advisory committees with the ACS. Mary and Albert Lasker also served as trustees of the Memorial Sloan-Kettering Cancer Center (MSKCC), the other major recipient of federal and ACS funding for cancer research. The committee recommending the War on Cancer to Congress was chaired by the leader of MSKCC and included board members of the ACS. One of these board members was also chairman of a pharmaceutical company that held patents on various anti-cancer drugs.

Lasker and Bobst built the ACS into the most powerful force in the cancer business. They seated representatives on its board of trustees from the biggest names in banking and industry. Most cancer research funded by the government and the ACS involves drugs for which private companies hold the patents. Since drug testing has grown prohibitively expensive, taxpayer financing means an enormous windfall to pharmaceutical companies in a position to obtain it. The most likely recipients are drug companies represented on the MSKCC and ACS boards.[126]

## The National Cancer Institute and the War on Cancer

*Like the AMA and the ACS, the NCI is a venerable organization that has done much that is commendable. But it, too, has its critics. I read . . .*

The NCI was created in 1937 to funnel taxpayer funding into cancer research. Prompted by heavy ACS lobbying, its federal budget has risen spectacularly since. While the NCI and the ACS vigorously discourage patients from pursuing unproven treatments outside the cancer establishment, they actively encourage enrollment in establishment-sponsored trials of the unproven. The drug companies represented at MSKCC and the NCI, where these clinical drug tests are carried out, stand to reap enormous profits from the tests. Taxpayer-financed studies can mean fortunes for the holders of viable cancer drug patents.

By the time the War on Cancer was officially declared in 1971, the NCI had already spent $500 million in government funds and had tested 170,000 toxic chemicals on nearly as many cancer patients. The vast majority of these chemicals proved useless, and many of the patients they were tested on underwent the drugs' terrible side effects without their full knowledge and consent. The argument advanced was that most of these patients were terminal anyway, and that they suffered in the cause of science. But later investigation showed that many of them would have had a good chance of survival without the drugs.[127]

Today, half of all cancer patients undergo cytotoxic chemotherapy, despite increasing questions about the drugs' effectiveness.[128] More than 100 billion dollars are poured annually into cancer research and treatment.[129] Yet the results of that massive investment have been disappointing. A 1991 issue of Science reported, "Overall death rates from many common cancers remain stubbornly unchanged -- or even higher -- than when the war began."[130] The outlook for most cancer patients has stayed the same since the fifties, while overall cancer incidence has increased since then by more than a third. Lung cancer in men has tripled. The incidence of breast cancer increased in two decades from one in twenty women to one in nine, while the death rate from that cancer hasn't changed in fifty years. Half of all breast cancer victims continue to die within ten years of being diagnosed, and twenty-five percent die within five years. For patients whose cancers of all types have metastasized to distant areas of the body, the survival rate is much worse.[131]

Then how is it that the NCI keeps reporting advances in the cancer cure rate? According to a report by the General Accounting Office, the NCI has manipulated data in order to "artificially inflate the amount of 'true' progress."[132] The reported gains in survival have evidently been a desperate attempt to make a desperate situation look good, in order to justify continued massive federal and private funding. As Nobel Prize winner James Watson cynically observed, "Today the press releases coming out of the National Cancer Institute have all the honesty of the Pentagon's." An editorial in the New England Journal of Medicine concluded, "The vast and ill-conceived undertaking that we created by the National Cancer Act of 1971 has inevitably spawned a monolithic bureaucracy with a heavily supported public-relations apparatus that is simply misleading the American public on a dreadfully serious subject."[133]

## *The Manipulation of Statistics: the NCI and Dr. Bross*

*The NCI's manipulation of statistics was addressed by NCI statistician Dr. Irwin Bross in the 33-page position paper he forwarded to the Keller defense team. He called the NCI's coverup "criminal fraud" and "genocide." But he said he hadn't meant to go that far . . .*

Dr. Bross had hoped for a quiet arbitration of charges he felt compelled to make against a top-level NCI official who was also a personal friend. Dr. Peter Greenwald, head of NCI Cancer Prevention, had claimed in the December 1989 Saturday Evening Post that "cancer deaths can be cut in half by the year 2000." Since cancer deaths had been inexorably increasing ever since the government's "War on Cancer" got underway in the early 1970s, this statement appeared to Dr. Bross to be scientifically outrageous. Other statisticians had been objecting to such claims for years, but their polite dialogue in medical journals had failed to influence public policy. Stronger action seemed necessary.

Dr. Bross requested NCI documents under the Freedom of Information Act (FOIA), intending to document a simple request for retraction of the NCI's claims in a popular magazine. But the information he got in response to his FOIA request revealed a fraud of such alarming proportions that the polite charge of "error" no longer seemed warranted. When the NCI brushed off Dr. Bross's private letter of intent, he was forced into open confrontation. In his position paper exposing the coverup, he stated, "my FOIA request for NCI documents connected with the claims of cancer reduction produced unexpected evidence that . . . revealed an NCI game plan that would lead to genocide" -- the deaths of great masses of Americans by public policies designed to protect private interests. Dr. Bross estimated that cancer deaths for which the government itself is responsible would total a million over the next decade.

He began his position paper by pointing out that cancer death rates have been steadily increasing over the past 15 years. From 1973-74 to 1985-86, they increased by 12.3 percent. In 1986, there were 100,000 more new cancers than in 1973-74. What caused this unprecedented increase? Additional human exposures to "mutagens" -- those chemical and radioactive agents that can produce biochemical lesions in human DNA. And what caused these new exposures? Radioactive fallout, leaking of toxic chemicals at dumpsites, environmental pollutants, and the very x-rays and mutagenic drugs used by the medical industry ostensibly to "cure." All of these exposures are from "mutagenic technologies" -- the businesses that control the economy and the government. In its twenty-year "War on Cancer," Dr. Bross observed, the NCI has taken virtually no action to prevent exposure to these mutagens. Worse, it has used fraudulent statistical methods to cover up the fact that they are hazards, and it has actively suppressed research proving that they are. This was often done by cutting off funding, a point for which Dr. Bross cited the Congressional Record. The NCI has also actively promoted "prevention" programs that actually increase the death rate from cancer. One example is its push for mass screening for breast cancer in women over forty (a point Dr. Bross would expand upon later).

The NIH Office for Scientific Integrity responded to Dr. Bross's letter of intent with the stock defense that Dr. Greenwald's statements were mere opinions. At most, they were "scientific error." Dr. Bross countered that in response to his FOIA request, he had received a monograph that was more than mere opinion. It was an official NCI document, Cancer Control Objectives for the Nation: 1985-2000 (P. Greenwald and E. Sondik, editors, NCI Monographs No. 2). And it was used for more than public relations. It was the basis for the NCI's "Final Report to the Senate

Appropriations Committee" in 1989, the report through which the agency got its funding. "When 'scientific errors'. . . are made in an NCI <u>budget</u> request," Dr. Bross maintained, "there is a reasonable presumption that they were <u>not</u> innocent errors. Instead, it seems likely that they were made by NCI in an attempt to deceive Congress about the performance of the NCI's prevention programs with the specific purpose of obtaining taxpayer dollars for these programs. . . . [T]here is solid documentary evidence that the fraudulent claims concerning reduction in cancer mortality have been used to obtain taxpayer dollars under false pretenses. Consequently, the scientific fraud here is also criminal fraud in the usual legal sense."

In support of his contentions about the hazards of breast cancer screening, Dr. Bross pointed to a large-scale Canadian study reported in the <u>London Times</u> on June 2, 1991. Titled "Breast Scans Boost Risk of Cancer Death," the article began, "Middle-aged women who have regular mammograms are more likely to die from breast cancer than women who are not screened, according to dramatic new research." The article discussed the Canadian National Breast Screening Study (NBSS), the largest study of its kind done anywhere in the world. The NBSS tracked 50,000 Canadian women aged 40 to 49 during the period 1980-88. Half were given mammograms every 12 to 18 months. The other half were given only a single physical exam. Alarmingly, at the end of the eight-year period, deaths among the group getting regular mammograms were significantly <u>higher</u> than in the group getting none. Worse, the mammograms themselves were not what was found to accelerate the death rate. Rather, <u>the failures seemed to be in the conventional cancer treatment that followed</u>.

The director of the study observed, "[O]ne potential problem was that surgery, the anaesthetic and radiotherapy involved in treating women with breast cancer were interfering with immunity." As a result, "the initial radiation and surgery to remove tiny breast lumps discovered by mammograms may make secondary cancers elsewhere grow faster. . . . You may find the cancers earlier (with mammography), but the women are still going to die. <u>Modern treatment does not work for these early cancers</u>."

Ironically, it was the <u>early</u> cancers that the cancer establishment had been saying modern treatment <u>does</u> work for. The late cancers -- the ones that have metastasized -- are the ones for which Dr. Bross testified in court that all treatments are essentially placebos. When the results of the NBSS were finally published in December of 1992, the increased risk of death from breast cancer for women undergoing mammography was reported to be a full 36 percent.[134]

Other data confirm Dr. Bross's contention that the government and the industries controlling it are themselves responsible for increasing the death rate from cancer. One disturbing article reported that more nuclear-weapons tests have been carried out in the United States than in any other area of the world. Besides its visible above-ground testing, the U.S. military has detonated 900 underground nuclear bombs within its borders. Of these, the Department of Energy has admitted that 100 underground explosions have "leaked." Underground testing is now estimated to be responsible for 15 to 50 percent of total radiation emissions. These emissions have been blamed for an epidemic of cancers, particularly among unsuspecting residents near the test sites who turned out regularly to watch. Concluded one doleful victim, "We have met the enemy, and he is us."[135]

# Appendix B

## Supporting Letters And Affidavits

The defense kept copies of more than 350 letters and affidavits sent to the U.S. District Court in Brownsville in support of Jimmy Keller and his clinic. The following excerpts are not complete. They are just some that struck me as I read through them.

### Excerpts from 1991 Letters to the Court

*"I have been a member of the Legislature for 20 years. My friendship with Jimmy began when we worked together to get legislative approval for the use of Laetrile treatment for cancer victims in the late 1970's. Jimmy himself has suffered terribly from cancer and had been diagnosed as incurable. When his life was saved thru the treatments he received, he committed his life to helping others who were suffering too. Jimmy is the kind of man who has always reached out to people that others have given up on. I do not believe he would ever do anything intentionally to hurt another human being."*

—*Rep. Louis (Woody) Jenkins,*
Louisiana House of Representatives, Baton Rouge, Louisiana

*"I have seen Jimmy pull . . . 'two weeks to a month to live' cases out of the jaws of death and give them back full and healthy lives . . . . Unknown to many is that he has also successfully treated two AIDS cases. . . . [H]e holds valuable pieces of the equation to both of these epidemics."*

—*Gary Beem,*
a computer consultant
from Burbank, California

*"Most of [the patients] were terminal when they arrived, couldn't eat or sleep, in pain, often couldn't walk, being carried in by friends. Some had fast recoveries, showing improvement within days or almost instantly. I saw people who had not been able to eat for months become*

able to hold food and even regain their appetite. Their color improved, they could walk again and had hope. Others showed slow but sure progress. We all watched as obvious tumors shrank before our eyes each day."

—*Beatrice B. Burns,*
Vista, California

"My wife had a 20 year history of excruciating headaches. She had been to numerous doctors and specialists without any lasting relief. When she was treated by Mr. Keller she got the first lasting relief ever -- without having to take drugs. He charged us only a minimal amount, far less than the treatments even cost him, with an understanding that we would pay when we could. I saw many others who were helped by Mr Keller when no help or hope was supposed to be possible. I saw a man dedicated to helping others and saving lives working with little sleep under oppressive conditions doing his best to help. I don't know what he was found guilty of, but I do know that Jimmy Keller is one of the most unselfish helpers of man it has been my honor to have met. Probably his biggest crime was in not looking out for his own well-being because he was so concerned for others."

—*Joseph P. Hochman,*
Studio City, California

"While down there I witnessed many people improving with their diseases, and in the sadder situations where [they] had failed with medical procedures to improve and were close to death, he made their last days more comfortable and less painful. . . . Mr. Keller always showed nothing but willingness to do what was needed to help including an 18-20 hr per day schedule when needed."

—*Annette Hochman,*
Studio City, California

"I live in Florida and travel[ed] to see him 5 times in the last 5 years. Despite the fact that I could not afford as many treatments that was needed, he never turned me away and treated me lovingly and made me feel alive once more. Isn't it unfair for people who have never encountered a near death experience to take away our choice of treatment?"

—*Miriam Aaronberg,*
Tamarac, Florida

"Prior to seeing Mr. Keller, I did a fair amount of research into the methods he used for treatment. I found that they were widely used with excellent results in Scandinavia, Europe, Japan and South America. They involved natural substances with little or no side effects, and improved the body's immune system to the point where it could combat injuries and diseases without the use of drugs. It seems his biggest crime was in becoming famous, and in using phones to conduct his business. I personally met over a hundred people at his clinic whose lives he had saved. His methods rehabilitated my injury in six weeks . . . . I know that many patients were given treatments at no cost."

—*Robert K. Baird,*
Vice President,
Investments,
Paine Webber,
San Diego, California

". . . I lost a 5 year old daughter in 1968, and my mother at age 59 in 1975 to cancer, and both endured long suffering from the ravages of surgery, radiation, and chemotherapy. Conversely, I have a 19 year old daughter who at age 14 was diagnosed with 40% arterial blockage; an 84 year old father who suffered a stroke and 7 years ago was repeatedly recommended for arterial surgery; and a wife who was diagnosed with breast and lymphatic cancer 6 years ago; all of whom are very alive and very well and all of whom received treatment from Jimmy Keller exclusively since their diagnosis.

". . . It is unconscionable to acknowledge that surgery, radiation, and chemotherapy do not cure cancer and then to legally bind sufferers to no alternative selections. . . . [We] continue to pour billions into dead end and economic driven research, chasing mythical, technological, one pill cures while persecuting those who . . . with true compassion are genuinely healing."

—*Ernest R. Lindo,*
Marina del Rey, California

". . . [K]nowing some people with serious conditions . . . I mentioned Jimmy to them and they went to see him . . . . The first man had one leg and was about to lose the other one, due to an apparent incorrectible circulation problem. He was facing amputation of his second leg, when he visited Jimmy Keller. That must have been close to 10 years ago, and he still has his leg.

"The other person was a man with cancer who had been sent home to die. His pain was so great that morphine would no longer stop it. After seeing Keller for a few weeks, I got a phone call from his wife. She spoke through tears of joy, as she told me that her husband's color was back, he'd gained 14 pounds and [was] down to only 2 aspirin a day for pain, instead of morphine.

"Granted, healing cancer and saving legs without being a doctor is illegal -- but is it really wrong? . . . Regardless what the charges are, and regardless what [illegible] statements you may have heard from pro-AMA and FDA sources, healing cancer, and doing it cheaply by comparison, is his crime."

—*Bob Norma,*
Terry, Mississippi[136]

"I say in all truth that I owe my life to him. . . . My treatment at St. Jude's caused my tumor to disappear completely, and to this day, I am free of any cancer in my body, as witness a copy of my most recent PSA . . . . Jimmy is a caring, loving and spiritual man who has been completely selfless in his dedication to all of us who were fortunate enough to come under his care."

—*John B. Macomber,*
Santa Ana, California

"I have known the above named defendant for over 20 years. I have known Jimmy's mother, daddy, and most of his family for about the same time. He comes from a very devout family. Jimmy has always been sincere in helping others, even when he knew they did not have the money to pay him."

—*Charles V. Pearce,*
Baton Rouge, Louisiana

". . . I met Jimmy Keller as a cancer patient through my mother and father, Charles and Dot Pearce, whom he had effectively lead to health . . . . I did not take conventional medical treatment and I am fine after many years. . . . I personally know that when something good happens to you, you have an evangelistic zeal to share it with others . . . and I know he was not doing what he was for the money involved because he has helped many with no compensation whatsoever."

—*Darlene Runfalo*

"I was a patient of Jimmy's in Mexico when the F.B.I. closed in on him in Rosarito here a few years ago. I wasn't able to finish my treatments because of his having to go into hiding. . . . As a widow I couldn't afford what others were paying and he helped me by letting me help the others at the Clinic. . . . I think it is terrible that our freedoms are being taken from us."

—*Ruth Christiansen,*
Pocatello, Idaho

". . . [I]t was on that morning on March 18th that men came and forcibly took him away. . . . I saw that one had a gun and threatened to use it. . . . [M]any . . . with whom I keep in touch desperately miss and need the treatment Jimmy Keller has to offer. I saw a 29 year old woman with lung cancer delighted after 3 weeks treatment that her signs of cancer were gone. . . . Jimmy knew that my present situation prevented me from having the money to pay him and accepted my promise to pay later. We just received our itemized statements on Saturdays. No one to my knowledge was required or even requested to pay 'up front.' . . . Most people who go to him are already terminal, so why is he blamed because some die? It is remarkable that so many live. What happens to doctors who administer highly toxic drugs and questionable treatments which make a patient miserable during his remaining time? . . . He is a God fearing, honest, gifted, sympathetic, generous man who deeply loves and cares about people in need. He himself has been there, knows what it is like and wants to be able to offer hope and life to others. To how many members of the jury could that previous sentence apply?"

—*Mrs. Patricia Davis,*
Santa Ana, California

" . . . He carried the heavy responsibility of trying to change [his patients'] lives of depression to an attitude of believing life was worth living. A heavy burden of responsibility which he willingly assumed. I don't believe money could motivate any man to take on such a voluntary assignment. I saw and heard patients talking and encouraging other patients on how Jimmy's therapy had helped them and gave them great moral and physical support."

—*Max Barlow,*
author and doctor of botanical medicine

"I had been diagnosed two different times by the medical doctors, after chemo and radiation, as having, probably, three months to live. . . . I am known as a medical miracle in this area . . . . I know that I am not a medical miracle but a Jimmie Keller miracle."

—*Arlene Torgesen,*
Soda Springs, Idaho


". . . Your decision regarding Jimmy Keller is more far reaching than its effect on his personal welfare. Alternative physicians, health practitioners and those of the public that are knowledgeable about what has been taking place in America are praying that you and others in your position will see the full scope of the problem. Freeing Jimmy Keller will provide a much needed stimulus at this important time in American medicine."

—*George E. Meinig,*
dentist, author, columnist
from Ojai, California


"I had cancer of the lymph glands. . . . Jimmy helped me out of my darkest hour. That was a year and a half ago. Jimmy has been a friend to many others in their darkest hour. I have seen him work long hours and help many. He would treat patients even if they could not afford it, myself included. Jimmy let me pay what I could afford. I never saw him turn anyone away who asked for help, regardless of their financial condition."

—*Gloria Tinney,*
Santa Monica, California


"I met Jimmy Keller in February of 1990 after I had been diagnosed as having Invasive Cervical Squamous Cell Carcinoma. The surgery and possible radiation that had been recommended to me by my doctor seemed a bit drastic to me, so I sought an alternative form of treatment which would heal the causes, not just remove the symptoms. I had not been able to work because of the cancer, did not have any medical insurance, and live alone. . . . Jimmy took me as a patient anyway. . . . I truly believe that I would not be alive today if it were not for Jimmy Keller and the treatment which he so lovingly gave to me."

—*Rev. Karen Paris,*
North Hollywood, California

"I had been diagnosed with testicular cancer. Mr. Keller accepted me at his clinic and when I had financial difficulty and could not pay him, he treated me for free for several months. . . . Mr. Keller has treated many people for free. . . . Jimmy Keller provided rational advice for me at a time when I was under considerable emotional upset and unsure of what I should do about my own illness. I don't believe that these are the characteristics or operating modes of a quack. . . . I am presently in superb health."

—*Brian McCaffrey,*
Astoria, New York

"My family and I have had my Grandmother two years longer than the doctors said. My family and I pray to have Jimmy Keller released, so he can continue to help others live longer, as well as my Grandmother. I thank the Lord for Jimmy Keller because I still have my Grandmother. It breaks my heart to see Jimmy Keller in jail for helping people live longer."

—*Alyssa Quijano Bostrom,*
granddaughter of Olga Quijano

"My wife and myself had been going to Dr. Elizabeth Huntly in La Crescenta on a nutrition program. Dr. Huntly who has her PhD. in nutrition happened to comment that on four (4) occasions she had sent patients with cancer to Jim Keller . . . . She said all four were cured. . . . I spoke with a number of patients . . . . Some had come in with large and/or painful cancers and spoke of how their cancer had shrunk or disappeared altogether. The previously sick had been cured by Jim Keller and would annually make the trek to St. Jude's for maintenance therapy. . . . He made you feel that the two of you were going to attack this thing together. There were no promises but there was no negativity either. At the end he would give the patient a hug and say 'God Bless You.' . . . What this guy has accomplished is really exciting and I hope the start of a new approach to cancer treatment -- one that involves love and the willingness to utilize drugs which have been found effective in other parts of the world in actually curing patients without having to use surgery, chemotherapy or radiation -- cut, poison, or burn."

—*Dan W. Foster,*
Port Hueneme, California

"Many times the patient waited too long, usually out of the panic of the diagnosis, to come to Jimmy. Other doctors gave up on these patients, but not Jimmy. These people that are alive today are literally 'living testimonies' to his gift of healing . . . . Jimmy Keller's sole concern was not power, fame, or fortune, but the health and welfare of every individual that walked, or was carried, into his clinic."

—*Clete Keith,*
an actor and writer from
Studio City, California

"I have found in my dealings with Mr. Keller that his sole purpose in life is to help others. He has done this without regard for the other person's ability to pay. . . . From my observation he spent 12-16 hours a day working at helping people in need, and regularly got little sleep -- much less than the normal eight hours a night. . . . From my viewpoint, Mr. Keller is a very dedicated healer and his knowledge of nutrition and vitamins is a very valuable asset to society. It would be a great shame to lose or waste this knowledge by sentencing Mr. Keller to a prison term."

—*Arthur Krowitz,*
a computer systems analyst
from Los Angeles

"He has helped many, many people -- among them myself, who my California doctor said I only had three months to live. That was nearly seven years ago. I went to Jimmy Keller in Tijuana and received his treatments. I am alive and well today because of him."

—*Ms. Vivian Miltimore,*
Lakewood, California

"His treatments work. I wish he could practice in America, so that I could see him more often."

—*Astrid Orrell,*
Rio Rancho, New Mexico

"I never heard Jimmy promise any cure nor did he promise any specific results from his treatment. . . . I have also seen him turn away several potential clients by stating he knew he could NOT help their particular condition. This is not the attitude of a so-called 'bilker' or

'schemer' to defraud individuals of fortunes or millions of dollars. . . .
[T]he law without a heart, without understanding and consideration of
true intent leaves us all in a sad state of flux not knowing where truth
and integrity abide. . . . This is a man who thought he was going to die
22 years ago, found life through alternative treatment and dedicated
his life to helping others. You will never know as I do the extra hours
and weekends he gave up for darn little money to help others."

—*Paul M. Hamilton, D.C.,*
Santa Monica, California

"I told him I did not have the funds to pay for his services. He told
me not to worry. By the end of six days I felt like a new person. My
strength, vitality and the will to live had returned. I can honestly say I
don't think I would be in good physical health today if it were not for
Jimmy Keller's help."

—*Stella Como*

"I talked with the accountant and told him I'd like to stay more
than the three days which I had planned, but since I was on Social
Security, and didn't have much money, I wouldn't be able to. The
accountant said to me, 'Don't worry about the money. As long as you
are here, stay and if you can, at a later date, you can send some money.'
So I stayed 2-1/2 weeks, and received health benefits. While I was
there I met other people who were not paying anything."

—*Marjorie Raucher, R.N.,*
Santa Monica, California

"[I]t was never necessary for him to call anyone to get them to go to
his clinic, he had all the people he could treat without calling anyone to
come to the clinic."

—*Annie Laura Wheeler Williams,*
Bush, Louisiana

"I have observed him on many occasions . . . help those without
Health Coverage, without money, or Underwriters protection of any
kind. No one was turned away . . . . This man should be honored
rather than trampled. Please help to restore the faith in what we teach
as our Criminal Justice system by aiding Mr. Keller to be FREE."

—*Mrs. Thelma Peoples,*
former California educational administrator

*"I accepted treatment at Jimmy's clinic at a time when I was unable to pay him. He knew this and he treated me anyway at great cost to him. I felt better afterwards than I ever felt in my life and am doing very well today."*

—*Jane Millan,*
Walnut Creek, California

*"Jimmy surely seemed to be quite candid and conservative, so I was surprised and disappointed that he had been found guilty of fraud. I feel sure that he could produce many more favorable witnesses than the opposition; but I understand many of his were not called to testify even though they made the long and expensive trip there for that purpose. . . .*

*"[Since] Jimmy had as many patients as he could possibly handle, so did not need to resort to subterfuge, I would imagine that he must have been a victim of a very few disgruntled and vindictive patients because Jimmy's treatments did not help them and they disregarded his initial statement to them.*

*". . . [W]e personally saw huge tumors on necks and bodies greatly reduced or disappear . . . and many previously forlorn people developed new hope and vigor as the treatments began having effect. . . . I am considerably saddened and disconcerted over Mr. Keller's recent arrest . . . . He was given no time to handle his affairs in Mexico, leaving many ill people in his clinic unattended."*

—*Alfred Lippman,*
Metairie, Louisiana
(formerly General Director of Research
at Reynolds Metal Company)

*"His sole purpose in life, despite incredible and crippling opposition, seems to be to help others. Even when threats were made on his life, . . . even after being beaten with a lead pipe, Jimmy kept getting up in the morning and serving others' needs. He couldn't let his patients down. I have been a patient of Jimmy's and he has . . . greatly helped me. I have referred dozens of people to him and ALL have benefitted, one for one."*

—*Carol R. Austin,*
Los Angeles, California

"*I know that the law takes into account the <u>intent</u> behind any act. Surely, any one who knows Jimmy Keller or who has heard his story, or had the benefit of his help, as I have, would know his intent was always to help and not hurt.*"

—*Sara Sherman, Ph.D.,*
Malibu, California

"*Jimmy was not only instrumental in saving my life, he taught me how to live. He helped me psychologically, spiritually and was the person who told me I could do anything I wanted to.*"

—*Sally Greer,*
Orange County, California

"*[I am a] builder and developer, with 40 years experience building. We have built numerous hospitals, both general and convalescent, with many churches, shopping centers, custom homes, etc. My wife Dorothy has spent 30 years in the medical field . . . . We have seen literal miracles happen at Jimmie Keller's Clinic! . . . My best friend, Dwight, an associate builder for 40 years, was sent home to die, from Loma Linda U. Medical Center. . . . At his request, we took this man to the Mexican Clinic, and stayed 3 weeks with him and his wife. We saw him able to [get] up out of his deathbed and walk. He became able to laugh and talk with us again, and enjoy life. What a change!*

"*Another dear friend, from Sonora, California, Betty, had been given 3 months to live; she had three brain tumors, and a huge tumor covering her liver. We took Betty and her husband in our motor home . . . . Prior to going there, she could not use her left hand, or control her left foot. . . . [A]fter her treatments in Mexico she was able to use left arm and leg, could play the piano, and walk. That was 3 years ago.*

"*A year ago we took an 82-year old friend, Adolph, with bladder cancer. His color was grey, and he walked with a cane. Now his color is normal, he doesn't know where his cane is, and he is out driving his tractor. . . .*

"*We know of cases, who couldn't afford to pay for their treatments in Mexico, who were treated <u>Free</u>! How many doctors and clinics here would do that?? Not many. We earnestly pray to God in Heaven, that you will deal kindly with this fine man, who <u>we</u> feel really deserves the NOBEL PEACE PRIZE for his Humanitarian efforts to help his fellow man.*"

—*Robert A. And Dorothy J. Schaefer,*
Yucaipa, California

"On two occasions I personally talked with family members who had brought their loved ones to the clinic for evaluation. They were sorely disappointed when Jimmy told them he felt he he could not help them. When they suggested trying, he said they would be wasting their money.

"Shortly after my arrival at Jimmy's clinic, I informed him I was living on disability income and could only afford to pay a fixed sum each week, an amount significantly below his usual charge. He accepted this immediately and without questioning. In the following weeks he added many expensive medications to my treatment program in an attempt to help me, knowing that he would not be reimbursed for them. I have talked with several other patients who had comparable experiences."

—*Bernadine Prince, M.D.,*
Jacksonville, Florida


"I believe the most important inalienable freedom we have is FREEDOM OF CHOICE. Whether Jimmy Keller is guilty or innocent of the charges against him seems less important to me than the effect his punishment will have not against Jimmy but against Freedom of Choice, and against this whole country once Jimmy's story is brought to nationwide and worldwide attention . . . . His story is bound to provoke heated debate in the near future."

—*Martin Zweiback,*
a screenwriter from
Beverly Hills, California

## Excerpts from 1984-1985 Letters

". . . We decided to go to Matamoros, Mexico for treatment in July 1983. When we talked to Maxine Louder about the treatment she told us there were no guarantees and she couldn't promise we would get well . . . . My condition was diagnosed as terminal with no hope of a cure . . . . I went back to the doctor who found the cancer originally for a physical examination. He could find no tumor in my lung and felt that I had been cured. He took several x-rays." [The medical records for this examination were attached. They showed "history of tumor, no evidence for recurrence at present time."]

—*Alan Freeland,*
Salt Lake County, Utah

"We saw a great many things happen when we were at the clinic. A young man came in who had a brain tumor. His leg was dragging and he could not raise his arm. In three days he could put his arm over his head and by the time he went home he was running. We saw an exposed tumor actually drip away. We saw pain leave after the first shot, and all this without any signs of any side effects. . . . We believe totally in Tumorex, and if any of our children should develop cancer we would take them to the clinic. If it should be closed, we would go wherever necessary to find it. We feel strongly that we should be able to choose what treatment we wish to be given."

—*Dawn Freeland,*
Salt Lake County, Utah

"I was treated at Jimmie Keller's clinic for breast cancer the latter part of last year. The cancer was eliminated and I had no ill effects from the treatment. I found him to be a very kind and gentle person who only thought of helping other people. He succeeded in doing this for a number of people while I was there. Everyone of those people only had good things to say about Jimmy Keller and his clinic."

—*Dorothy Ard,*
Port Arthur, Texas

"[My mother] had received radiation every day for 33 times (her neck looked like raw meat). After going through this painful ordeal, which by the way inhibited her ability to swallow because of the continuous sore throat and destruction of the salivary glands, she was asked to receive chemotherapy indefinitely.

"Being a nurse myself, I knew what they were offering: only doom. I begged her not to continue during the fifteen weeks she went. I could see her dying each time I'd come for a visit with the rapid weight loss. Five specialists offered her expensive medical bills. After hearing about Jimmy Keller, she asked my dad if he would drive her down to Mexico. The decision was hers alone . . . . She told me after her first treatment she became very hungry, which was remarkable, since she [had lost] her appetite for over a year. She returned home after several herbal treatments and is doing remarkable.

"Our whole family thanks God and Jimmy Keller . . . . I believe Jimmy has devoted his life for the sole purpose of helping others recover from the deadly disease called cancer. He never claimed to be a healer,

but uses herbs which God put on this earth to use and not poisonous
chemicals."

—*Karen Zak*

"I have been diagnosed as having lung cancer and told that nothing
could be done. Jimmy Keller has treated me with Tumorex and really
did help me. As far as I am concerned, Jimmy is a caring and thoughtful
individual and has sincerely helped me in my fight against cancer."

—*Edith Moon*

"[W]e were not promised a cure by Jimmy Keller or any of his
staff. . . . Several days into the treatment, Jimmy Keller offered to
return our money because he felt my son was not benefiting from the
treatment. We chose to stay and Jimmy Keller and his associates
expended considerably more time and effort on my son than would
have been expected."

—*Donna Birdseye,*
Santa Clara, California

"I have seen and know a number of people who have been treated
by Mr. Keller and have benefited greatly, especially in gaining hope
for living, which the medical doctors could not give them. It is ridiculous
to know that he is being accused of fraud, criminal intent and malicious
conduct. It is a blotch on the image of a free country that dying and
suffering people have no freedom to choose alternative methods of
treatment or therapy. A country founded on godly principles and human
rights is freedom deficient when a union-like medical establishment
and government oppress and persecute those who pioneer and promote
new ideas and modalities not approved by the orthodox establishments."

—*Robert S. Overstreet,*
Indialantic, Florida

# APPENDIX C

## FOR MORE INFORMATION

Information on currently available non-traditional treatments may be obtained from the Cancer Control Society at 2043 North Berendo, Los Angeles, CA 90027; telephone 213-663-7801.

For a comprehensive guide to alternative cancer therapies, see the Alternative Medicine Definitive Guide to Cancer (Tiburon, California: Future Medicine Publishing, Inc., 1997), by W. John Diamond, M.D., and W. Lee Cowden, M.D., in collaboration with Burton Goldberg and a long list of M.D. contributors. Other excellent guides are Dr. Ralph W. Moss's Cancer Therapy: The Independent Consumer's Guide (New York: Equinox Press, 1992); and Richard Walters' Options: The Alternative Cancer Therapy Book (New York: Avery Publishing Group, 1993).

For an international directory of alternative cancer therapy centers, see John M. Fink's Third Opinion (Garden City Park, New York: Avery Publishing Group Inc., 1988).

To keep abreast of developments in the alternative health care field, see the Townsend Letter for Doctors, 911 Tyler Street, Port Townsend, WA 98368-6541. Other excellent journals are Dr. Julian Whitaker's Health & Healing 7811 Montrose Road, Potomac, MD 20854; Dr. David Williams' Alternatives, P.O. Box 829, Ingram, TX 78025; and the journal of the Life Extension Foundation, P.O. Box 229120, Hollywood, FL 33022. For a listing on the Internet of many other journals, along with studies, political updates, and an electronic database of over 10,000 holistic health care providers, see the Alternative Medicine Connection, ARxC Web Site: http://arxc.com.

I am not a doctor and cannot give medical advice, but if you have information on this subject that you would like to share, correspondence may be addressed to P.O. Box 504, St. Helena, CA 94574.

# NOTES

1. K. Ausubel, Hoxsey: Quack Who Cures Cancer? (film) (Santa Fe, New Mexico: One West Media, 1987).

2. A. Lang, "Cancer patients organized against FDA violations," Townsend Letter for Doctors (May 1988), pages 178-80.

3. J. Wallach, M. Lan, Let's Play Doctor! (Rosarito Beach, Baja-California, Mexico: Wholistic Publications, 1989), at pages 76-78, 109-13.

4. A. Barbul, "Arginine: Biochemistry, physiology, and therapeutic implications," Journal of Parenteral and Enteral Nutrition 10(2): 227-38 (1986).

5. Y. Cho-Chung, et al., "Arrest of mammary tumor growth in vivo by L-arginine," Biochemical and Biophysical Research Communications 95(3):1306-13 (1980).

6. J. H. Weisburger, et al., "Prevention by arginine glutamate of the carcinogenicity of acetamide in rats," Toxicology and Applied Pharmacology, vol. 14 (1969).

7. H. Beard, "The effect of parenteral injection of synthetic amino acids upon the appearance, growth and disappearance of the Emge sarcoma in rats," Archives of Biochemistry 1:177-86 (1943).

8. R. Houston, "Sickle cell anemia and the metabolites of vitamin B17," reprinted in G. E. Griffin, World Without Cancer: The Story of Vitamin B17 (Westlake Village, California: American Media, 1974), pages V-XXVI.

9. S. Benton, "Patients swear by treatments," Baton Rouge Morning Advocate (February 4, 1981), pages 1 ff.

10. K. Ausubel, op. cit.; E. Mullins, Murder by Injection (Staunton, Virginia: National Council for Medical Research, 1988). The Hoxsey formula has now been published. See M. Kulawiec, "Hoxsey formula elaborated," The Townsend Letter for Doctors 148:86 (November 1995).

11. U.S. v. Hoxsey Cancer Clinic, 94 F. Supp. 464 (N.D. Tex. 1950).

12. U.S. v. Hoxsey Cancer Clinic, 198 F.2d 273 (5th Cir. 1952).

13. See, e.g., the case of In re George A. Guess, 393 S.E.2d 833 (1990), in which Charles Guess, M.D., a North Carolina family physician, lost his medical license for using homeopathic remedies in his practice. The remedies were not only legal but were available without a prescription; but since no other M.D. was using them in North Carolina, Dr. Guess

was found guilty of not conforming to "prevailing medical practice" as required by statute.

14. This broad definition of a "drug" is set forth in 21 United States Code Secs. 321(g)(1), 331.

15. B. Inglis, R. West, The Alternative Health Care Guide (New York: Alfred A. Knopf, 1983), pages 209, 259.

16. Personal conversation with Mr. Crane in 1990. See also B. Lynes, The Cancer Cure That Worked! (Queensville, Ontario: Marcus Books, 1987). R. Atkins, M.D., Dr. Atkins' Health Revolution (Boston: Houghton Mifflin Co., 1988).

17. R. Atkins, M.D., Dr. Atkins' Health Revolution (Boston, Houghton Mifflin Co., 1988).

18. E. Hodgson, "Restrictions on unorthodox health treatment in California: A legal and economic analysis," UCLA Law Review 24(3):647-96 (February 1977).

19. U.S. v. Rutherford, 442 U.S. 544, 99 S. Ct. 2470 (1979).

20. R. Moss, Cancer Therapy (New York: Equinox Press, 1992), pages 267-68.

21. "The Krebiozen affair," New England Journal of Medicine 269(10):531-32 (1963). See also R. Houston, "Repression & reform in the evaluation of alternative cancer therapies, Part II," Townsend Letter for Doctors 59:222 (June 1988).

22. See R. Houston, "Misinformation from OTA," Townsend Letter for Doctors (August/September 1990), page 600; J. Weese, et al., "Do operations facilitate tumor growth?", Surgery 100(2):273-77 (1986) (surgery and anesthesia enhance the implanting of tumors and facilitate metastasis); J. Stjernsward, "Decreased survival related to irradiation postoperatively in early operable breast cancer," Lancet (November 30, 1974), pages 1285-86; R. Moss, The Cancer Industry: Unravelling the Politics (New York: Paragon House 1989), pages 59-72.

23. I. Bross, "To the editor," New England Journal of Medicine 307(2):118-20 (1982).

24. C. L. McCormick, "Respected M.D. targeted by 'Medical Gestapo,'" Freedom (June 1986), pages 16-20.

25. B. Halstead, M.D., "William Jarvis' conspiratorial 'innocence' & related matters," Townsend Letter for Doctors 47:116 (May 1987). See also "Dr. Halstead, free on appeal, hits 'libel & slander,'" Townsend Letter for Doctors 112:936 (November 1992).

26. See N. Clarke, et al., "Treatment of occlusive vascular disease with disodium ethylene diamine tetra-acetic acid (EDTA)," American Journal of Medical Science 239:732 (1960); N. Clarke, et al., "Treatment of angina

pectoris with disodium ethylene diamine tetra-acetic acid," ibid. 232:645 (1956); C. Lamar, "Chelation therapy of occlusive arteriosclerosis in diabetic patients," Angiology 15:379 (1964).

27. See W. Blumer, et al., "Ninety percent reduction in cancer mortality after chelation therapy with EDTA," Journal of Advancement in Medicine 2:183-188 (1989).

28. M. Walker, "DMSO," Townsend Letter for Doctors (Aug./Sept. 1993), pages 830-34; M. Walker, D. Sessions, Coping with Cancer (Devin-Adair Publishers, 1985). On the ruby laser, see R. Moss, Cancer Therapy, op. cit., page 388; and R. Gerber, Vibrational Medicine (Santa Fe, New Mexico: Bear & Co., 1988), page 339.

29. M. Walker, "DMSO," op. cit. Dr. Walker wrote that after seeing films and interviewing patients, he was convinced that hematoxylon in combination with DMSO, administered intravenously, was indeed curing Dr. Tucker's patients of malignancies.

30. See M. Natenberg, The Cancer Blackout (Los Angeles: Cancer Book House, 1974), pages 73-86; G. Borell, The Peroxide Story (Delano, Minnesota: ECHO, 1988), page 74.

31. See M. Browne, "Controversial report in Nature supports homeopathy," Townsend Letter for Doctors (August/September 1988), page 378; D. Ullman, "Recent homeopathic research startles scientists," ibid., page 335.

32. See G. Bodey, "Infections in cancer patients," Cancer Treatment Review 2:89-128 (1975); R. Moss, The Cancer Industry, op. cit., pages 73-74.

33. Similar possibilities are being explored by American medical researchers. See R. Coxeter, "Will fetal cells bring new life to old hearts?", Business Week (April 11, 1994), page 115; "Something new in mind" [fetal cells for Parkinson's disease], The Economist (March 22, 1997), page 99.

34. The PLM, the Central American equivalent of the Physician's Desk Reference, describes isoprinosine as an anti-viral and immune system stimulant particularly recommended for herpes and viral influenza. See PLM: Diccionario de Especialidades Farmaceuticas (Panama: Panamericana del Libros de Medicina, S.A., 1994), page 670.

35. The National Cancer Institute later issued an alert stating that levamisole should be part of the standard management of Dukes's C colonic cancer. The annual U.S. cost of the treatment -- $1,267.35 -- was touted as a 90 percent savings over that for major bowel surgery, which tallied in at $13,377.20. Levamisole was recommended although the researchers admitted they didn't know why it worked. The recommendation was subsequently withdrawn, when later test results

weren't as good as earlier ones. Arguably the researchers, not knowing why the drug worked, were giving too much. See D. Cunningham, et al., "Important progress in treatment," British Medical Journal 310:247 (1995); 1995 Physicians GenRx (Riverside, Connecticut: Denniston Publishing Co.); R. Moss, Questioning Chemotherapy (Brooklyn, New York: Equinox Press, 1995).

36. E. Russell, Report on Radionics: Science of the Future (Essex, England: C. W. Daniel Co. Ltd., 1973), pages 41-49. See also D. Tansley, Dimensions of Radionics (Essex, England: C.W. Daniel Co. Ltd., 1977); D. Tansley, Radionics -- Interface with the Ether Fields (Essex, England: C.W. Daniel Co. Ltd., 1975); A. Westlake, M.D., The Pattern of Health (Berkeley, California: 1973).

37. E. Russell, op. cit.

38. B. Inglis, R. West, op. cit., pages 257-64.

39. E. Russell, op. cit., pages 83-87.

40. R. Gerber, op. cit., pages 143-53.

41. Ibid., pages 39-40.

42. This work was later discussed by Dr. Hunt in her book Infinite Mind: The Science of Human Vibrations (Malibu, California: Malibu Publishing Co., 1995), and in a 1993 video called "The Human Energy Field." See J. Klotter, "Linking science and spirit," Townsend Letter for Doctors & Patients (January 1996), pages 124-26.

43. B. Inglis, R. West, op. cit., pages 116-18.

44. J. Diamond, M.D., Your Body Doesn't Lie: How to Increase Your Life Energy Through Behavioral Kinesiology (New York: Warner Books, 1979), page 32.

45. See P. Lisa, The Great Medical Monopoly Wars (Huntington Beach, California: International Institute of Natural Health Sciences, Inc., 1986), pages 7-10; B. Lynes, The Healing of Cancer, op. cit., page 33.

46. S. Haught, Cancer? Think Curable! (Bonita, California: Gerson Institute, 1983), page 137; B. Lynes, The Healing of Cancer, op. cit.; E. Mullins, op. cit., pages 39-40, 61-66; R. Moss, The Cancer Industry, op. cit., pages 46-47, 390-99.

47. K. Napier, "Unproven medical treatments lure elderly," FDA Consumer (March 1994), page 32.

48. "House bill to outlaw all 'unproven medical remedies,'" Townsend Letter for Doctors 20:201 (October 1984); M. Salaman, "The nefarious post office 'thought police' bill," Townsend Letter for Doctors 26:112 (May 1985); P. Lisa, op. cit., pages 7-10.

49. California Health and Safety Code, Section 1707.1.

50. C. Barfield, "Cancer and quackery: Jailing of Tijuana clinic owner underscores debate," San Diego Tribune (September 16, 1991), page A-1.

51. M. Onstott, "In the name of consumer protection," in J. Morgenthaler, et al., eds., Stop the FDA: Save Your Health Freedom (Menlo Park, California: Health Freedom Publications, 1992), pages 81-82.

52. W. Nolan, McQueen (New York: Congdon & Weed, Inc., 1984), pages 202-15.

53. E. Mullins, op. cit., page 100.

54. See B. Inglis, Natural Medicine (William Collins Sons & Co., Ltd., 1979), pages 167-68: "Perhaps the commonest of all causes of disruption . . . are personality clashes. Any individual who has made a success of his career in what until quite recently was a depressed area of therapeutics is likely to have done so by force of personality and through faith in his own theories and practices. He is consequently apt to feel that anybody who favours some rival theory or practice must be wrong, and perhaps dishonest."

55. The conventional definition of "response to treatment" includes regression of tumors for as little as a month. See R. Wittes, M.D., Manual of Oncologic Therapeutics 1991/1992 (Philadelphia: J.B. Lippincott Co.), Appendix C.

56. L. Harter, "Malignant seeding of the needle track during sterotaxic core needle breast biopsy," Radiology 185:713-14 (1992); F. Roussel, et al., "Evaluation of large-needle biopsy for the diagnosis of cancer," Acta Cytologica 39:449-52 (1995); F. Roussel, et al., "The risk of tumoral seeding in needle biopsies," Acta Cytologica 33(6):936-39 (1989); K. Denton, et al., "Secondary tumour deposits in needle biopsy tracks: An underestimated risk?", Journal of Clinical Pathology 43:82-84 (1990); J. Fortner, "Inadvertent spread of cancer at surgery," Journal of Surgical Oncology 53:191-96 (1993). In December of 1995, CNN reported that a new form of sonogram may soon make biopsies obsolete.

57. U. Abel, Chemotherapy of Advanced Epithelial Cancer (Stuttgart: Hippokrates Verlag GmbH, 1990), summarized by R. Moss in "Chemo's 'Berlin Wall' Crumbles," Cancer Chronicles (December 1990), page 4. Dr. Abel observed that for breast cancer, there is no direct evidence that chemotherapy prolongs survival, making its use "ethically questionable." His work was reviewed in the popular German magazine Der Spiegel in 1990.

58. G. Mead, "Chemotherapy for solid tumours: Routine treatment not yet justified," British Medical Journal 310:246 (1995).

59. G. Borell, op. cit., page 30.

60. See I. Tannock, "Treating the patient, not just the cancer," New England Journal of Medicine 317(24):1534-35 (1987).

61. "Substantial evidence" is defined as "adequate and well-controlled investigations . . . on the basis of which it could fairly and responsibly be concluded . . . that the drug will have the effect it purports or is represented to have under the conditions of use prescribed, recommended, or suggested in the labeling or proposed labeling thereof." 21 United States Code Sec. 355(d). Despite this legal requirement, the U.S. Office of Technology Assessment has reported that "Only 10%-20% of all procedures currently used in medical practice have been shown to be efficacious by controlled trial." Office of Technology Assessment, U.S. Congress, Assessing Efficacy and Safety of Medical Technology (Washington D.C.: OTA 1978).

62. R. Oye, et al., "Reporting results from chemotherapy trials: Does response make a difference in patient survival?", JAMA 252(19):2722-25 (1984).

63. See G. Mead, op. cit.; I. Tannock, op. cit.; U. Abel, op. cit.

64. See R. Houston, "Misinformation from OTA," op. cit., page 600; J. Weese, et al., "Do operations facilitate tumor growth?", Surgery 100(2):273-77 (1986) (surgery and anesthesia enhance the implanting of tumors and facilitate metastasis); J. Stjernsward, "Decreased survival related to irradiation postoperatively in early operable breast cancer," Lancet (November 30, 1974), pages 1285-86; R. Moss, The Cancer Industry, op. cit., pages 59-72.

65. R. Walters, in Options: The Alternative Cancer Therapy Book (Garden City Park, New York: Avery Group Publishing Co., 1993), page 13, observes that as early as 1953, Benedict Fitzgerald, special counsel for the Department of Justice, presented studies to Congress showing that patients who received no radiation lived longer than those who were irradiated.

66. J. Cuzick, et al., "Overview of randomized trials of postoperative adjuvant radiotherapy in breast cancer," Cancer Treatment Reports 71(1):15-29 (1987).

67. J. Cairns, "The treatment of diseases and the war against cancer," Scientific American 253(5):51 (1985).

68. See R. Walters, op. cit., pages 9-11.

69. B. Culliton, "The rocky road to remission," Science 244:1432 (June 23, 1989).

70. H. Muss, et al., "Interrupted versus continuous chemotherapy in patients with metastatic breast cancer," New England Journal of Medicine 325:1342-48 (1991).

71. Early Breast Cancer Trialists' Collaborative Group, "Systemic treatment of early breast cancer by hormonal, cytotoxic, or immune therapy," Lancet 339(8785):71-85 (1992).

72. The recommendation was based on a series of 1989 studies finding a "significant prolongation of disease-free survival" from drug treatment. However, the studies did not find a significant increase in actual survival. "Disease-free survival" was a term of art meaning a period of time without new tumors. See B. Fisher, et al., "A randomized clinical trial evaluating sequential methotrexate and fluorouracil in the treatment of patients with node-negative breast dancer who have estrogen-receptor-negative tumors," New England Journal of Medicine 320(8):473-78 (1989); Ludwig Breast Cancer Study Group, "Prolonged disease-free survival after one course of perioperative adjuvant chemotherapy for node-negative breast cancer," New England Journal of Medicine 320(8):491-96 (1989); E. Mansour, et al., "Efficacy of adjuvant chemotherapy in high-risk node-negative breast cancer," New England Journal of Medicine 320(8):485-90 (1989). The same year, the General Accounting Office issued a report on the effectiveness of chemotherapy in breast cancer. It focused on patients with cancers of the type thought to benefit most from the drugs. The GAO found no detectable increase in the survival of these patients, despite a threefold increase in the use of chemotherapy since 1975. See "GAO report on breast cancer," World Research Foundation News (3rd & 4th quarter 1990), page 7.

73. R. Walters, op. cit. See also H. Vorherr, "Adjuvant chemotherapy of breast cancer: Reality, hope, hazard?", Lancet (December 19/26, 1981), pages 1413-14: "Data on five-year survival [show] the benefit from adjuvant [independent] chemotherapy of breast cancer is only 4% . . Mortality due to chemotherapy may be as high as 4.4% . . In view of the many uncertainties and controversies about adjuvant chemotherapy, which itself has serious health hazards, no patient should be routinely subjected to this kind of 'treatment.'"

74. See W. Irons, "Arginine-arginase relationship in regeneration, repair and development of neoplasms," Journal of Dental Research 25:497 (1946).

75. Hearings, Senate Subcommittee on Administrative Practice and Procedure, 1965, quoted in O. Garrison, The Dictocrats' Attack on Health Foods and Vitamins (New York: ARC Books, 1970), page 49.

76. See G. Mead, op. cit.: "[M]ost cancers are incurable once metastatic and often respond poorly to chemotherapy, which can result in side effects, inconvenience, and financial costs without improvements in symptoms or survival."

77. L. Horowitz, Emerging Viruses: AIDS and Ebola -- Nature, Accident or Genocide? (Tetrahedron Publishing Group, 1996). For similar theories and supporting data, see J. Rappoport, AIDS Inc. (San Bruno, California: Human Energy Press, 1988), pages 209-41; T. Bearden, AIDS: Biological Warfare (Greenville, Texas: Tesla Publishing Co., 1988), pages 11-17.

78. K. Park, et al., "Stimulation of lymphocyte natural cytotoxicity by L-arginine," Lancet 337:645-46 (1991).

79. K. Park, op. cit.; J. Daly, et al., "Immune and metabolic effects of arginine in the surgical patient," Annals of Surgery (October 1988), pages 512-23; A. Barbul, et al., "Arginine enhances wound healing and lymphocyte immune responses in humans," Surgery 108:331-37 (1990). The Petri dish study focused on by the defense in closing argument was Y. Cho-Chung, et al., "Growth arrest and morphological change of human breast cancer cells by dibutyryl cyclic AMP and L-arginine," Science 214:77-79 (1981).

80. See Office of Technology Assessment, Unconventional Cancer Treatments (Washington D.C.: U.S. Congress, 1990), page 99: "As a possible cytotoxic agent, DMSO has been studied in human tumor cell lines and in human tumor model systems in animals, and in each case, DMSO demonstrated no activity. . . . One of the properties of DMSO is that it is absorbed very rapidly through the skin and cell membranes, carrying along almost anything else [that is] dissolved in it that would not otherwise be able to cross those barriers. . . . DMSO was found to increase the activity of some [cytotoxic] agents in tumor-bearing rats. DMSO has been tested experimentally for antitumor effects, both in various tissue culture and in animal systems, and was found to be inactive."

81. See C. Bird, The Divining Hand (Atglen, Pennsylvania: Schiffer Publishing, 1993); P. Tompkins, C. Bird, The Secret Life of Plants (New York: Harper and Row, Publishers, 1973).

82. R. Chesemore, "FDA evaluation of amino acid supplements underway," Townsend Letter for Doctors (June 1991), page 402; D. Pearson, S. Shaw, "The war over health freedom in America approaches a turning point," in J. Morgenthaler, et al., Stop the FDA, op. cit., pages 67-79.

83. See B. Leibovitz, "Nutrition: At the crossroads," Journal of Optimal Nutrition 1(1):69-83 (1992), reprinted in Stop the FDA, op. cit., pages 13-40.

84. See "Human growth hormone: The fountain of youth?", Harvard Health Letter 17(8):1-3 (1992); G. Cowley, "Can hormones stop the clock?", Newsweek (July 16, 1990), page 66; "Growth hormone in elderly people," Lancet 337:1131-32 (1991); K. Schmidt, "Old no more," U.S. News & World Report (March 8, 1993), pages 66-73.

85. S. Moncada, et al., "Biosynthesis of nitric oxide from L-arginine," Biochemical Pharmacology 38(11): 1709-15 (1989); A. Barbul, et al., "Wound healing and thymotropic effects of arginine: A pituitary mechanism of action," American Journal of Clinical Nutrition 37:786-

94 (1983); J. Daly, et al., "Effect of dietary protein and amino-acids on immune function," Critical Care Medicine 1990 (supp. 2):86-93.

86. See "Cancer kid's mom jailed," New York Post (June 1, 1989), page 1; "'We had to kidnap our son from the hospital,'" Good Housekeeping (October 1989), page 144; G. Cowley, "Does doctor know best?", Newsweek (September 24, 1990), page 84; J. Feron, "Mother apparently wins bid to block surgery," New York Times (December 13, 1990), page B5; P. Chowka, "Chad Green: A matter of life, death, and freedom," New Age (January 1980), page 31.

87. See E. Hodgson, op. cit., pages 652-53.

88. The government claimed more deaths by 1991, but the 1985 survey was the last that was relevant for purposes of determining "cure," assuming the official definition: five years' disease-free survival. Dixon testified before the grand jury that the number of patients he counted in his survey in 1985 dropped from 93 to 89 when four patients were eliminated because their cancers were "unproven;" e.g., they refused to speak to the FBI. How many more of Keller's two hundred 1983 patients were alive in 1985 but were eliminated simply because they refused to speak to the FBI was undetermined, but trial testimony indicated that the government was aware of other survivors who, for unstated reasons, were not included in the FBI survey.

89. S. White, Across the Unknown (Columbus, Ohio: Ariel Press, 1987), pages 188-89 [originally published in 1939].

90. B. Leibovitz, op. cit.

91. See D. Manders, "The curious continuing ban of L-tryptophan: The serotonin connection," Townsend Letter for Doctors (October, 1992), pages 880-81.

92. See S. Kent, "January phone protest against FDA terrorism," Townsend Letter for Doctors 138:4-8 (January 1995).

93. "Reno clinic raided: Patients' lifeline cut," Nevada Sentinel, quoted in Townsend Letter for Doctors (December 1993), page 1244.

94. S. Kent, op. cit.

95. D. Mouscher, "The FDA's vendetta against Dr. Burzynski," Life Extension Magazine (September 1995), pages C1-C4.

96. J. Whitaker, M.D., "The FDA's latest abuse of power," Townsend Letter for Doctors and Patients (January 1997), pages 105-06.

97. See B. Leibovitz, "Hatch-Richardson passes: No time to celebrate," Townsend Letter for Doctors 137:1306 (December 1994); "FDA Raid Report: The FDA kills Americans by denying them lifesaving information," op. cit., page 3.

98. C. Russell, "Gaining ground as the world's no. 1 killer," Washington Post (March 27-April 2, 1995), page 8.

99. M. Culbert, "Apricot power: Laetrile as the Marine Corps of the 'Alternative' Revolution," Townsend Letter for Doctors (June 1995), pages 71-82.

100. See, e.g., N. Fabris, et al., Thymus 19(supp. 1):S21-S30 (1992) (oral arginine supplementation significantly increased the functional activity of the thymus in patients with cancer of all types); J. Brittenden, et al., "L-arginine stimulates host defenses in patients with breast cancer," Surgery 115:205-12 (1994) (ten grams of L-arginine given orally three times a day to women with breast cancer significantly enhanced their immune function); J. Brittenden, et al., "L-arginine and malignant disease: A potential therapeutic role?", European Journal of Surgical Oncology 20(2):189-92 (1994); J. Brittenden, et al., "Nutritional pharmacology: Effects of L-arginine on host defences, response to trauma and tumour growth," Clinical Science 86:123-32 (1994).

101. J. Brittenden, et al., "L-arginine stimulates host defenses . . .," op. cit.

102. R. Moss, The Cancer Industry, op. cit., pages 46-47, 390-99. See also E. Mullins, op. cit., pages 61-66.

103. U.S. v. Allied Chemical & Dye Corp., U.S. District Court of New Jersey, May 14, 1942.

104. R. Moss, The Cancer Industry, op. cit., page 395.

105. New York Times (October 21, 1945), Sec. I, pages 1, 12.

106. Flynn, God's Gold: The Story of Rockefeller and His Times (New York: Harcourt Brace & Co., 1932), page 58.

107. W. Hoffman, David: Report on a Rockefeller (New York: Lyle Stuart, Inc., 1971), page 24.

108. G. E. Griffin, op. cit., pages 248-52, 256, 329-41, 350-51, 501-02.

109. H. Ambruster, Treason's Peace (New York: Beechhurst Press, 1947), page vii, quoted in G. E. Griffin, op. cit., page 247.

110. Dr. W. Douglass, "CODEX: A German proposal to outlaw all supplements," Townsend Letter for Doctors and Patients (January 1998), page 132. Details are available from Advocates for Health Freedom, Attn: John Hammell, 2411 Monroe St. #2, Hollywood, FL 33020, fax 954-927-8795; web site http://www.pnc. com.au/ ~ cafmr/hammell/index.html. See also the web site of the Life Extension Foundation, http://www.lef.org.

111. H. Piffard, "The status of the medical profession in the State of New York," New York Medical Journal 37:401 (April 14, 1883).

112. See H. Coulter, Divided Legacy: A History of the Schism in Medical Thought (Washington D.C.: Wehawken Book Co., 1973-77); M. Kaufman, op. cit; K. Goss, The Complete Book of Homeopathy (New York: Bantam Books, 1982); B. Inglis, Natural Medicine, op. cit.

113. G. E. Griffin, op. cit., pages 369-82; K. Ausubel, op. cit.

114. American Journal of Law and Medicine, vol. 9, page 263.

115. E. Mullins, op. cit.

116. K. Ausubel, op. cit.

117. E. Mullins, op. cit., pages 25-33, 50-51.

118. E. Mullins, op. cit., pages 120-21.

119. Decision by Administrative Law Judge Ernest G. Barnes, docket No. 9064, dated November 13, 1978, quoted in B. Halstead, op. cit.

120. The suit was brought by chiropractors a decade after the AMA had formally resolved that chiropractic was an "unscientific cult." A memo uncovered in the suit stated: "Since the AMA board of trustees' decision . . . to establish a Committee on Quackery, your committee has considered its prime mission to be, first the containment of chiropractic and, ultimately, the elimination of chiropractic." Memo dated January 4, 1971 from H. Doyl Taylor, head of the AMA department of investigation, to the AMA board of trustees, quoted in P. Lisa, op. cit., pages 1-2.

121. P. Lisa, op. cit., pages 1-7, citing the now-published "Operating Procedures" of the CCHI and minutes of its meetings. Lisa's work was updated and expanded in his later book, The Assault on Medical Freedom (Norfolk, Virginia: Hampton Roads Publishing Co., Inc., 1994).

122. P. Lisa, The Assault on Medical Freedom, op. cit., page 45.

123. P. Lisa, Monopoly Wars, op. cit., pages 15-16, 33, 37-38; E. Mullins, op. cit., pages 36-37.

124. P. Lisa, Monopoly Wars, op. cit.; The Assault on Medical Freedom, op. cit., pages 52-66.

125. O. Garrison, The Dictocrats' Attack on Health Foods and Vitamins (New York: Arc Books, 1970), pages 322-23.

126. R. Moss, The Cancer Industry, op. cit., pages 399-406; E. Mullins, op. cit., pages 61-62, 76-102.

127. R. Moss, The Cancer Industry, op. cit., pages 406-11; O. Garrison, op. cit., pages 270-74.

128. See, e.g., J. Cairns, op. cit.; H. Vorherr, op. cit.; I. Tannock, op. cit.; U. Abel, op. cit.

129. B. Thomson, "Surviving cancer," Natural Health (March-April 1993), page 74.

130. E. Marshall, op. cit. See also B. Ingram, "Cancer strides challenged: Establishment's therapeutic claims overstated, says activist coalition," Medical Tribune 33:1 (1992).

131. See R. Bazell, "Cancer warp," The New Republic (December 18, 1989), pages 12-14; D. Davis, J. Schwartz, "Trends in cancer mortality: U.S. white males and females, 1968-83," Lancet (March 19, 1988), pages 633-35; American Cancer Society, Cancer Facts & Figures -- 1990 (Atlanta, Georgia: American Cancer Society, 1990); A. Lang, op. cit.; R. Moss, "Breast cancer on the rise," Cancer Chronicles 2(2):2 (Autumn 1990); E. Marshall, "Breast cancer: Stalemate in the war on cancer," Science 254:1719-20 (1991); "Risk of breast cancer increase to 1 in 9," Townsend Letter for Doctors (May 1991), page 302; R. Walters, op. cit., pages 9-11.

132. A. Lang, op. cit.

133. D. Greenberg, "'Progress' in cancer research -- don't say it isn't so," New England Journal of Medicine 292(13):707-08.

134. A. Miller, et al., "Canadian National Breast Screening Study: 1. Breast cancer detection and death rates among women aged 40 to 49 years," Canadian Medical Association Journal 147(10):1459-76 (1992).

135. A book on this subject was published by Carole Gallagher through the MIT Press in 1993. My data comes from an article in Spin Magazine titled "How the West was lost," but the date is missing from my xeroxed copy.

136. Last name was difficult to decipher and may be incorrect.